Nutrition in Adolescence

Nutrition in Adolescence

L. KATHLEEN MAHAN, M.S., R.D.

Nutritionist, Pediatric Pulmonary Disease Center;
Lecturer, School of Nutritional Sciences, University of Washington;
Consulting Nutritionist, Private Practice,
Seattle, Washington

JANE MITCHELL REES, M.S., R.D.

Nutritionist, Division of Adolescent Medicine;
Lecturer, School of Nutritional Sciences, University of Washington,
Seattle, Washington

With **75** illustrations

TIMES MIRROR/MOSBY College Publishing

St. Louis • Toronto • Santa Clara   1984

Editor: Julia Allen Jacobs
Assistant editor: Catherine H. Converse
Editing supervisor: Judi Wolken
Manuscript editor: Cliff Froehlich
Design: Diane Beasley
Production: Carol O'Leary, Barbara Merritt, Teresa Breckwoldt

Cover photo by Four by Five Inc.

Copyright © 1984 by Times Mirror/Mosby College Publishing
A division of The C.V. Mosby Company
11830 Westline Industrial Drive, St. Louis, Missouri 63146

Printed in the United States of America

Library of Congress Cataloging in Publication Data

Mahan, L. Kathleen.
   Nutrition in adolescence.

   Bibliography: p.
   Includes index.
   1. Youth—Nutrition.   I. Rees, Jane Mitchell.
II. Title. [DNLM: 1. Nutrition—In adolescence.
QU 145 N97404]
RJ235.M33 1984   613.2'088055   83-9124
ISBN 0-8016-3070-3

AC/VH/VH 9 8 7 6 5 4 3 2 1   01/A/002

To
Carlin and Robert
John and Mike

Contributors

LEONA L. EGGERT, M.A., R.N.
School Nurse, Bellevue Public Schools; Assistant Clinical Professor, Department of
Psychosocial Nursing, School of Nursing; Ph.D. candidate, Speech Communication, University
of Washington, Seattle, Washington

MARGARET L. McINTYRE, M.S., R.D.
Clinical Dietician, Department of Dietetics,
Children's Hospital National Medical Center, Washington, D.C.

ROBIN H. ROSEBROUGH, Ph.D., R.D.
Formerly Assistant Professor, Department of Pediatrics, University of Maryland School of
Medicine; Nutrition Consultant, Women, Infants, and Children Program, Maryland Department
of Health and Mental Hygiene; Nutrition Consultant, Good Shepherd Center, Residential
Psychiatric Treatment Facility for Adolescents, Baltimore, Maryland

MARY STORY, Ph.D., R.D.
Nutritionist, Adolescent Health Program; Assistant Professor, Public Health Nutrition, School of
Public Health, University of Minnesota, Minneapolis, Minnesota

BONNIE WORTHINGTON-ROBERTS, Ph.D.
Chief, Nutrition Section, Child Development and Mental Retardation Center; Professor, School
of Nutritional Science, University of Washington, Seattle, Washington

LANITA S. WRIGHT, M.D.
Formerly Clinical Associate Professor of Pediatrics, Division of Adolescent Medicine,
University of Washington, Seattle, Washington

Continued

Foreword

It is an honor to write a few words of introduction to this important book on adolescent nutrition. The publication is timely, coming as it does when increasing numbers of youth, parents, and professionals are concerned with adolescent health care and the difficulties encountered in assisting youth to achieve maturity. There is a great deal of information on the market today in the area of adolescent health care related to nutrition. It is supplied in abundance by our media and available to all. It is becoming a great challenge for all those involved in providing services and advice to sort out sound scientific information from the myth or fads of the moment.

It is fitting that L. Kathleen Mahan and Jane Mitchell Rees should write this book to meet the increasing demand and need for sound nutritional information. Both authors not only are accomplished professionals in the field of nutrition but also have the unique experience of clinical practice in an interdisciplinary setting where all aspects of physical, psychosocial, and nutritional growth and development are considered in providing comprehensive health care to youth. Their work is based on the experience of nutritionists who for over 20 years have been an integral part of an adolescent program. As a result, their book not only discusses the theoretical basis of nutritional issues in adolescence but also contains practical information about providing nutritional care and helping teenagers change their eating habits.

As we approach the end of the twentieth century, we can look back over many achievements in the health care of adolescents. This book represents an outstanding contribution to those achievements in the field of nutrition, and it is with pleasure that I introduce it to you.

Robert W. Deisher, M.D.
Professor of Pediatrics
Director, Division of Adolescent Medicine
University of Washington
Seattle, Washington

Preface

If the principles of nutrition are to be viewed as significant beyond the classroom and research laboratory, students must learn to apply these principles in specialized areas of health care. We have developed *Nutrition in Adolescence* primarily for students majoring in nutrition, dietetics, and nursing who have a basic knowledge of nutrition and who are interested in the application of that knowledge to the adolescent age group. It serves as a text for a one-quarter or one-semester course devoted to the study of adolescent nutrition. It is also a unique and valuable resource for life-cycle nutrition courses of one quarter or greater length. The full resources for such a life-cycle course are available if this book is used in combination with other Times Mirror/Mosby nutrition texts (Worthington-Roberts's *Nutrition in Pregnancy and Lactation* and Pipes's *Nutrition in Infancy and Childhood*). In clinical settings health practitioners working with adolescent populations, especially dietitians, nutritionists, nurses, and physicians, will find the text a useful clinical handbook.

OBJECTIVE

The main objective of the book is to focus on the nutritional aspects of a phase of the life cycle that has been puzzling to health professionals and to help students and practitioners to recognize the characteristics and needs of this special group, thus developing in them a greater appreciation both for teenagers in general and for those they may serve as health-care providers. The material is presented in a fashion intended to help the student of nutrition develop a comprehensive understanding of nutritional issues by integrating knowledge from other disciplines in the physical and social sciences.

SCOPE AND SEQUENCE

To lead to a comprehensive understanding, the book addresses a wide range of nutritional aspects, incorporating background material related to the developmental processes and characteristics of adolescents. It presents not only theoretical discussions of the specific topics but also clinical protocols in which results from controlled studies are synthesized to derive solutions to long-term problems arising in uncontrolled "real life" situations.

Chapters 1 and 2 describe the physical and psychological characteristics of growth and development that are unique to adolescents. Chapter 3 presents the theoretical basis for current nutritional recommendations and clinical methods for nutritional assessment in individual adolescents. The section of Chapter 3 focusing on assessment of height/weight proportions and body composition is especially significant to the student of nutrition today. Chapter 4 explores typical eating habits, taking environment, life-style, and developmental factors into consideration. These initial chapters thus set the stage for the main body of the book, which discusses nutritional support for growth and development in eating disorders (Chapter 5), fitness and competitive sports (Chapter 6), chronic disease (Chapter 7), and pregnancy (Chapter 9). Chapter 8 discusses nutrition and behavior and evaluates the theories and myths concerning the influence of nutritional factors on adolescent behavior in light of current research. Chapter 10 is an introduction to counseling techniques that are useful in helping adolescents—and, indeed, other individuals—improve their nutritional practices as suggested in any of the specific areas.

Students will find a compilation of material in this book that for the first time has been collected and presented with an orientation toward practical application of theoretical principles. The material has been chosen to provide the student with an in-depth knowledge of adolescent nutrition. The authors, as clinical practitioners associated with academic institutions, have written *Nutrition in Adolescence* with the expectation that it constitutes a basis for increased knowledge and improved nutritional care for adolescents.

ACKNOWLEDGMENTS

Many people have helped us in the preparation of this book, but certain people deserve recognition for the time they spent in reviewing parts of the manuscript. We would like especially to thank Diane Stein, M.D., Carol Bach, M.D., Theus L. Doolittle, Ph.D., Janet Edlefson, M.S., James Farrow, M.D., Marie Root, Ph.D., and Christopher K. Varley, M.D. Those who reviewed the entire manuscript gave us valuable ideas regarding the scope and focus of the book. They are the following:

Virginia Beal, University of Massachusetts
Felix Heald, University of Maryland
Kathryn Kolassa, Michigan State University
Virginia Lee, Colorado State University
Marjorie Dibble, Syracuse University
Deborah McNeill, Wayne State University

We would also like to thank the many colleagues of various disciplines who have contributed to our understanding of clinical work with adolescents and the friends, family, and associates who have supported us in developing this book. We want to give a very special thank you to Janelle Douglas, whose devotion to preparing the manuscript pulled us through some hard times to meet deadlines.

L. Kathleen Mahan
Jane Mitchell Rees

Contents

Chapter 1

Physiological Development in Adolescence

LANITA S. WRIGHT

What is happening? Where is that helpful 10-year-old who was here last week? Why has the milk bill sky-rocketed this summer? Why does the slightest sugges-tion from mother cause a reaction second only to Mt. St. Helens? The shoes purchased only 3 months ago are too small!

What is this lump under my nipple? Do I have cancer? I can't go to school today because my hair is a stupid mess! I wish that I were bald! I'm such a klutz! No one wanted me on the volleyball team in P.E. today. I don't use drugs or smoke and I'm a wimp! Why are all the stoners bigger than I am?

Sound familiar? To anyone who has any asso-ciation with adolescents or their parents it should sound very familiar.

Adolescence is a period of dynamic change. These changes occur in all spheres of development of the human potential—physical, emotional, in-tellectual, and even spiritual. In a span of 2 to 4 years, linear height increases as much as 25 cm (10 in) for males and 22.5 cm (9 in) for females. The average teen may gain as much as 22.5 kg (50 lb) during the 3 years of peak weight-gain velocity. To put it another way, during the total 5 to 7 years of adolescent growth, 20% of linear height and 50% of ideal body weight are gained. Skeletal mass, heart, lungs, liver, spleen, kidneys, pancreas, thyroid gland, adrenal glands, gonads, phallus, and uterus all double in size during this time.[1]

At this same time, society is demanding more of the individual. Responsibility, independence, and sexual pressures all seem to become issues. Yet legally and practically, adolescents remain de-pendent with few rights. Magnified by the adoles-cent's internal hormonal activity, these external pressures may result in a stormy period that, even in the best of circumstances, may be painful for both the adolescent and his or her family.

Definition of Terms

What does the term *adolescence* include, and is there a difference between adolescence and pu-berty? Adolescence is the time period that begins with the onset of puberty, which is the appearance of secondary sexual characteristics. Adolescence continues through the completion of pubertal de-velopment, resulting in functional reproductive organs, and the attainment of final physical growth. Psychosocial maturation occurs simul-taneously. In adolescence we see the prepubertal child develop a physically mature adult body and a psychosocially maturing young adult mind.

Developmental Stages of Adolescence

It is useful to divide adolescence into three stages: early, middle, and late. Early adolescence includes the onset of puberty and usually occurs by the ages of 10 to 12 years in girls and 11 to 13 years in boys. Middle adolescence continues through the ages of 12 to 15 years in girls and 13 to 16 years in boys. Late adolescence completes the process of somatic growth through the ages of 16 to 21 years in both sexes.

Psychological Aspects of Adolescence

Psychologically, early adolescents are concerned mainly with the physical and physiological events of body change. They focus on sexual development and awareness and establish an identity in relation to those changes.

Middle adolescents are finding places for themselves as individuals in the community. They become somewhat accustomed to their new bodies and now begin to question the societal norms in the hope of establishing answers for themselves. They alternate between the old and the new.

In late adolescence the psychological problems of forming a sexual identity, attaining independence, and choosing a vocation theoretically are resolved. A productive adult is the result.[2]

These psychological and emotional aspects of adolescent development are dealt with in detail in Chapter 2.

ASPECTS OF GROWTH

Although this chapter is concerned with the adolescent age period, to adequately understand growth during adolescence we must review the changes that preceded it. Fetal growth and growth during infancy are discussed elsewhere and will not be covered in detail here.[3]

Growth in Childhood

Weight increases during the first year of postnatal life at the rate of 20 gm/day (0.7 oz/day) for the first 6 months and 15 gm/day (0.5 oz/day) for the second 6 months. Length increases 25 to 30 cm (10 to 12 in) (at least 17 cm [6.8 in] in females and 16 cm [6.4 in] in males) in the first 6 months but only 8 cm (3.2 in) during the second 6 months. Appetite often falls off at 10 months and may continue to decrease in the second year. During the second year, the child adds more height than

weight—11 cm (4.4 in) for females and 10 cm (4 in) for males with an average weight gain of 2.5 kg (5.5 lb). School age children grow approximately 6 cm/yr (2.4 in/yr) (at least 5 cm [2 in]) and gain 3 to 3.5 kg/yr (6.6 to 7.7 lb/yr).[4]

Differences in Growth Between Males and Females

There are sexual differences in growth rates. Halfway through fetal life, the female skeleton is 3 weeks more advanced than the male. At birth the difference is even greater, with the female skeleton being 4 to 6 weeks more advanced. Some other organ systems also show greater physiological maturity in females at birth. These differences may be the reason why more females survive at birth.[3]

The actual steps and order of sequence in the maturing process are the same for the male and female until puberty. During puberty, the female usually matures earlier. For example, permanent teeth erupt earlier in females, and centers of skeletal ossification in the elbow and other regions appear earlier in females. This earlier maturation in females follows for most organs.[3]

Although boys are slightly larger at birth, size difference in childhood is small until the female accelerates her growth during adolescence. At that time girls are temporarily taller. Most boys continue prepubertal growth for 2 years longer than girls, and this results in an additional 8 to 10 cm (3.2 to 4 in) in height for boys. Leg growth in the prepubertal years is relatively faster than trunk growth for boys; therefore boys have longer legs. Height added during the growth spurt is only 3 to 5 cm (1.2 to 2 in) greater in boys than in girls, but the final difference in height is 13 cm (5.2 in). Thus the difference in overall body size between males and females primarily results from the boy's longer period of growth before the growth spurt of adolescence.[3-5]

Fig. 1-1 illustrates velocity of growth in boys and girls. As shown, typical girls are slightly shorter than boys of the same age until adolescence. Shortly after the age of 11 years the girl

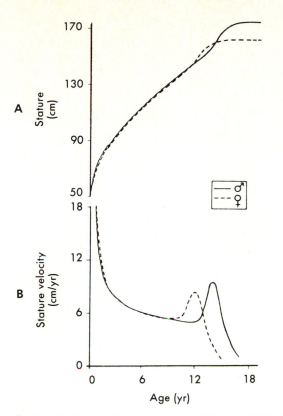

Fig. 1-1. A, Growth in stature of typical boy *(solid line)* and girl *(interrupted line).* **B,** Growth velocities at different ages of typical boy *(solid line)* and girl *(interrupted line).* (From Marshall, W.A.: Clin. Endocrinol. Metab. **4:**4, 1975.)

becomes taller because of her growth spurt. By the age of 14 years, boys experience their growth spurt, and the average girl is passed in height. Weight also is equal in childhood, but girls at about the age of 9 years become heavier than boys. Girls remain heavier until approximately the age of 14½ years when boys surpass them.[3-5]

In the year just preceding the adolescent growth spurt, the gain in height velocity reaches its lowest point in males. That year only 3.5 to 5 cm (1.4 to 2 in) is gained. In girls, because their spurt is sooner, the velocity in the year preceding does not slow down quite so much.

The processes of growth and differentiation are self-stabilizing. The ability to stabilize and return to a predetermined height growth curve following a period of growth arrest persists throughout the entire period of growth. However, it appears that regulation in canalization (the tendency to return to the original height growth channel when factors have caused a change in the growth channel) is better in females than in males. For example, females recover from growth arrest more quickly than males and are slowed less by such factors as atomic radiation and undernutrition.[3]

PUBERTY

Growth during puberty is dramatic not only because of added height and weight but also because of changes in habitus and the functioning of specific organs. These changes are related to profound hormonal events.

Initiation of Puberty

What causes the upsurge in hormonal activity that initiates pubertal development? Current radioimmunoassay techniques allow the measurement of hormonal concentrations that previously were below the sensitivity limits of earlier assays. This allows the hormonal changes to be measured as they occur chronologically. However, even with the development of these refined laboratory techniques, the exact factor or combination of factors that initiates the onset of these changes is unknown at present.[6-8]

The interaction between the hypothalamus, the pituitary, and the gonads in the hypothalamic-pituitary-gonadal (HPG) axis includes the major hormonal changes occurring during puberty. Since this system does not respond in children as it does in adults, it is obvious that during the period of puberty gradual changes take place in the HPG axis ultimately resulting in mature adult function.

Gonadotropin-releasing hormone (GnRH) is secreted by the hypothalamus. This hormone acts on

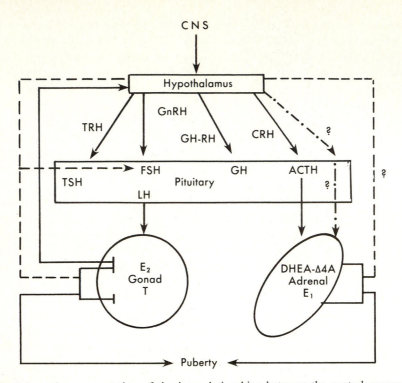

Fig. 1-2. Schematic representation of the interrelationships between the central nervous system *(CNS)*, the hypothalamus *(TRH, thyrotropin-releasing hormone; GnRH, gonadotropin-releasing hormone; GH-RH, growth hormone–releasing hormone; CRH, corticotropin-releasing hormone)*, the pituitary gland *(GH, growth hormone; TSH, thyroid-stimulating hormone; FSH, follicle-stimulating hormone; LH, luteinizing hormone; ACTH, adrenocorticotropic hormone)*, the gonads (E_2, estradiol; *T*, testosterone), and the adrenal glands *(DHEA, dehydro-3-epiandrosterone; Δ4A, Δ4-androstenedione; E_1, estrone). Interrupted line, negative feedback; continuous line, positive feedback; ?, hypothetical stimulatory or inhibitory pathway.* (From Sizonenko, P.C.: Clin. Endocrinol. Metab. **4:**174, 1975.)

the pituitary causing it to release follicle-stimulating hormone (FSH) luteinizing hormone (LH). FSH and LH in turn travel via the bloodstream to the gonads (ovaries and testes) and stimulate germ cell maturation and hormone synthesis as shown in Fig. 1-2.

Before puberty the HPG axis is minimally functional because the amounts of GnRH are kept very low by an unknown system.[7] At puberty this unknown system gradually changes. Many theo-

ries have been suggested to explain the change. One popular theory proposes that there is a "gonadostat," an area in the brain that is extremely sensitive to sex steroids (estrogen, testosterone, progesterone). GnRH release causes the pituitary to release LH and FSH that stimulate the gonads to release small amounts of sex steroids. These sex steroids are sensed by the gonadostat. The gonadostat stops the release of GnRH and inhibits the cycle until the blood level of the sex steroids is below some unknown amount. The process then begins again only to be shut down again. Just before puberty, however, at 8 to 10 years of age, this inhibition gradually is removed by some unknown means, and the GnRH is allowed to be secreted in increasing amounts. Pulsatile and episodic secretion of gonadotropins occurs at levels of 1 to 5 IU/ml. No differences between sleep and wake measurements are noted. The increased levels of GnRH result in the release of increased amounts of LH and FSH. This change appears to be accompanied by maturation of the gonads, which includes an increased response of the gonads to LH and the beginning of puberty.[6,9-11]

Frisch and her co-workers[12] relate pubertal onset to a change in body composition. They observed an association between menarche and the attainment of a critical body weight in North American and most European girls. They theorize that the achievement of the critical body weight of 47.8 kg (105 lb) causes a change in metabolic rate that triggers menarche and initiates the adolescent growth spurt in girls. Frisch further states that the attainment of a minimal level of body fatness of 17% of body weight is necessary for the onset of menstruation. However, this theory has been analyzed critically. Other researchers acknowledge an association between change in body composition and the onset of menarche, but they do not view it as a triggering factor of puberty.[12-15]

As described, the HPG axis is the main system involved with pubertal development, but other hormones also play a part. Fig. 1-2 illustrates the complex interrelationships involved in the endocrine system at puberty.

Hormonal Activity and Physical Changes of Puberty[6-11,16]

Very Early Puberty. Although no physical maturation is evident in very early puberty, there is an increase in the release of gonadotropins and sex steroids from 1 to 5 IU/ml up to 5 to 10 IU/ml. This rise occurs during sleep. Adrenal sex steroids also increase.

Early Puberty. In early puberty sleep augmentation of gonadotropins continues, and sex steroid concentrations increase. Some increase in growth hormone and change in thyroid function may occur.

Physical changes also begin to occur. In females the increased secretion of gonadotropins and sex steroids that occurred previously results in breast budding, enlargement of ovaries, and estrogenization of the vaginal mucosa. The uterus begins to enlarge, and the distribution of body fat begins to change.

In males the epididymis, seminal vesicles, prostate gland, and testes enlarge. Testicular volume greater than 3 ml indicates puberty has begun. The scrotum begins to redden and change in texture.

Middle Puberty. By middle puberty physical changes are definite. Males experience enlargement of penis length, and pigmented straight pubic hair appears around the base of the penis. During this stage, hair spreads over the symphysis, becomes coarser and more pigmented, and begins to curl. Facial hair develops on the upper lip. No axillary hair is present, but increased axillary sweating is noted. Arm and leg hair may become coarser. Enlargement of the areolae occurs, and breast tissue enlargement (gynecomastia) may be noted. Usually this breast tissue enlargement regresses spontaneously 1 to 2 years after its appearance. Testes and scrotum continue to enlarge, and the voice begins to change. The growth spurt may begin toward the end of middle puberty.

In females middle puberty brings the enlargement of ovaries and the separation of breast and areolar tissue. The uterus increases substantially in size, with the corpus becoming longer than the cervix. Pubic hair appears. Toward the end of this stage, there is a moderate amount of coarse curly pubic hair on the mons pubis and labia majora. Most girls attain peak height velocity in this stage, usually before menarche. Change in distribution of body fat is definite, with females adding more body fat than males. Once peak height velocity is reached, there is a dramatic increase in the accumulation of fat, particularly in the hips and breasts.

Activity of the sebaceous glands increases in both sexes, and acne may become a problem.

Hormonally, there are increasing concentrations of gonadotropins and sex steroids during wakeful periods, although sleep values still exceed wakeful values. Growth hormone may be seen during wakeful periods, but sleep values are higher and more frequent. Goiters may occur, but no change in the concentrations of thyroid hormones accompanies them.

Late Puberty. During late puberty in males, the penis continues to enlarge in length and breadth. Testes, prostate gland, and seminal vesicles continue to enlarge, and scrotal skin becomes pigmented. Mature sperm are contained in the ejaculate, and seminal fluid volume increases. Pubic hair is curly, coarse, and abundant and may extend up the abdominal midline. Axillary hair develops, and facial hair develops on the upper part of the cheek and the midline below the lower lip. Voice change continues. Muscle mass increases, and peak height velocity occurs if it has not occurred in middle puberty.

In females breast enlargement continues, but the areola remains separate from the breast. Internally, the vagina elongates, and the uterus assumes adult size and shape. Increased vaginal secretion is noted. Menarche occurs if it has not already occurred in middle puberty. Growth slows and in most girls is complete within 2 years after menarche.

Sleep augmentation of gonadotropins and secretion of growth hormone are maximal. A positive feedback system develops in which higher levels of estrogen stimulate instead of stop GnRH secretion.

In females a rapid rise in the sex steroid estradiol during the middle of the menstrual cycle stimulates either the hypothalamus to release GnRH or the pituitary directly to release LH. This LH rise is seen with ovulation. This positive feedback loop may be seen as early as late middle puberty. Some studies have suggested that in the first 2 postmenarcheal years 55% to 82% of the cycles are anovulatory. By 5 years postmenarche, only 20% of cycles are anovulatory.[8] Maturation is almost complete.

Adulthood. By adulthood all physical changes have been completed. Gonadotropins and sex steroids are at adult levels, and sleep augmentations no longer occur. Growth hormone sleep augmentation is still present but with lower peaks. Secretion of growth hormone occurs less frequently during wakeful hours.

SEQUENCE AND STAGES OF PUBERTAL GROWTH

Sexual Maturity Stages

Chronological age is not always helpful in discussing adolescent growth because of great individual variations in beginning and completing the growth sequences. A more useful way of describing pubertal development is to divide pubertal growth into stages of breast and pubic hair development in girls and genitalia (penis and testes) and pubic hair development in boys. Table 1-1 and Figs. 1-3 and 1-4 summarize these stages. Table 1-2 relates the pubertal stages to chronological age.

The sequence of pubertal events tends to follow a similar pattern in most normal adolescents and allows for the prediction of future events. In males, for example, a height spurt will follow about 1 year after testicular enlargement is first noted. Peak height velocity usually is reached in approximately 1 more year, when the penis is at its maximal rate of growth and pubic hair is stage 3 or 4.

However, as Table 1-2 illustrates, the range of chronological ages at which each event takes place is wide. For instance, acceleration of penis growth may begin as early as 10½ years or as late as 14½ years, with most males noting growth by 12½

Table 1-1. Stages of sexual maturation

Boys	Pubic Hair	Genitalia
Stage 1	None	No change from childhood
Stage 2	Small amount at outer edges of pubis; slight darkening	Beginning penile enlargement; testes enlarged to 5 ml volume; scrotum reddened and changed in texture
Stage 3	Covers pubis	Longer penis; testes 8-10 ml; scrotum further enlarged
Stage 4	Adult type; does not extend to thighs	Larger, wider, and longer penis; testes 12 ml; scrotal skin darker
Stage 5	Adult type; now spread to thighs	Adult penis; testes 15 ml

Girls	Pubic Hair	Breasts
Stage 1	None	No change from childhood
Stage 2	Small amount; downy on labia majora	Breast bud
Stage 3	Increased; darker and curly	Larger; no separation of nipple and areola
Stage 4	More abundant; coarse texture	Increased size; areola and nipple form secondary mound
Stage 5	Adult type; now spread to thighs	Adult distribution of breast tissue; continuous outline

Modified from Tanner, J.M.: Growth at adolescence, ed. 2, Oxford, 1962, Blackwell Scientific Publications, Ltd.

Table 1-2. Mean ($\pm$ SD) ages (years) of the various pubertal events in American adolescents

Pubertal Event*	Females	Males	Pubertal Event*	Females	Males
Br 2	11.2 ± 1.6		PH 3	12.7 ± 0.5	13.9 ± 0.9
G 2		11.9 ± 1.1	Voice change		14.1 ± 0.9
PH 2	11.9 ± 1.5	12.3 ± 0.8	Acne	13.2 ± 0.5	14.3 ± 1.3
G 3		13.2 ± 0.8	G 4		14.3 ± 0.8
Gynecomastia		13.2 ± 0.8	Regular menses	13.9 ± 1.0	
Voice break		13.5 ± 1.0	PH 4	13.4 ± 1.2	14.7 ± 0.9
Peak height velocity	12.5 ± 1.5	13.8 ± 1.1	Br 4	13.1 ± 0.7	
Peak weight gain	12.4 ± 1.4	13.9 ± 0.9	Facial hair		14.9 ± 1.1
Axillary hair	13.1 ± 0.8	14.0 ± 1.1	Br 5	14.5 ± 1.6	
Br 3	12.4 ± 1.2		G 5		15.1 ± 1.1
Menarche	13.3 ± 1.3		PH 5	14.6 ± 1.1	15.3 ± 0.8

Reprinted by permission of the publisher from "Normal ages of pubertal events among American males and females," by P.A. Lee, J. Adolesc. Health Care **1**(1):28. Copyright 1980 by Elsevier Science Publishing Co., Inc.
*Br, Breast; G, genital; PH, pubic hair.

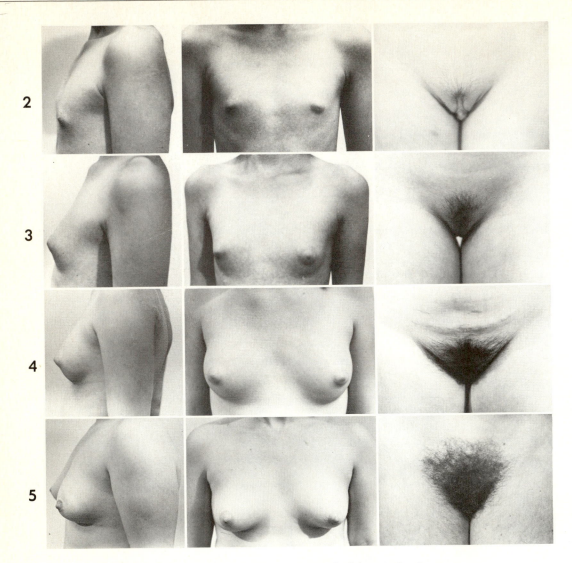

Fig. 1-3. Female adolescents in all stages of adolescent development.

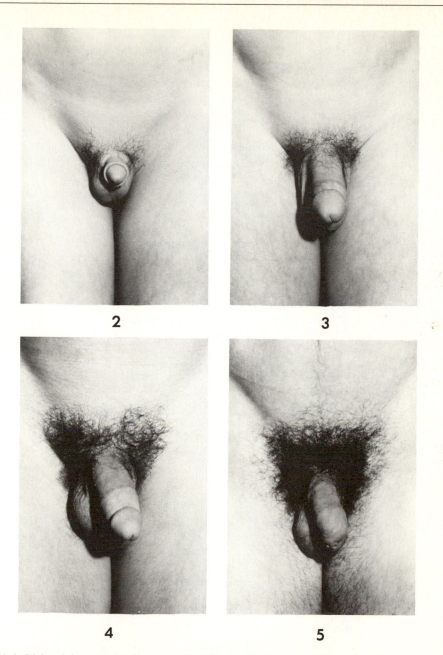

Fig. 1-4. Male adolescents in all stages of adolescent development. (From Farrow, J.A.: Semin. Fam. Med. **2**[3]:146-153, 1981. By permission of Grune & Stratton, Inc.)

years. Fig. 1-5 illustrates this phenomenon well.

Individual differences also occur in the rapidity with which an individual completes a sequence once it has started. Average boys have 1 year between genitalia stage 2 and genitalia stage 3 and 3 years between genitalia stage 2 and genitalia stage 5, but others progress from genitalia stage 2 to genitalia stage 5 in 2 years. This variation added to the variation in the age of pubertal onset explains the great differences in size and development of boys in junior high locker rooms. Boys of the same

chronological age range physically from childhood development and stature through advanced development and almost adult stature (Fig. 1-6). With the great concern and focus on body image at this time of life, consider the problems a young male encounters when he enters puberty but moves through it at a snail's pace as compared with a more rapidly maturing peer. This variation has implications for the planning of sports competition for adolescents.

Females manifest the same variability in age at

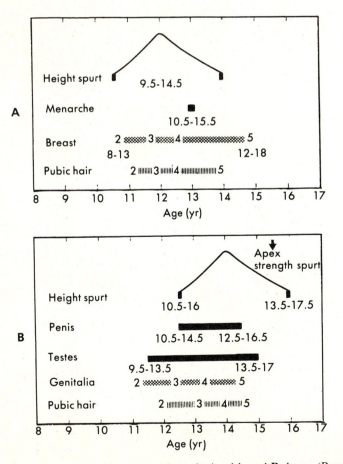

Fig. 1-5. Diagram of sequence of events at puberty in **A,** girls and **B,** boys. (Reprinted by permission of The New England Journal of Medicine. Marshall, W.A., and Tanner, J.M.: Arch. Dis. Child. **45:**13, 1970.)

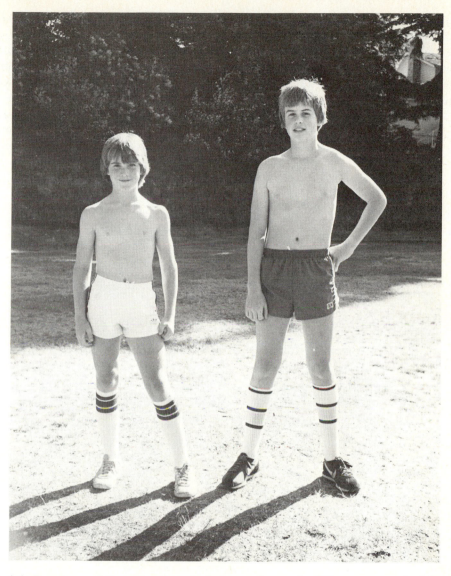

Fig. 1-6. Two boys of the same chronological age who are in different stages of adolescent development.

onset and time required for completion of each stage. The first event to be noticed usually is breast budding at an average age of 10.6 years. The range of normal ages is 9 to 13 years. Pubic hair usually develops later, but in one third of all girls pubic hair appears before breast development. The average time elapsed from breast budding to breast stage 3 is 1 year. Average time elapsed before reaching adult breast development is 4 years.

Some young women complete all phases in 1½ years, and others take 5 or more years.

Menarche occurs relatively late within the sequence of pubertal development. The mean ages at menarche for North American and European white females range from 12.8 to 13.2 years. (Table 1-3 gives the mean ages in other races and countries.) Menarche is largely independent from other pubertal characteristics and seems to relate most

Table 1-3. Heredity and environment in the control of growth*

Europe		Near East and India	
Oslo	13.2	Bagdad (well-off)	13.6
Stockholm	13.1	Istanbul (well-off)	12.3
Helsinki	13.2	Tel Aviv	13.2
Copenhagen	13.2	Iran (urban)	13.3
Netherlands	13.4	Tunis (well-off)	13.4
North-east England	13.4	Madras (urban)	12.8
London	13.0	Madras (rural)	14.2
Belgium	13.0		
Paris	13.2	**Asiatics**	
Zurich	13.1	Burma	13.2
Moscow	13.0	Singapore (average)	12.7
Warsaw	13.0	Hong Kong (well-off)	12.5
Budapest	12.8	Japan (urban)	12.9
Romania (urban)	13.3	Mexico	12.8
Carrara, Italy	12.6	Yucatan (well-off)	12.5
Naples (rural)	12.5	Eskimo	13.8
European-descended		**Africans**	
Montreal	13.1	Uganda (well-off)	13.4
USA, all areas	12.8	Nigeria, Ibadan (university-educated parents)	13.3
Sydney	13.0		
New Zealand	13.0	South Africa (urban)	14.9
Pacific		**African-descended**	
New Zealand (Maori)	12.7	USA, all areas	12.5
New Guinea (Bundi)	18.0	Cuba, all areas	13.0
New Guinea (Megiar)	15.5	Martinique	14.0

Reprinted by permission of the publishers from Foetus into man, by Tanner, J.M., Cambridge, Mass.: Harvard University Press, Copyright © 1978 by J.M. Tanner.
*Mean ages of menarche (years) in various population groups. All data refer to period between 1960 and 1975: status quo data with means calculated by probits or logits.

closely to skeletal age. Most young women are in breast stage 4 at menarche, but one fourth are in breast stage 3. A very small percentage will menstruate before breast stage 3. Similarly, most young women menstruate during pubic hair stage 3 or 4, a few in stage 5, and fewer still in stage 1. The relationship to height spurt is also close. All females menstruate when their height-gain velocity is decreasing, and the average menarche occurs at the time when the velocity is dropping most rapidly.[3,7,17-19]

Maximal height velocity occurs earlier in the growth sequence in females than in males. Postmenarcheal height gain is only about 6 cm (2.4 in), and the amount of this growth does not relate to early or late onset of menarche.

There appears to be a secular trend over the past 100 years for children living in industrialized countries to have increased height and weight.[3] This may be in part the result of earlier maturation. In industrialized countries the trend is stopping slowly. More recently, the trend has been observed in underdeveloped countries.[3]

A secular trend of decreasing menarcheal age (at a rate of 0.3 yr/decade between 1830 and 1960) also has been reported.[3] Recently, however, there have been questions raised concerning the accuracy of this interpretation of these data. Although the menarcheal age has decreased to some degree, the suggestion has been made that the change is not of the magnitude previously described.

Longitudinal studies that determine mean menarcheal ages of specific ethnic groups presently are unavailable. One researcher, using cross-sectional data, reported mean menarcheal ages of Puerto Rican, black, and white girls living in a large East Coast city to be earlier than 12.8 years.[20] A larger study of class-homogeneous Oriental, Spanish-American, black, and white women in a West Coast city found no significant difference in mean menarcheal ages.[21] Menarcheal age appears to be more closely related to socioeconomic class variables, such as nutrition, than to ethnicity. Recent hormonal studies of white and Bantu girls supported the relationship of inadequate nutrition to delayed adrenal maturation.[22] They also showed that delay in reaching critical body weight/fat ratio resulted in delayed menarche.

Magnitude and Areas of Growth

The growth spurt is under the joint hormonal control of androgens and growth hormone, and height gained during the growth spurt seems to be somewhat independent of previous growth. The hormonal control of skeletal maturation is not completely understood, and maturation may depend on different hormones at different times. Testosterone, other androgens, and estrogen exert an effect on linear growth and accelerate skeletal maturation (closure of epiphyses). Growth hormone, thyroid hormone, and sex hormones are all necessary for proper growth during adolescence.

For the average male, there is an expected increase of 7 cm (2.8 in) in the first year of the growth spurt, 9 cm (3.6 in) in the second year, and 7 cm (2.8 in) in the third year. The spurt increases trunk length more than leg length, and leg length growth peaks 6 to 9 months before trunk length growth. This difference in leg and trunk growth, coupled with muscles that have not fully developed, may result in a 6-month period during which the adolescent will experience balance problems.

Because the farthest part of a limb begins to grow first, a practical sign of the onset of the growth spurt is a rapid change in shoe size. The complaint from young adolescents that hands and feet seem too large relates to this growth. Since shoulders and chest are the last to reach growth peaks, young men stop outgrowing their jeans before their jackets.

During adolescence, skull bone thickness increases by 15% and scalp tissue grows, thus enlarging head diameter. Definite facial changes are noted, particularly in males. Brow ridges and air sinuses grow, resulting in a more prominent forehead. The jaws grow forward and facial muscles develop. However, these changes are individualized, and some young men may show little if any change in facial dimension.[3]

The greatest sexual difference of pubertal skeletal growth is between male and female shoulder and hip growth. This difference is caused by the specific response to estrogen in the female hip joint cartilage and the specific response to testosterone in the male shoulder joint cartilage. In final size, the female skeleton is smaller than the male skele-

ton with the exception of the hips. The female skeletal hip growth spurt equals that of young men, and this, combined with the smaller skeletal structure of females, gives the larger hip appearance. The male skeletal shoulder, on the other hand, has a marked pubertal spurt that results in the broad-shouldered adult male.

During adolescent growth, the female pelvic outlet, which is already wider than the male, widens further. This, along with the increased hip

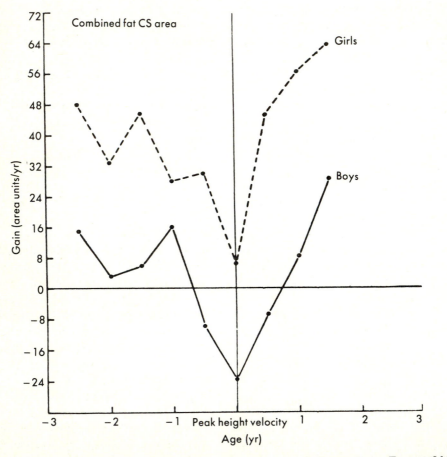

Fig. 1-7. Subcutaneous fat growth in upper arm and calf at adolescence. (From Tanner, J.M.: Radiographic studies of body composition. In Brožek, J., editor: Human body composition: approaches and applications, Oxford, 1965, Pergamon Press, Ltd.)

width, provides room for prenatal fetal growth should there be a pregnancy. Conception before this growth is complete conceivably could result in restriction of the fetal growth process.

Both male and female experience a muscle growth spurt—an increase in muscle mass and strength. The somewhat earlier though smaller spurt in females results in a short period of time during which girls have more muscle than boys. Ultimately, however, the muscle mass increase in males is much greater than in females. This muscle size increase is accompanied by a marked increase in strength. Males also develop larger heart and skeletal muscles and experience an increase in blood pressure and a decrease in resting heart rate. Power, skill, and endurance increase steadily throughout adolescence.[3,23]

Subcutaneous fat deposition takes an opposite course. During adolescence, girls accumulate more fat. In males the fat deposition decreases and actually reaches a negative velocity (Fig. 1-7). This results in body composition of higher percentage fat in females as shown in Fig. 3-1. Methods for determining percentage of body fatness are discussed in Chapter 3.

Knowledge of pubertal development and growth can be used to prepare adolescents and to reduce their anxiety over these changes. Discussion about what is happening to their bodies by a caring professional is usually of keen interest to adolescents and is well accepted.

MEASUREMENT OF DEVELOPMENTAL AGE

Because bones pass through the same various stages and result in the same final state of maturation in all individuals, skeletal maturity or bone age is the most accurate measurement of developmental age at any chronological age. Skeletal age can be used to determine remaining growth potential and to estimate ultimate height.

To determine skeletal age, accurate height is measured and chronological age obtained. Roent-genograms then are taken of bone growth centers, and skeletal age is determined by comparing these centers to a standardized atlas of roentgenograms compiled by Greulich and Pyle or by using the bone-scoring method of Tanner and co-workers.[24] The difference if any between the skeletal age and chronological age is determined. By using this information in the formula presented in Appendix A, adult height can be predicted.

Although skeletal growth continues until about age 30 by apposition of bone to upper and lower surfaces of the vertebral bodies, for practical purposes growth is considered to have ceased when the epiphyses of the long bones completely fuse. This happens at an average age of 17.75 for males and 16.25 for females.[25]

Advanced or delayed bone age that differs from the chronological age by 3 or more years suggests the possibility of an endocrine imbalance, and a complete medical evaluation should be pursued.

PROBLEMS ASSOCIATED WITH PUBERTAL GROWTH

Short Stature

Chronic systemic disease in nonendocrine systems is the most common pathological reason for short stature. Many disorders fit into this category (for example, inflammatory bowel disease, chronic renal disease, chronic lung disease, diabetes, liver disease, and heart disease). Malnutrition resulting from chronic malabsorption and hormonal regulation resulting from hypoxemia and/or acidosis have been suggested as possible causes for growth retardation in these disorders. Any suggestion that systemic disease may be present should be followed with a complete medical evaluation.

Skeletal and chromosomal abnormalities are commonly associated with short stature, but short stature is rarely the only manifestation of these disorders. Turner's syndrome and its variants are one group that may be characterized by short stature in females with delayed onset of pubertal development.

For usually unknown reasons, children who are mentally retarded or severely emotionally disturbed frequently display poorer growth than peers of the same age.[26] Catch-up growth may be seen if the emotional deprivation is reversed.

Endocrine disorders are the least frequent causes for short stature and usually can be specifically treated. Disorders of the gonads or the pituitary, thyroid, or adrenal glands may result in short stature. Diagnosis can be made by using thorough physical and laboratory evaluations.[26]

The most frequent cause of short stature is constitutional delay in growth and development. No sign of secondary sexual development will be seen in an otherwise normal 13-year-old female or 14-year-old male affected by constitutional delay. The rapid growth of most adolescents during puberty makes the lag these youngsters experience appear even more severe. The cause for this condition is unknown, but 60% of these teens will have a family history of similar growth patterns.

An example of a short stature problem caused by constitutional delay would be a 16-year-old male whose height is similar to an average 12½-year-old male. He has no sign of chronic disease and has grown slowly but steadily throughout childhood. His father entered puberty at 16 years of age and grew until 19 years of age. Laboratory studies reveal normal levels of growth hormone and/or somatomedin and normal thyroid function. At 16 years of age, he shows definite concern over his lack of growth. His problem is intensified if he has a brother or sister who is growing at a more accelerated rate and is the same height at a younger age. Evaluation includes a careful history emphasizing parental size, growth patterns, and age at pubertal onset; actual growth records since early childhood; nutritional status; and any significant disease process. Typically, the physical examination will reveal the body of a 12-year-old male with beginning testicular enlargement at genitalia stage 2. Bone

age will be 12½ to 13 years. An adult height prediction can be made using Appendix A. For many young men, reassurance and the knowledge that they will reach a normal height is sufficient. However, if the psychological impact of pubertal delay is extreme and reassurance is not enough, treatment with a synthetic steroid such as oxandrolone (Anavar), which will act to accelerate linear growth, may be indicated. If oxandrolone is used, the clinical effects of its use should be monitored carefully at frequent intervals. Bone age should be monitored every 6 months, and therapy should be discontinued if no catch-up growth occurs, if epiphysial maturation accelerates too rapidly, or if unacceptable virilization occurs. Oxandrolone will not increase the ultimate height.[27]

Familial short stature occurs less frequently than delayed adolescence. These adolescents tend to be short from birth. They are healthy youngsters whose growth, although below the 3rd percentile, follows a normal curve. Their adolescent growth spurt and pubertal development are on schedule and normal. Bone age is equal to chronological age. Although the adolescent growth spurt is of average duration, ultimate height remains near the 3rd percentile.

In idiopathic intrauterine growth retardation, there is no family history of similar growth patterns. Some of these infants manifest rapid catch-up growth and continue in a normal growth pattern. Others remain small during early childhood but catch up later. Another group remains small while growing at a normal rate. The pattern of adolescent growth for these teens ranges from the early end of normal to a pattern similar to that of constitutional delay. The latter group, like adolescents with constitutional delay, would be considered for treatment with anabolic steroids.

Adolescent males or their parents exhibit the most concern over short stature. Occasionally, young women have a similar complaint. These young women usually are below the 150-cm (5-ft) mark and are concerned that they will remain be-

---

Causes of Short Stature

Constitutional delay in growth and pubertal development

Familial short stature

Intrauterine growth retardation

Chronic systemic disease in nonendocrine organs

Endocrine disorders

Chromosomal abnormalities

Skeletal abnormalities

Mental retardation

Emotional deprivation (psychosocial dwarfism)

---

low 150 cm in height. In addition to the approach described in the evaluation of young males, if the young woman has not menstruated, a chromosome analysis (karyotyping) should be obtained to rule out abnormalities of the X chromosome that could affect height growth potential.[26]

The causes of short stature are summarized in the box above.

Tall Stature

In contrast to the short male, young women complain more often about being too tall. Young women with this complaint, however, are fewer in number than the short males, perhaps because the definition of excessive tallness is varied and individually made. Body image and the heights of parents and peers are involved in whether a young woman considers herself excessively tall. Treatment usually is not considered unless adult height prediction is above 180 cm (71 in). The approach to diagnosis is the same as with a short stature problem and includes a family history, a record of past growth, and a review of systems (including careful attention to the onset of breast development and menarche). Physical examination, laboratory studies of growth hormone and thyroid function, and bone age films for height prediction complete

the evaluation. Ninety-five to ninety-eight percent of children who complain of tallness are normal. Organic diseases that cause tallness are summarized below:

Marfan's syndrome

Homocystinuria

Pituitary tumor

Cerebral gigantism

Untreated hyperthyroidism

Sexual precocity

Testicular feminization syndrome

XXY or XYY karyotype

Treatment of constitutional tall stature is controversial. The current method of treatment, large doses of estrogen, induces premature puberty in a young patient. The earlier treatment is started, the greater the reduction of adult height attained. Most clinicians will wait until a young woman is near menarche (bone age of 12½ to 13 years) before initiating treatment. Frequently, the young woman will not seek advice until after maximal height velocity has been reached, and this will affect the evaluation and treatment. Although the benefits may be less in postmenarcheal girls, treatment is still offered by some endocrinologists. Because tall stature is not a disease and estrogen therapy may have unknown long-term side effects, treatment continues to be controversial. Careful consideration of side effects versus possible benefits must be made before treatment is suggested.[28-30]

Males rarely complain of tall stature. However, if a male of tall stature has poor testicular development, an organic disorder must be considered. In constitutional tall stature, a mature height of 195 cm is used as a minimal height prediction before treatment is offered. Treatment consists of testosterone administered intramuscularly.[28]

Delayed Puberty

Delayed puberty or variation in the time needed to complete pubertal development can also create problems. The delayed onset of menarche, in particular, may be a problem for young women. If menarche does not follow within 4 years of initial breast development, an evaluation is in order. In addition to attention to family patterns of pubertal development, childhood growth, and history of disease and emotional stress, the possibility of eating disorders such as anorexia nervosa should be explored (see Chapter 5). Extreme physical exercise combined with the stress of performance and competition can influence menarche in some adolescents (for example, serious ballet students, runners, and swimmers). The exercise alone or in combination with diets intended to keep body fat below 20% can delay menarche. On the other hand, a recent large weight gain can also be significant. A thorough physical examination (including accurate measurements of height and weight, a determination of breast and pubic hair stages, and a pelvic examination to rule out anatomical reasons for delayed puberty such as an imperforate hymen or absent uterus) should follow. Thyroid screening and laboratory studies to determine bone age and LH, FSH, and prolactin levels should be done. If there is any suggestion that Turner's syndrome (ovarian dysgenesis) could be present, a chromosomal analysis should be done.[11,29]

Sports Participation

Sports may present a possible problem during adolescent growth. Chronological age and sex commonly are used to group children for participation in sports programs. Some programs include weight in their criteria. As previously stated, the range of individual variation in physical structure and maturation is greatest between the ages of 10 and 16 years. Boys at the same chronological age can vary by as much as 60 months in skeletal age. That difference can result in a height difference of 37.5 cm (15 in) and a weight difference of 40.5 kg (90 lb). Muscle mass and strength will also vary. These differences should be considered when organizing boys for athletic competition.

Although young women experience a brief period of time in early puberty when they may be larger and stronger than young men of the same chronological age, once puberty is complete the average male will be larger and stronger than the average female. For this reason, some experts oppose unisex competition after puberty in sports that require speed, strength, and endurance.

Adolescents experience other sports-related problems because peak height velocity causes ligaments to slacken and become more elastic. This can result in major trauma from twisting, turning, and jumping activity in sports.

It would be helpful if these factors would be taken into consideration when planning sports programs for adolescents. Parents should be made aware of the possible hazards to their children and should be encouraged to promote skill building over extreme competitiveness.[22,31]

Gynecomastia

Gynecomastia is often a significant event to young men. During puberty, 30% or more of normal males will develop some discrete breast tissue. This is usually bilateral and nontender. Twenty percent will have unilateral development, and some will be tender. Gynecomastia ordinarily recedes spontaneously within 18 to 24 months after its appearance. Should it persist for more than 24 months, surgical correction may need to be considered to prevent psychological distress in the adolescent.[32]

Early breast development in the normal female may occur unilaterally. Usually the inequality in size disappears with further growth. Since surgical biopsy of a breast bud in its early stages of growth could remove the entire bud, it is important to recognize the possibility of unilateral development and avoid hasty treatment.[33]

Use of Sexual Maturity Stages

The sexual maturity stages for breasts, pubic hair, and genitalia can be useful in alerting the

Table 1-4. Common conditions at various stages of sexual maturity

Event	Sexual Maturity Stage
Hematocrit rise (male)	2-5
Adolescent hormonal levels (rise in estrogen for females and testosterone for males)	3
Peak height velocity (male)	3-4
Peak height velocity (female)	2-3
Short male with growth potential	2
Short male with limited growth potential	4-5
Usual appearance of menarche	Late 3 or early 4 (1-3.6 yr after stage 2)
Slipped capital femoral epiphysis (obese)	2-3
Rapid progression of scoliosis	2-4
Osgood-Schlatter disease	3
"Normal" gynecomastia	2-3
Acne	2-3
Decreased serous otitis	2-3

Modified from Greydanus, D.E., and McAnarney, E.: J. Curr. Adolesc. Med. **2**(2):21, 1980.

health professional, teacher, and parent to possible commonly seen physical problems. The stages can help predict situations that will need to be attended to in health screening and guidance. Table 1-4 illustrates this well.

SUMMARY

Physical growth during the adolescent years is great. The end result is an adult physique that falls within the genetic, environmental, nutritional, and cultural norms of each individual. This result is reached by a definite sequence of events. The chronological age of onset, the length of time required to complete each sequence, and occasionally the events within the sequence vary. It is important for persons dealing with the adolescent to be aware of the changes that occur and of the resulting problems that may develop. This knowledge helps either to avoid the problems or to prepare for and plan to solve the problems.

Attempts have been made to relate emotional and behavioral changes in adolescence to hormonal changes. Unfortunately, no one has successfully studied normal adolescent development by comparing emotions and hormones longitudinally. Such research would be valuable.

The following chapters will relate the nutritional needs of the adolescent to the aspects of growth and development summarized in this chapter.

REFERENCES

1. Barnes, H.V.: Physical growth and development during puberty, Med. Clin. North Am. **59**:1305, 1975.
2. Marks, A.: Aspects of biosocial screening and health maintenance in adolescents, Pediatr. Clin. North Am. **27**:155, 1980.
3. Tanner, J.M.: Foetus into man, Cambridge, Mass., 1978, Harvard University Press.
4. Vaughan, V.C., McKay, R.J., and Nelson, W., editors: Nelson textbook of pediatrics, Philadelphia, 1975, W.B. Saunders Co.
5. Frasier, S.D.: Growth disorders in children, Pediatr. Clin. North Am. **26**:1, 1979.
6. Finkelstein, J.W.: The endocrinology of adolescence, Pediatr. Clin. North Am. **27**:53, 1980.

7. Grumbach, M.M., and Grave, M., editors: Control of the onset of puberty, New York, 1974, John Wiley & Sons, Inc.

8. Apter, D., and Vihko, R.: Serum pregnenolone, progesterone, 17-hydroxyprogesterone, testosterone and 5-dihydrotestosterone during female puberty, J. Clin. Endocrinol. Metab. **45:**1039, 1977.

9. Sizonenko, P.C.: Endocrinology in preadolescents and adolescents. I. Hormonal changes during puberty, Am. J. Dis. Child. **132:**704, 1978.

10. Reiter, E.O., and Root, A.W.: Hormonal changes of adolescence, Med. Clin. North Am. **59:**1289, 1975.

11. Odell, W.D.: Symposium on adolescent gynecology and endocrinology. I. Physiology of sexual maturation and primary amenorrhea, West. J. Med. **131:**401, 1979.

12. Frisch, R.E., and McArthur, J.W.: Menstrual cycles: fatness as a determinant of minimum weight for height necessary for their maintenance or onset, Science **185:**949, 1974.

13. Frisch, R.E.: Fatness of girls from menarche to age 18 years, with a nomogram, Hum. Biol. **48:**353, 1976.

14. Frisch, R.E.: Menarche and fatness: reexamination of the critical body composition hypothesis, Science **200:**1506, 1978.

15. Crawford, J.D., and Osler, D.C.: Body composition at menarche: the Frisch-Revelle hypothesis revisited, Pediatrics **56:**449, 1975.

16. Faulkner, F., and Tanner, J.M., editors: Human growth, vol. 2, New York, 1978, Plenum Press.

17. Greydanus, D.E., and McAnarney, E.R.: The value of the Tanner staging, J. Curr. Adolesc. Med. **2**(2):21, 1980.

18. Bullough, V.L.: Age at menarche: a misunderstanding, Science **213:**365, 1981.

19. Lee, P.A.: Normal ages of pubertal events among American males and females, J. Adolesc. Health Care, **1:**26, 1980.

20. Litt, I.F., and Cohen, M.I.: Age of menarche: a changing pattern and its relationship to ethnic origin and delinquency, J. Pediatr. **82:**288, 1973.

21. Weir, J., and others: Race and age at menarche, Am. J. Obstet. Gynecol. **111:**594, 1971.

22. Hill, P., and others: Diet and menarche in different ethnic groups, Eur. J. Cancer **16:**519, 1980.

23. Smith, N.J., editor: Sports medicine for children and youth. Report of the Tenth Ross Roundtable on Critical Approaches to Common Pediatric Problems, Columbus, Ohio, Dec. 1969, Ross Laboratories.

24. Tanner, J.M., and others: Assessment of skeletal maturity and prediction of adult height, London, 1975, Academic Press, Inc., Ltd.

25. Kelley, V.C., editor: Practice of pediatrics, rev. ed., New York, 1981, Harper & Row, Publishers, Inc.

26. Fisher, M., and others: Growth problems in adolescence. I. Short stature, J. Curr. Adolesc. Med. **2**(10):24, 1980.

27. Moore, D.C., and others: Studies of anabolic steroids. V. Effect of prolonged oxandrolone administration on growth in children and adolescents with uncomplicated short stature, Pediatrics **58:**412, 1976.

28. Fisher, M., and others: Growth problems in adolescence. II. Tall stature, J. Curr. Adolesc. Med. **2**(11):23, 1980.

29. Davajan, V., and Kletzky, O.: Symposium on adolescent gynecology and endocrinology. II. Secondary amenorrhea: hirsutism in adolescents and the clinical consequences of stilbestrol exposure in utero, West. J. Med. **131:**516, 1979.

30. Bailey, J.D., Park, E., and Cowell, C.: Estrogen treatment of girls with constitutional tall stature, Pediatr. Clin. North Am. **28:**501, 1981.

31. Faiget, H.C.: A developmental approach to adolescence, Pediatr. Clin. North Am. **21:**353, 1974.

32. Penny, R.: The testis, Pediatr. Clin. North Am. **26:**107, 1979.

35. Dewhurst, J.: Breast disorders in children and adolescents, Pediatr. Clin. North Am. **28:**287, 1981.

Chapter 2

Psychosocial Development in Adolescence

LEONA L. EGGERT

Who am I? What will I do with my life? What do I value? How do I find myself? How do I go about building meaningful relationships?

Adolescents search for answers to these and other questions like them even though they rarely express them as such. For the majority of youth, adolescence is a time for enjoying many successes; others experience certain times of particular stress; and still others find the whole transition into adulthood to be full of uncertainties, instabilities, and many, many surprises. For all adolescents, however, the task of finding a sense of identity is of primary importance. No other 10-year period in life contains as many requirements and momentous changes as adolescence. It is helpful to remember that although the conflicts met in adolescence vary widely from one person to another, they all serve to prepare the adolescent for the subsequent developmental tasks of young adulthood.

One purpose of the study of adolescent development is to aid adults in facilitating the transition of adolescents from childhood to adulthood. Since our youth are often viewed as the hope and future of our nation, it is important that the phenomenon of adolescence be understood clearly. This understanding comes from examining adolescents' psychosocial development: what it is, when it occurs, and what forces influence and shape it.

SPAN OF ADOLESCENCE

"Adolescence." . . . It sounds just like some disease!

—*a 16-year-old*[1]

The developmental period called adolescence, although often set apart from other periods in life for the convenience of academic discussion, is in reality intimately related to the preceding period of childhood and the following period of young adulthood. Adolescence, derived from *adolescere,* the Latin verb meaning "to grow into maturity," is the time between the onset of puberty and adulthood. The phenomenon is firmly rooted in both physiological facts, the times, and the culture.

Social scientists interested in human development disagree about the definition, characteristics, patterns, and meaning of adolescence. However, there seems to be a relative consensus among current scholars about some observations: (1) Psychologically, adolescence is a period of multiple physiological changes requiring many personality adaptations toward more adultlike behavior and responsibilities. It is a time of cognitive awakening when expanded ways of thinking become possible. (2) Sociologically, adolescence is a transition period marked by a cyclical progression away from the dependent state of a child and toward the independent state of an adult. Acceptance of the role responsibilities and status of an adult is the goal. (3) Anthropologically, adolescence is a cultural invention, a transition period sanctioned by a society to give an individual time to become initiated into adulthood. In some cultures, initiation rites are granted at puberty, thus promoting an individual *directly* from childhood into adulthood. In our society, no such distinct initiation rites exist, and adolescence is a diffuse interval.

Arriving at a precise age range for the period of adolescence is difficult in our society. Although it generally is agreed that adolescence begins with puberty, there is less agreement on when it ends. One of the difficulties is that many believe full adulthood is not assumed until people are completely independent of their parents. With increasing numbers of youth continuing on in college for many years, economic emancipation from parents is delayed. This delay accounts for the belief by some that adolescence is overly long. Another reason it is difficult to determine adulthood in our society is that adult status and privileges are granted at different ages for different tasks. For example, although young men must register for the draft and are considered ready to fight in a war at 18 years of age, they cannot buy liquor until 21 years of age. Adolescence thus has a biological beginning and a psychological and sociocultural ending.

As summarized in Chapter 1, adolescent development, both psychological and physical, is often divided into three stages: early, middle, and late. The various aspects of psychosocial development progress along their own continuums and can be studied independently.

COMPONENTS OF ADOLESCENT DEVELOPMENT

People tend to have tacit preconceptions about adolescence derived from their own teenage years within a particular culture. To attain greater objectivity, a study of theories related to adolescent development is necessary. Professionals from the fields of psychology, psychiatry, anthropology, sociology, and education have contributed concepts developed from their perspectives on the developmental processes of adolescence. Some of these concepts are summarized in the following discussion.

Changes in Body Image

Blos[2] claimed that puberty *causes* adolescence and results in multiple changes in virtually every aspect of life for the adolescent. He contended that these changes help the adolescent to accomplish one major task: *the modification of former ideas about body and image*. Blos said, ''A change of one's body image and a re-evaluation of the self in the light of new physical powers and sensations are two of the psychological consequences of the change in physical status.''[2] The changes, being so highly evident and marked, cause adolescents continually to compare and contrast their progress and status with that of their peers. Variations in breast and genital development, voice changes, pimples, facial hair, and all other kinds of physical changes and differences cause concern among self-conscious adolescents. Obesity of varying degrees frequently leads to experimenting with diets in search for an instant cure. The hope of all adolescents is that they are not significantly different from their peers, since there is comfort and stability in being the same. But this hope is incongruent with the highly variable progression of physical development among adolescents.

Cognitive Awakening

According to Piaget,[3-5] one of the fundamental differences that exists between children and adolescents is their cognitive capability. Before adolescence, children are in the period of *concrete operations*. During this time, children learn to think logically, but they find it difficult to go beyond what can be imagined in relatively concrete terms. During adolescence, the teenager enters the period of *formal operations*. In this period, individuals acquire the ability to deal with the hypothetical as well as the concrete or the actual. They learn to reason about what is possible in imagined settings and develop the ability to be idealistic. Adolescents learn to recognize that many of the world's problems are not just accidental and that human creations could have been created differently. They are capable of profoundly feeling the injustice, the inequity, and, in some cases, the stupidity that led to the world's problems. In contrast, they can also feel awed by human nature and the forces that shape our destiny. They can be moved to organize in an attempt to eliminate the injustices or to change the state of affairs that they now recognize.

Also during this time, the conscience, the set of rules that governs behavior, is thoroughly reexamined. Rules enforced by parents (or other authorities) and rules that made sense in terms of peer interaction are examined, tested, modified, discarded, or accepted. Rules are individualized to fit the adolescent's own sense of morality.[6]

Inhelder and Piaget[3] discussed two distinct stages within the formal operations period. Stage A, occurring approximately between 11 and 13+ years of age, is characterized by transitions. During this stage, cognitive capacity is still expanding. Stage B, occurring approximately between 13 and 15+ years of age, is characterized by final restructuring of the mind. In this stage, the mind realizes full potential, and there is movement away from the concrete toward forms of experimentation, hypothesis testing, analysis, synthesis, and evaluation. Exploratory ideas and abstract, reflective, self-generated thoughts dominate.

Table 2-1 summarizes the periods of cognitive development as defined by Piaget.

Although able to think abstractly, adolescents probably will still learn best through their own concrete actions and experiences with the support and limit setting of important adults. They are novices in the process of learning when it comes to thinking out all the possibilities, combinations,

and determinants that one must cope with in making decisions about the future or resolving interpersonal problems in the present.

The capacity for formal operational thought permits adolescents to conceptualize not only what they think but also what others think. They often become obsessed with the idea that others are as concerned with them as they are themselves. According to Elkind,[7] "This belief that others are preoccupied with their appearance and behavior constitutes the egocentrism of adolescents." The two mental configurations Elkind[8,9] described as being a consequence of adolescent egocentrism are an *imaginary audience* and the *personal fable*. Frequently adolescents anticipate the reactions of other people in light of their own perceptions; in this sense, they are continually playing to an imaginary audience. Another way that adolescents fortify themselves is by creating a story, a personal fable, that they tell themselves and want to believe. By 16 or 17 years of age, however, adolescents are cognitively able to differentiate between their thoughts and those of others.

Simply because an adolescent has grown several inches in height, it does not follow that his or her thinking ability has expanded at the same rate or at the same time. The tall boy and the well-developed girl are not necessarily more mature thinkers or better learners. The more complex thinking capabilities acquired during adolescence occur in different ways and at different times in different individuals. Thus it is important to realize in working with adolescents that their mental capabilities with regard to problem solving are in differing stages of refinement. The adolescent's skill will depend on individual state of development and on the opportunities the adolescent has received for exercising the mind in the use of these new skills.

Certainly the ability to do effective personal and interpersonal problem solving and decision making is one important outcome of intellectual development. Mentally acting on or reacting to life's problem situations constitutes much of adult thought.

Table 2-1. Comparison of Erikson's and Piaget's developmental models

Approximate Age (yr)	Erikson	Piaget
0-1	**Stage I** Basic trust versus mistrust	**Sensorimotor Period** Learning through senses and manipulation
1-4	**Stage II** Autonomy versus shame and doubt	**Preconceptual Period** Classification by a single feature (e.g., size); no concern for contradictions
4-8	**Stage III** Initiative versus guilt	**Initiative Thought Period** Intuitive classification (e.g., awareness of conservation of mass concept)
8-12	**Stage IV** Industry versus inferiority	**Concrete Operations Period** Logical thought development; learning to organize
12-20	**Stage V** Ego identify versus role confusion	**Formal Operations Period** Comprehension of abstract concepts; formation of "ideals"
20 onward	**Stage VI** Intimacy versus isolation	—
Middle adulthood	**Stage VII** Generativity versus stagnation	—
Late adulthood	**Stage VIII** Integrity versus despair	—

The adolescent is in the process of developing skills for intelligently approaching problem-solving situations by exercising problem-solving skills. The adolescent is learning to distinguish between facts and hypotheses in a situation, to synthesize the validity and relevance of information, and to evaluate everything as it relates to the problem situation. By 16 to 18 years of age, the adolescent usually has developed intellectually to where his or her thought processes are like those of an adult.

Evaluation of personal weaknesses and strengths and development of individualized values and attitudes are now possible and become integrated with self-identity, interpersonal communication, and decision making.

Social and Cultural "Fit"

Sociologically, the major task to be accomplished during adolescence is learning to accept and fit adult roles in society. Adolescence is a time

Qualifying as an Adult: What Does It Take?

Some Requirements for Adulthood in the United States	A	P	L	R	S	$*
Are granted the right to vote	X		X			
Can answer the question, "Who am I?"					X	
Are capable of supporting self						X
Have reached full physical maturation		X				
Have chosen a vocation and defined congruent goals for achievement					X	
Have achieved procreative family status (learned a sex role)				X	X	
Can legally buy liquor			X			X
Are required to register for the draft	X		X			
Have organized a value system to guide actions throughout life					X	
Have achieved full development of intellectual skills		X			X	
Can obtain a driver's license	X		X			X
Have become legally responsible for own actions			X		X	X
Have become a contributing member of society	X		X	X	X	X
Have become emancipated from parents (left home)				X		X
Have become 18 years of age or 21 years of age	X					

*A, Requires a specific age. P, Requires physical changes. L, Requires legal rights. R, Requires relationship changes. S, Requires increased self-awareness. $, Requires self-support or money.

when individuals within a society are no longer perceived as children but have not yet been accorded the status of adults. From the sociological viewpoint, adolescence thus is not determined by the biological changes of puberty. Rather, the form, substance, duration, and onset of adolescence are variously determined in different cultures and societies. Hollingshead[10] concluded that psychological facts about adolescence are often dependent on sociocultural realities.

Mead[11-13] emphasized the importance of cultural factors and social institutions in a young person's development. In contrast to less complex cultures, our American culture presents youth with a myriad of choices and forces them to consider a whole series of different and conflicting opinions, practices, and values when making those choices. In our society, youth also are faced with conflicting realities, for they view extensive violations of every code we have in almost every newspaper, magazine, film, and TV program. Compounding the burden of choice that our youth must face is the fact that various members of the same extended or even immediate family may hold contradictory beliefs and opinions. In sum, adolescents in our society are faced by countless groups, each believing and advocating something different. In each of the groups, some friend, relative, or trusted or admired adult may be trying to influence the adolescent in his or her decisions. Thus critical decisions that arise for youth are made difficult by the presence of conflicting standards; the resulting pressure can be overwhelming.

During adolescence, individuals mature toward adulthood by learning to act like adults, by preparing for life's work, and by developing a sense of responsibility. The box above lists some of the criteria that usually are used to define adulthood.

The list is not exhaustive and is subject to changes in laws and traditions. It serves to illustrate the complex way we inform adolescents about how and when they are accorded adult status in our society.

Question of Identity

Erikson[14-16] modified psychoanalytical theory in accord with the findings of cultural anthropology. He divided psychosexual development into eight progressive stages of development from birth to death as shown in Table 2-1. The stage of development that corresponds with adolescence is labeled "Ego Identity versus Role Confusion." The adolescent's search for an identity is the major focus of contemporary American youth and is a consequence of the way our society shapes their lives. The task is made more difficult because of the myriad of choices adolescents face and the discontinuity in learned values and behavioral expectations they experience throughout their total child development.[16,17]

Identity, according to Erikson, is the capacity to see yourself as having continuity and sameness. He regards adolescence as a developmental stage during which a positive ego identity is to be established. If ego identity is not effectively established at this time, there is the danger of role confusion. Adolescents need to come to know themselves in a new way made possible by their expanded intellectual capabilities. They need to believe that others see them as they see themselves. Of principal importance is the adolescent's need to develop a real sense of uniqueness. Erikson's primary theme regarding identity seems to be this notion of uniqueness. He wrote:

Identity includes, but is more than, the sum of all successive identifications of those earlier years when the child wanted to be, and often was forced to become, like the people he depended on. Identity is a unique product, which now meets a crisis to be solved only in new identifications with age mates and with leader figures outside of the family.[16]

A *sense of identity* includes knowing what you want and what you can and cannot do. It involves a willingness and ability to fit goals and talents to the possibilities afforded by the surroundings. The essence here is the development of potential. This development of the self involves an awareness and appraisal of skills and aptitudes. The adolescent must find a place in the network of social roles that includes work, procreation, and function in society. The adolescent must come to some sense of what life means, decide what rules shall guide behavior, and discover what intrinsic worth he or she is to have.

A *negative identity*, on the other hand, is characterized by individuals being in rebellion against themselves and against all those with whom they ordinarily would be expected to have good relations. There are strong feelings of hostility and of being totally isolated and left out. Adolescents react negatively or even self-destructively to new situations.

Identity diffusion exists when individual adolescents have no clear concept of who they are or what they want to be but are not overwhelmed by negative factors or hostility. For many, this period of time or condition is a preliminary phase to the development of a true identity.

An *identity crisis* is a term Erikson used to indicate an intense, though not pathological, state during which adolescents reexamine their basic values, their vocational choices, and their entire approach to the business of living. The behavioral picture for individuals in this state is predictable: they may find it difficult to direct their energies and may feel the need for taking some "time out" to let their souls catch up with their bodies.

For many American youth, their identity search becomes an identity crisis because of the multiple choices they face regarding future occupation, religious conviction, political affiliation, marriage, life-style, and so forth. All of these decisions ultimately contribute to the adolescent's sense of identity in our culture. Unlike some other societies, however, American culture expects the majority of these decisions to be made during the second decade of life, thus contributing to a culturally determined adolescence.

To ease the crisis situation, Erikson proposed a moratorium on decision making so that at least part of adolescence would be a time when decisions are deferred and experimentation is permitted. Erikson claimed that an opportunity to test many alternatives before decision-making would enhance a firm sense of self. He also suggested that *meaningful frustration* serves to challenge, direct, and facilitate learning for adolescents; it is meaningless frustration that results in neurosis. He contended further that there is a psychological need for adolescents to establish firmly a sense of identity before intimacy can be achieved. Thus marriage should not be considered before the establishment of ego identity.[14-16]

SOCIETAL DEFINITIONS OF MATURITY

Right now, getting out of school and becoming my own man. . . . Establishing my own roots and establishing myself, period, as a successful black man. . . . That's what's very important to me right now.[18]

Society's expectations for adolescents have great impact on the developmental process. The tasks that Havighurst[19] and other theorists[10] have identified for adolescents represent society's goals for individuals. These tasks become the criteria by which society judges the relative maturity of individuals. Fig. 2-1 presents the tasks, the customary age range when teens are focusing on the tasks, and the ways teens might express the tasks.

An additional aspect of developmental task theory is that mastery of the tasks is sequential. That is, progression of development through task mastery ordinarily is continuous, and mastery of earlier developmental tasks in childhood is often a prerequisite for mastery of later tasks. Havighurst

believed that there is usually a critical stage when developmental tasks are most easily mastered and should be accomplished. For example, adolescents who do not establish the kinds of close relationships with others that are expected of them during adolescence may experience greater difficulty attempting to do so during later periods of life. Further, this difficulty in accomplishing the task of intimacy in late adolescence may be the result of a lack of mastery of trust in early childhood. Hence there is real purpose in the adolescent years.

Adolescence permits major changes or transformations of personality. Because of this, adolescence is a time for optimism, since it is rather like a second chance to work through the tasks of earlier stages. It is analogous, in some respects, to "upsetting the egg basket," examining the contents, perhaps doing some rearranging, adding or subtracting, and then returning the eggs to the basket. A challenging, responsive, and confirming environment is important in this process. Parents and other important adults who provide these challenges, responsive interactions, and messages of confirmation can enable the adolescent to undo damage done in earlier stages. Wounds of inconsistency, deprivation, or ignorance can be healed, and the adolescent can then move beyond these scars to responsible and satisfying adulthood.

Hence the manner in which a sense of identity is achieved and movement into adult roles is made depends greatly on what is happening in the society or in the social circle and environment of the adolescent. Social context has a profound influence on the results of events that are likely to occur and on the reactions that the adolescent is likely to have in the process of forming a stable identity.

THE ADOLESCENT'S WORLD

If the adolescent leaves the home with a feeling of warmth and worth, the rest of the way will be that much easier.[1]

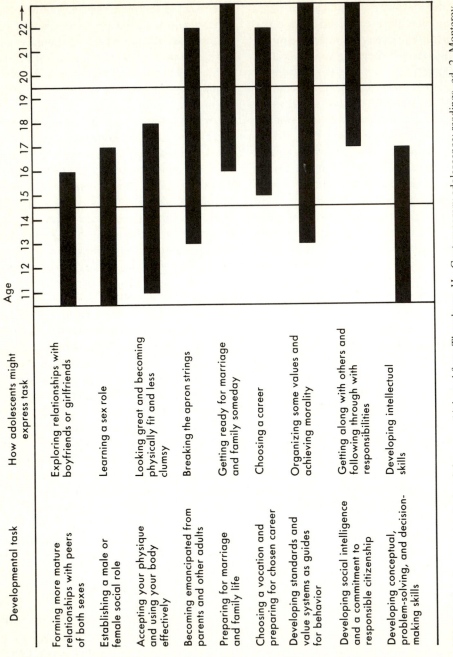

Fig. 2-1. Developmental tasks in adolescence. (Adapted from Thornburg, H.: Contemporary adolescence: readings, ed. 2, Monterey, Calif., 1975, Brooks/Cole Publishing Co.)

Adolescents and Their Families

There is an old Chinese proverb that states, "Nobody's family can hang out a sign, 'Nothing matters here.'" In our society the family is the cornerstone. Many people believe that the strength of our nation is dependent on the strength of the family. Likewise, many believe that the nature of adolescents' identity crises are dependent on the kinds of relationships they have with their parents. The better the relationship, the less likely the teen is to develop an identity crisis of serious proportions. The family has the primary responsibility for enabling the adolescent to establish a personal identity, to develop independence, and to attain sexual maturity. Paradoxically, the family also experiences a demise in its relative influence over the adolescent. Other groups and values compete with the family and become highly relevant to the adolescent. The family remains, for the most, the predominant reference group, but it no longer has the field to itself.

Changing Relationships. Campbell[20] described the changing relationship between adolescents and their parents in terms of two related dimensions: "There is a shift from power to companionship, and from instructing to advising." The shift may be anything from smooth to trying to stormy, but it is gradual; often adolescents and parents are unaware of the process.

The shift in power is described in terms of resources. In childhood there is a dependency on parents, and even though a child's opinions and involvement are sought out, parents make the decisions for their children. This is because parents have the bulk of resources (that is, money, strength, experience, knowledge, and community support) for acting in the best interests of their children. Shortly after the onset of adolescence, there are beginning attempts to move toward greater independence and a power balance. Adolescents mature and broaden their knowledge and experiences; they often equal or surpass their parents in physical strength. Since the majority earn money

or have an allowance, there is less dependence on the parents for buying power. With regard to community support, parents still have authority over adolescents, but this is juxtaposed with community support for adolescent autonomy. For example, in health care systems adolescents may have the right to contraceptive information and supplies and abortion without parental consent or knowledge.

The second dimension of change that Campbell described is a shift from an instructing to an advising mode. Although the emotional bonds remain and often grow stronger and shift to more mature forms of affection, the parents' responsibility for the individual ends at some point, and the adolescent becomes personally and legally responsible for him or herself. Parents now offer advice to their offspring, and the offspring have the freedom to "take it or leave it"; they are not compelled to "do as their parents say," which was implied in the earlier instruction mode.

The important point in this process of changing relationships is that the whole family system changes. Not only do the roles of the adolescent and the parent change, the role system changes. Since there is a change in the family role system during adolescence, some theorists refer to this developmental period as a family experience. The family is important not only because it gives emotional support and provides for physical needs but also because it transmits highly significant cultural values and societal functions.

In helping adolescents mature and achieve independence, a sense of identity, and sexual maturity, the goal of parents is to strengthen and to confirm adolescents in their environment without making them feel dependent.

Parents err when they either try to maintain total control through power or abandon all involvement or limits. In both child-rearing styles, the adolescent's development of a sense of autonomy can be inhibited. Baumrind[21] noted that a proper blend of explicit warmth and caring with firm discipline is likely to aid the adolescent in developing self-reliance, self-control, and adequate self-esteem. Bronfenbrenner[22] concluded that discipline and authority from the father is important to the development of a sense of responsibility in males. Paternal discipline, however, inhibits or is negatively associated with the development of responsibility in adolescent young women.

Teenagers need parents who know themselves: who they are, what their principles and values are, and what their hopes are. Parents should (1) serve as models or examples to either emulate or reject (living examples to test or knock against), and (2) represent stability (people to be sure of in a world that suddenly has become fraught with complexity and full of choices and decisions).

Generation Gap. Much research has been conducted in recent decades to explore the generation gap to discover the extent to which adolescents and their parents are in conflict. Coleman[23] and Friedenberg[24] both have researched the topic but have reached opposite conclusions. Coleman asserted that adolescents are developing a subculture of their own. Friedenberg, on the other hand, argued that conflicts and disparity of values between parents and adolescents have been exaggerated and are not as prevalent as media reports would have us believe. Mead[17] concurred with Friedenberg, and his conclusions probably are more representative of current trends. The findings of the *Youth 1976* survey[25] showed that

many young people accept traditional values and tend to live in conventional ways. However, many other young peole continue to be forerunners in the women's liberation movement, in the emergence and expansion of a new focus on self-fulfillment, and in changing work ethics that emphasize job satisfaction and the psychological benefits of work. This considerable minority, remaining critical of our society's institutions, politics, and lifestyles, comprises a major force for change.[25]

As Laycock[26] concluded, each investigator in this area "points to a danger that cannot be ignored if social health is to be maintained—on the one hand, that of stultification of the drive and energy with which adolescents challenge the shibboleths of previous generations, and on the other hand, that of the alienation of adolescents from the adult world."

Adolescents and Their Peers

There is little question that the peer group is extremely important during adolescence and serves as a major socializing agent. Hamacheck[27] modified the seven basic functions of the peer group as identified by Ausubel[28] in light of recent research findings. These functions, along with their value to the adolescent, are summarized below*:

1. *A replacement for family.* Status, or lack of it, and objective feedback from the peer group provide invaluable preparation for adulthood.
2. *A stabilizing influence.* The peer group becomes a stabilizer during a time of rapid change and transition—endocrinological developmental and social. There is comfort in knowing that others are also going through the stage of pimples and jitters.
3. *A source of self-esteem.* Becoming important to someone outside the family builds self-esteem. Unfortunately, the reverse is true for the adolescent who is isolated or made a scapegoat.
4. *A source of behavioral standards.* Recent research indicates that the peer group supplements rather than replaces the family as an important source of influence regarding behavioral standards. The family continues to be more influential on important issues such as future status, crucial values, and satisfaction of needs. Evidence indicates that the strongly peer-oriented child is such more by default and less by choice as a result of parental disregard.
5. *There is security in numbers.* In addition to persuading, the universal plea that "everyone else is going (or doing it, or whatever), why can't I?" serves to

---

*Modified from Hamachek, D.E.: Psychology and development of the adolescent self. In James F. Adams, Understanding adolescence: current developments in adolescent psychology, Fourth Edition. Copyright © 1980 by Allyn & Bacon, Inc. Reprinted with permission.

insulate and protect the adolescent from potential adult coercions.

6. *Opportunities for practice by doing.* The peer group serves as self-proclaimed critics ready to point out flaws in performance as adolescents practice by doing in dating, extracurricular activities, getting together to talk, and all other important rehearsal experiences. Sometimes the feedback is unmerciful, but it provides the necessary cues for modifying and refining adolescents' maturity concepts of who they are as persons.

7. *Opportunities for modeling.* Peers can serve as models. They offer a psychosocial mirror that many parents cannot provide, particularly in relation to moral development.

We can see clearly that the peer group serves an important socializing function by aiding the adolescent to develop independence. The objective feedback of the peer group serves to help the adolescent establish a personal identity.

The peer group also aids the adolescent in attaining sexual maturity, the capacity to love and be loved by others outside the family, by offering the teen rehearsal opportunities to accomplish the developmental tasks related to intimacy and sexuality. There is usually a time lag between the biological force of sexuality and an understanding of how it fits with a person's total life. During this time lag, peers provide many interpersonal relationship opportunities that serve as prototypes for future adult relationships. In these relationships, adolescents learn to relate in new social situations and to experience closeness while maintaining their own dignity. They develop both sensitivity for other people's feelings and the communication skills necessary for expressing this empathy. Adolescents develop a more mature affection for their parents and learn to distinguish the different kinds of love in the process. Adolescents also clarify their values and actions in relation to the purpose of sexuality. Will sex be "coitus," a "disease," an expression of self, or "something to do"? Through highly significant peer group instruction, adolescents decide how far they will go with sex

and achieve some understanding of both the consequences and responsibilities of sexual behavior.

Hence the abilities to make and keep friends, to socially interact, and to develop personal relationships with others outside the family are crucial to the adolescent's development in our society. The adolescent who is denied friends is not only extremely lonely and often depressed but also is denied an important opportunity to gain the necessary skills for intimate adult relationships through social interaction with peers.

Friends and Peer Acceptance. Considering peer acceptance and the factors that affect and influence it helps in understanding the world of the adolescent. The following diary notation passionately and poignantly illustrates how important peer acceptance is in an adolescent's life:

Dear Diary:

Sept 10—Breakfast time—coffee tastes metallic—I am dreading second period. It's really a drag—teacher making me write this dumb diary. My mother begins to hassle me about not doing work around the house. I am aware that I am grinding my teeth, that my stomach is tight and I want to get out of the kitchen.

Lunch. As I walk to the lunch table where my friends are sitting, I am aware that the conversation drops off to nothing. I feel left out, insecure, lonely, talked about. The other kids don't look me in the eye but talk past me. I am very upset. I am aware that I have eaten my lunch without tasting anything. My hands are sweaty and I guess I'm scared.

After School. "j" comes up behind me and gives me a friendly rap on the shoulder. I feel good. He is smiling. I want to touch him. Physical contact seems reassuring. Why am I afraid to put my hand on his shoulder? Why is touching a taboo? Would he reject me if I did? Why don't I tell my friends how I feel? Why weren't my friends honest with me at lunch? Oh, to hell with it! I don't want to think about this anymore.[1]

School and Youth Cultures

The school is the adolescent's turf. Many teens come to school not because their driving force is to learn but because school belongs to them as a place to meet and to be with friends. One of the most devastating punishments of adolescents is to deny them the right to be on a school campus. Although adolescents often perceive a suspension from a particular class as rewarding because it gives them an open class period to "hang around" with their friends, suspending them from school entirely is devastating because it denies them the opportunity to meet daily with their group.[29] Students will even change their schedules to be in classes with their peers; little thought may be given to what is studied. Much discussion goes on to ensure that friends get classes together, and some teens refuse to take classes if no friends are present.

In the high school students dominate numerically and spend more time during the day and the year with people of their own age and with teachers than with family members. School provides adolescents with the time, the place, and the mass to build their own social world.[20]

The substantial literature describing youth culture[10,23,24,30,31] in schools and other settings provides a consensus on these prominent features: (1) a strong hedonistic quality (pleasure, fun, and new experiences are the emphasis); (2) a carefree character ("just fooling around" is virtuous); (3) a glorification of the body (athletics, glamour, and attractiveness to the opposite sex are emphasized); (4) humanism (a humanistic flavor characterizes friendship patterns and interpersonal interactions); (5) idealism (hypocrisy is regarded as terrible); (6) a community spirit (giving and receiving help gladly are attractive); (7) egalitarianism (power and authority are lateral rather than vertical with the power differential being narrowed as much as possible); (8) independence ("doing it on our own" without adult authority and interference is an ideal sought even when impractical); (9) a flirtation with immorality (immoral and improper acts, in fantasy or reality, are encouraged and tolerated as a way of learning more about the world and of demonstrating independence).[20]

Thus adolescent development—development of a personal identity, of independence, and of sexual maturity—occurs within the home, peer groups, and the school environment.

Family, Peers, and Youth Culture: At War?

It is often thought that parents and peer groups (or youth culture) are at odds with each other and are polar opposites. These assumptions have been found to be inaccurate by scholars studying adolescent development, however, and parents and adolescents are more compatible than is commonly acknowledged. Campbell[20] and Lefrancois[32] concur that parents are accepting of and responsive to peer groups and youth culture values for several important reasons. First, parents want their youth to be accepted by their peers. They recognize that happiness and personal adjustment frequently are dependent on being accepted by and receiving positive responses from friends. Second, it is in the best interests of both parents and their offspring that the developing adolescent learn to be independent and self-directing. Third, parents want to preserve a warm relationship with their adolescents, hoping that it will develop into a mature form of companionship rather than dissolving and disintegrating into estrangement.

NORMAL PATHWAYS THROUGH ADOLESCENCE

When we come out of adolescence, after feeling alone or left out and different, we'll learn to appreciate ourselves and learn to like ourselves more, and feel important, and not care as much what other people think of us. We'll know who we are and where we're at in life.[1]

Offer and his associates[33-35] found three developmental routes normal teenagers take through adolescence: continuous growth, surgent growth, and tumultuous growth. Teens in each group have characteristic types of adaptation responses and relationships with parents and peers.

Continuous Growth Pattern

Adolescents in this group basically experience rather smooth sailing through adolescence. They demonstrate little evidence of conflict or stress; move gradually, quietly, and comfortably toward adulthood; and remain relatively unscathed. They appear self-assured, have relatively high self-esteem, comfortably accept societal norms, and usually have successfully mastered earlier developmental tasks. Their relationships with parents are trust-filled, affectionate, and characterized by reciprocal respect. Relationships with peers are also good; they frequently are admired and liked and serve as role models for others. Many teenagers fit this picture.

Surgent Growth Pattern

Adolescents experiencing this pathway into adulthood have periods of smooth sailing and periods of rough times. They may experience crises but consciously work at overcoming and mastering them. The rough times seem related to less fostering of independence by parents or difficulties within the family. The troubles in the family often stem from situational crises like parental divorce, death of a parent, serious parental illness, or frequent moves and changes in schools. However traumatic these crises, this group of adolescents works at adapting to these changes. Characteristically they appear less confident than the continuous growth group: they engage in less introspection and appear to get less positive reinforcement from parents or important others in their life. Peer relationships are good and during rough times become important buffers and sources of emotional support.

Tumultuous Growth Pattern

The third normal pathway through adolescence is characterized by rough sailing most of the time. Youth in this pathway, however, differ from those youth categorized as delinquents in that they do not actually engage in delinquent, antisocial acts as a primary mode of adaptation. On the other hand,

they appear similar to delinquents in that their lives are filled with much discord, stress, and wide mood swings. They often express disappointment in themselves and others and mistrust in most adults. They differ from their peers in the continuous growth and the surgent growth groups in that their relationships with parents are not as comfortable. Peer relationships are treasured more, and earlier dating patterns occur as a means of breaking away from parents.

Regardless of the growth pattern that adolescents take, there are some common conflicts and sources of stress that most experience to some degree.

STRESS IN ADOLESCENCE

Many adolescents are not given the chance to succeed, so therefore many more don't and won't even try. With this society today and the attitude it carries towards the adolescent age, its a wonder that most adolescents haven't crawled into a hole and stayed there till they are adult and responsible, because they are given more problems on top of the ones they are already trying to handle.[1]

Most adolescents have some stress in their lives. Body image and sexuality conflicts; scholastic and athletic pressures; relationships with parents, siblings, and peers; decisions about current and future roles, careers, and finances; and ideological conflicts are some of the major common sources of stress. In addition, there is the continuation or exacerbation of earlier childhood conflicts that, if not resolved, are carried over into adolescence.

Stress is defined as physical, mental, or emotional strain or tension. It comes in various intensities and is different from minor hassles, nuisances, or irritants. Stress can be caused for adolescents by immediate situations or events—an exam tomorrow, the death of a parent—or by an ongoing circumstance—the desire to do well in school, worry about being overweight or skinny, pursuit of someone of the opposite sex who is out-of-reach. Stress resides not in the person or situation but depends on the interaction between the two: how a person chooses to define and respond to the situation. Learning to cope with stress and finding healthy ways to respond to it become highly important during adolescence. Ongoing stress may result in physical and emotional problems unless the adolescent learns to cope in appropriate ways. Coping with stress is part of the process of maintaining good health and of assuming responsibility for self.

Major conflicts involving sex and drugs are topics of particular concern to some adolescents and their parents. However, it is the visible minority who often attract the most attention, and it is usually a minority who experience serious conflicts with sex and drugs. Exploring these topics, however, provides an understanding of the problems occurring for those adolescents experiencing maladaptive responses.

Characteristic of most adolescents is their desire not only to conform to their peers but also to experiment with life and to rebel somewhat against "the establishment." Drugs, alcohol, sex, speeding in cars, and other forms of pushing the limits of authority appeal to these desires for experimentation, rebellion, and conformity. Some adolescents are more vulnerable to losing control of this experimentation than others.

Drugs

Today drugs represent a somewhat different problem than they did previously. Drugs are exceedingly available and are becoming a problem for increasing numbers of youth. The hysterical response of the 1960s to drug use did more to encourage experimentation than to deter it; young people turned deaf ears to adults when they found that the emotionally charged threats and warnings were unfounded. The 1980s have brought us face-to-face with the fact that the majority of youth have easy access to drugs of all kinds.[36]

However, there is no generation gap in many American homes and families when it comes to drug use. We are a society that consumes psychoactive drugs and alcohol at a staggering rate. Many adults, as well as youth, become dependent on amphetamines, barbiturates, tranquilizers, and sleeping pills without even being aware of it. The desire for a pill to solve problems and cope with stress—be it to lose weight, to quit smoking, to calm down, or to get high—is all too prevalent. Adults have served too well as role models for drug use.

Chapter 4 contains further discussion of teenage alcohol and drug use.

Sex

Increasing numbers of teenagers are sexually active at earlier ages. "Everybody is doing it" is the myth that leads many youth to engage in these activities. This is disturbing when the results of this activity are reviewed. Venereal disease among teenagers is on the rise. Lack of sexual and contraceptive knowledge among teenagers is astounding.[37] (Contraceptive use is further discussed in Chapter 9.)

Teenage pregnancy, something we tried to ignore in the hopes that it would go away, is increasing. The National Commission on Youth reported that

Of the approximately 1 million girls who become pregnant each year, 400,000 are 17 and under, 30,000 are 14 or under. Of these 1 million girls, 600,000 have their babies. Although more than 235,000 of these babies are born out of wedlock, 9 out of 10 unmarried mothers keep their babies.[38]

A nationwide survey revealed one legal abortion for every four live births. The average age of those obtaining abortions was 23 years. Three out of four of these women were not married.[39] Eight out of ten young women who become mothers by the age of 17 never finish high school. And of all children born out of wedlock, 60% end up on welfare.[40] (Teenage pregnancy is further discussed in Chapter 9.)

Youth in Turmoil: a Profile

What, then, are these troubled youth like in comparison to Offer's normal growth groups? Vorrath and Brendtro[41] have worked for years with adolescents who have experienced difficulty in society. They describe these youth as having three central problems: *low self-image, lack of consideration for others,* and *lack of consideration for self.* Nine other specific problems were identified and given behavioral descriptions, but all nine relate back to one or more the these three central problems. The definition of a problem is anything that damages yourself or another person. The twelve problems are as follows:

1. *Low self-image:* Has a poor opinion of self; often feels put down or of little worth
2. *Inconsiderate of others:* Does things that are damaging to others
3. *Inconsiderate of self:* Does things that are damaging to self
4. *Authority problem:* Does not want to be managed by anyone
5. *Misleads others:* Draws others into negative behavior
6. *Easily misled:* Is drawn into negative behavior by others
7. *Aggravates others:* Treats people in negative, hostile ways
8. *Easily angered:* Is often irritated or provoked or has tantrums
9. *Stealing:* Takes things that belong to others
10. *Alcohol or drug problem:* Misuses substances that could hurt self
11. *Lying:* Cannot be trusted to tell the truth
12. *Fronting:* Puts on an act rather than being real[41]

Some of the same observations were made in recent studies with students involved in class skipping and drug use in a high school.[28,36] The researchers found that the students engaged in rebellion by pushing at limits: skipping classes, abusing drugs on campus, and participating in routinized forms of pleasure to escape boredom.

Much of this behavior resulted from loneliness, the need to belong to a group, and a vulnerability to peer pressure to use drugs and become sexually involved. These students experienced school failure and estrangement from teachers and other students. Ultimately these problems led to poor communication with others in the school community. The adolescents experienced alienation as individuals and as a group, and they sought escape and belonging through chemicals and through sex, which they knew lacked any real intimacy or caring.

Implications

What are the implications of an increasing number of youth using drugs, experimenting widely with sexuality, conforming more to fads and religious cults, or using other self-destructive forms of experimentation? The concern expressed by many parents and adults working with teenagers is that these young people are using these means as a way of coping with the conflicts of normal adolescence. In doing so, they are failing to develop healthy methods of coping. Rather than acquiring skills in problem solving by taking a hard look at the alternatives open to them and weighing the consequences of each approach, these youth are developing habits of responding by escapism. They drop out, do not think about circumstances, and fail to acknowledge what this form of response is doing to them. Frequently, their great need for sociability and belonging leads them further and further into difficulties. Depression, poor interpersonal relationships, health problems related to alcohol abuse, socially unproductive lives, and suicide are the not inconsequential results.

Clearly there is a need to encourage youth to formulate informed opinions about what they are doing based on known facts instead of on peer fantasies and wishes. There is also a need to decrease the number of youth living sedated lives and the number facing the dangers of multiple drug use with all its potential health hazards. Finally, there is a need to encourage youth in discovering the meaning of an intimate and responsible relationship and in carefully considering the consequences of experimentation with superficial sexual involvement.

It is undeniable that an increasing minority of youth is in crisis and that the extent of this crisis is greater than it ever has been in the past. At the same time, there are also unequaled opportunities for dealing with the factors that are contributing to this crisis. The highly visible minority is not unimportant. Until there is commitment and action, the present trends will continue and become tomorrow's realities. Changes will not occur until new ways of helping adolescents realize their full potential are developed. Herein lies the challenge for those in the helping professions.

HELPING YOUTH TO COPE

"People are always claiming that
they want to help me— . . .
All tell me this, but I wonder what
they mean by help.
Is it to make me over to be like
them? This is not for me."[42]

Because of the individual changes of adolescence and changing societal influences, contemporary youth particularly need help in developing coping skills. To develop these skills, adolescents need the following:

1. *To receive and give affection*. Not only do adolescents need to receive affection, particularly from their family and peer group, they also need to be able to give and show affection. This is the time during which they are developing the skills necessary for intimate relationships with others outside the family.

2. *Opportunities for self-learning and decision making*. A natural curiosity arises in response to adolescent maturational changes. Adolescents are motivated to learn about what is happening to their bodies emotionally, sexually, and physically. This curiosity presents a need for learning opportunities, information, and participatory education. It affords a chance to exercise decision-making skills in choosing alternatives that fit with personal preferences and values.

3. *Self-responsibility and freedom*. Adolescents need to be free of excessive domination or interference with their own affairs. At the same time, they need to develop self-responsibility. They need greater opportunities to exercise concern for the family and community to nurture their sense of autonomy, individuality, and independence.

4. *Limit setting and discipline*. Paradoxically, the adolescent also needs limit setting and discipline. Since self-responsibility does not occur overnight, adolescents still need limit setting from persons they respect such as parents and other adults in authority. There is, however, a great need for this discipline to be administered in a friendly manner. It should be administered consistently but be flexible enough to change as the adolescent matures and develops his or her own standards.

5. *Authoritative, not authoritarian, adult relationships*. Adolescents need both personal and career role models. They want to know what the adults they respect think and value. The key here is that there is a need for a system of values to explore, rebel against, and "knock heads with" in the search for what fits. The adolescent should not be forced to accept without question the values of their parents or important adults.

6. *Changing relationships with family*. Achieving independence implies changing relationships with the family. This does not mean that adolescents must renounce their families or that the family becomes the enemy. Teens still need emotional support, and the family provides the kind of structure within which self-identity can grow. For example, although for many years adolescents were content to be introduced as "so-and-so's" son or daughter, they now abhor that because of their need to be recognized as separate persons rather than as just extensions of their parents.

At the same time, the adolescent's family is a vital source of support, and most families desire involvement. Some adolescents need assistance in securing this involvement and in communicating with the family when major conflicts are the issue.[43]

Persons working with adolescents, helping them to grow and change in some significant way, must understand and respect the adolescent's experience and the reciprocal associations between cognition, emotions, and behavior. Ultimately as helping persons, we must use ourselves and the relationship that develops between us and the adolescent as instruments of aid.[44]

SUMMARY

During adolescence, the child grows into a mature adult physiologically, psychologically, and socially. Social scientists disagree about many aspects of the adolescent process: what initiates it, what characterizes its nature, and what responses are considered normal versus maladaptive. However, most would agree that there are certain important developmental tasks to be accomplished during this part of the life span, for example, the establishment of self-identity and adult role responsibilities appropriate to the particular subculture. A successful passage through adolescence thus equips youth for successful adult lifestyles.

Adolescence is the ideal time in life for learning the skills necessary for meaningful interpersonal relationships and informed decision making. These skills affect life-long physical and mental health patterns.

All adolescents are candidates for health care. Those that are currently healthy can benefit from learning health-consumer skills that promote health throughout life. Adolescents that currently are sidetracked into self-destructive behaviors need help in changing their direction. Skills, caring, and heeding the advice of youth are needed for effective helping. Adolescents are testifying over and over of their need for information and education regarding sexuality, drug abuse, coping strategies for growth, and personal health care. There is ample evidence that the peer group is not the best source of accurate information regarding health needs. The challenge is ours together. More than anything else we need to provide leadership. We must be committed to creating new directions and new environments for youth.

REFERENCES

1. Eggert, L.L.: Notes from some teens: on what would make adolescence easier, Unpublished collection, 1978. Reprinted with students' permission.
2. Blos, P.: On adolescence: a psychoanalytic interpretation, New York, 1962, The Free Press.
3. Inhelder, B., and Piaget, J.: The growth of logical thinking, New York, 1958, Basic Books, Inc., Publishers. (Translated by A. Parsens and S. Milgran.)
4. Piaget, J.: Judgment and reasoning in the child, New York, 1928, Harcourt Brace.
5. Piaget, J.: Six psychological studies, New York, 1967, Random House, Inc.
6. Piaget, J.: The moral judgement of the child, New York, 1926, Harcourt Brace.
7. Elkind, D.: Children and adolescents: interpretive essays on Jean Piaget, New York, 1970, Oxford University Press, Inc.
8. Elkind, D.: Egocentrism in adolescence, Child Dev. **38:**1025, 1967.
9. Elkind, D.: Adolescent cognitive development. In Adams, J.F., editor: Understanding adolescence, ed. 4, Boston, 1980, Allyn & Bacon, Inc.
10. Hollingshead, A.: Elmtown's youth, New York, 1946, John Wiley & Sons, Inc.
11. Mead, M.: Coming of age in Samoa, New York, 1950, The New American Library, Inc.
12. Mead, M.: Growing up in New Guinea, New York, 1953, The New American Library, Inc.
13. Mead, M., and Macgregor, F.C.: Growth and culture, New York, 1951, Putnam.
14. Erikson, E.H.: Identity and the life cycle, Psychological Issues (monograph), vol. 1, no. 1, New York, 1959, International Universities Press, Inc.
15. Erikson, E.H.: Childhood and society, ed. 2, New York, 1964, W.W. Norton & Co., Inc.
16. Erikson, E.H.: Identity: youth and crisis, New York, 1968, W.W. Norton & Co., Inc.

17. Mead, M.: Culture and commitment: the new relationships between the generations in the 1970's, ed. 2, New York, 1978, Columbia University Press.

18. Black in white America, vol. 4, New York, 1974, Macmillan Publishing Co., Inc., Education Development Center.

19. Havighurst, R.L.: Developmental tasks and education, ed. 3, New York, 1972, David McKay Co., Inc.

20. Campbell, E.Q.: Socialization: culture and personality, Dubuque, Iowa, 1975, Wm. C. Brown Group.

21. Baumrind, D.: What research is teaching us about the differences between authoritative and authoritarian child-rearing styles. In Hamachek, D.E., editor: Human dynamics in psychology and education, ed. 3, Boston, 1977, Allyn & Bacon, Inc.

22. Bronfenbrenner, U.: Some familiar antecedents of responsibility and leadership in adolescents. In Petrullo, L., and Bass, B., editors: Leadership and interpersonal behavior, New York, 1961, Holt, Rinehart & Winston, Inc.

23. Coleman, J.: The adolescent society, New York, 1961, The Free Press.

24. Friedenberg, E.A.: The vanishing adolescent, Boston, 1959, Beacon Press.

25. Youth 1976: attitudes of young Americans fourteen through twenty-five towards work, life insurance, finances, family, marriage, life styles, religion, New York, 1976, Research Services, American Council of Life Insurance.

26. Laycock, A.L.: Adolescence and social work, London, 1970, Routledge & Kegan Paul, Ltd.

27. Hamachek, D.E.: Psychology and development of the adolescent self. In Adams, J.F., editor: Understanding adolescence, ed. 4, Boston, 1980, Allyn & Bacon, Inc.

28. Ausubel, D.: Theory and problems of adolescent development, New York, 1954, Grune & Stratton, Inc.

29. Eggert, L.L.: Speaking like a "skipper" in high school: an ethnography, Unpublished paper, Seattle, 1983, University of Washington.

30. Havighurst, R.L.: Subcultures of adolescents in the United States. In Adams, J.F., editor: Understanding adolescence, Boston, 1980, Allyn & Bacon, Inc.

31. Larkin, R.W.: Surburban youth in cultural crisis, New York, 1979, Oxford University Press, Inc.

32. Lefrancois, F.R.: Adolescents, ed. 2, Belmont, Calif., 1981, Wadsworth, Inc.

33. Offer, D.: The psychological world of the teen-ager, New York, 1969, Basic Books, Inc., Publishers.

34. Offer, D., and Howard, K.: An empirical analysis of the Offer self-image questionnaire for adolescents, Arch. Gen. Psychiatry **27**:100, 1972.

35. Offer, D.: Three developmental routes through normal adolescence. In Feinstein, S., and Fiovacchini, P., editors: Adolescent psychiatry, vol. 4, Developmental and clinical studies, New York, 1975, Jason Aronson, Inc.

36. Eggert, L.L.: Adolescent's metaphors for "usin' and dealin' drugs": a cultural analysis, Unpublished paper, Seattle, 1983, University of Washington.

37. National Assessment of Educational Progress: What students know and can do, Denver, 1977, Education Commission of the States.

38. National Commission on Youth: The transition of youth to adulthood: a bridge too long, Boulder, Colo., 1980, Westview Press, Inc.

39. Guttmacher Institute: Eleven million teenagers: what can be done about the epidemic of adolescent pregnancy in the U.S.? New York, 1976, Research and Development Division of Planned Parenthood Federation of America.

40. Richmond, J.: Adolescent pregnancy, Hearing before the Subcommittee on Select Education of the Committee on Education and Labor, House of Representatives, July 24, 1978, Washington, D.C., 1978, U.S. Government Printing Office.

41. Vorrath, H., and Brendtro, L.: Positive peer culture, Chicago, 1974, Aldine Publishing Co.

42. Konopka, G.: The adolescent girl in conflict, Englewood Cliffs, N.J., 1966, Prentice-Hall, Inc.

43. National Institute of Mental Health: Facts about adolescence, Department of Health, Education and Welfare, Publication (HSM) 73-9133, Washington, D.C., 1973, U.S. Department of Health, Education, and Welfare.

44. Eggert, L.L.: The therapeutic process with adolescents experiencing psychosocial stress. In Longo, D., and Williams, R., editors: Clinical practice in psycholosocial nursing: assessment and intervention, East Norwalk, Conn., 1977, Appleton-Century-Crofts.

ADDITIONAL READINGS

Adams, J.F.: Understanding adolescence, ed. 4, Boston, 1980, Allyn & Bacon, Inc.

Ausubel, D.P., and Ausubel, P.: Cognitive development in adolescence, Am. Ed. Res. J. **3**:403, 1966.

Bandura, A., and Walters, R.: Social learning and personality development, New York, 1963, Holt, Rinehart & Winston, Inc.

Benedict, R.: Patterns of culture, New York, 1950, New American Library, Inc.

Benedict, R.: Continuities and discontinuities in cultural conditioning. In Martin, W., and Stendler, C., editors: Readings in child development, New York, 1954, Harcourt, Brace & Co., Inc.

Block, H., and Niederhoffer, A.: The gang: a study in adolescent behavior, New York, 1958, Philosophical Library, Inc.

Douglas, J.D.: Youth in turmoil: America's changing youth cultures and student protest movements, Chevy Chase, Md., 1970, National Institute of Mental Health.

Freud, A.: The ego and the mechanism of defense, New York, 1946, International Universities Press, Inc. (Translated by C. Baines.)

Freud, S.: A general introduction to psychoanalysis, New York, 1953, Permabooks. (Translated by J. Riviere.)

Gallatin, J.: Theories of adolescence. In Adams, J.F., editor: Understanding adolescence, ed. 4, Boston, 1980, Allyn & Bacon, Inc.

Ginsberg, J., and Opper, S.: Piaget's theory of intellectual development: an introduction, Englewood Cliffs, N.J., 1969, Prentice-Hall, Inc.

Goodman, P.: Growing up absurd, New York, 1960, Random House, Inc.

Hall, G.S.: Adolescence, 2 vols., New York, 1904, Appleton-Century-Crofts.

Havighurst, R.L., and Dreyer, P.H., editors: Youth: the seventy-fourth yearbook of the National Society for the Study of Education, Chicago, 1975, University of Chicago Press.

Josselson, R., Greenberge, E., and McConochie, D.: Phenomenological aspects of psychosocial maturity in adolescence. I. Boys, J. Youth Adolesc. 6:25, 1977.

Josselson, R., Greenberge, E., and McConochie, D.: Phenomenological aspects of psychosocial maturity in adolescence. II. Girls, J. Youth Adolesc. 6:145, 1977.

Lewin, K.: Field theory in social science, New York, 1951, Harper & Row, Publishers, Inc. (Edited by D. Cartwright.)

Lynn, D.B.: The father: his role in child development, Monterey, Calif., 1974, Brooks/Cole Publishing Co.

Lynn, D.B.: Daughters and parents: past, present, and future, Monterey, Calif., 1979, Brooks/Cole Publishing Co.

Marcia, J.: Development and validation of ego-identity status, J. Pers. Soc. Psychol. 3:551, 1966.

Marcia, J.: Ego-identity status: relationship to change in self-esteem, general adjustment, maladjustment, and authoritarianism, J. Pers. Soc. Psychol. 35:118, 1967.

Marcia, J., and Friedman, M.L.: Ego-identity status in college women, J. Pers. Soc. Psychol. 38:249, 1970.

McClain, E.W.: An Eriksonian cross-cultural study of adolescent development, Adolescence 10:527, 1975.

Muuss, R.: Theories of adolescence, ed. 2, New York, 1968, Random House, Inc.

Siege, A.: Why adolescence occurs, Adolescence 6:337, 1971.

Sommer, B.: Puberty and adolescence, New York, 1978, Oxford University Press, Inc.

Thornburg, H.: Adolescent development, Dubuque, Iowa, 1973, Wm. C. Brown Group.

Thornburg, H., editor: Contemporary adolescence: readings, ed. 2, Monterey, Calif., 1975, Brooks/Cole Publishing Co.

Chapter 3

Nutritional Requirements and Nutritional Status Assessment in Adolescence

L. KATHLEEN MAHAN

ROBIN H. ROSEBROUGH

Because of the difficulty in studying adolescents as a group and the incomplete knowledge regarding the nutritional requirements of the adolescent growth spurt, the recommendations for nutritional requirements for teenagers are based on remarkably limited data.

At the same time that adolescents have large nutritional requirements, the strong psychological and cultural factors influencing what teenagers consume may sometimes adversely affect whether teens meet their requirements. (These factors are discussed in Chapter 4.) Thus the stage is set for young people to be at risk for nutritional inadequacies during their teen years. Sensitive measures of nutritional status are important as a basis for assuring optimal health, energy, and development of the adolescent. However, techniques for measuring some nutrients are imprecise; for other nutrients the standards for appropriate levels during the teen years are inadequate. Clinicians thus must interpret the nutritional requirements and status of a teen from as much information as is available.

CHARACTERISTICS OF ADOLESCENT GROWTH AS BASIS FOR NUTRITIONAL REQUIREMENTS

Since most nutritional needs parallel adolescent changes in body composition, the nutritional needs of adolescents are best understood in this context. Chapter 1 discusses these changes during adolescence. Nutritional requirements during this stage of life are more closely associated with physiological rather than chronological age. Since nutritional requirements are affected by growth and the alteration in body composition and physiology that occur as a result of maturation, recommendations for nutritional intake made according to chronological age only introduce more error in already tenuous estimates. These errors are largest for adolescents who mature very early or very late in relation to the reference population.

Period of Peak Growth Velocity

During the adolescent growth spurt, there is an acceleration in growth velocity for 18 to 24 months during which the growth rate is at its maximum. During this period, the nutritional requirements of the teen may be as much as double those during the rest of the period of adolescence. Table 3-1 shows the deposition of nutrients during this period as compared with the rest of adolescence. Unfortunately, it is not easy to determine exactly when this acceleration in the rate of growth will occur. It differs between males and females and among teens of the same sex. It also differs depending on the type of growth (for example, the spurt in weight growth precedes the spurt in height

Table 3-1. Daily increments in body content due to growth

		Average for Period 10-20 yr (mg)	At Peak of Growth Spurt (mg)
Calcium	M	210	400
	F	110	240
Iron	M	0.57	1.1
	F	0.23	0.9
Nitrogen*	M	320	610 (3.8 g protein)
	F	160	360 (2.2 g protein)
Zinc	M	0.27	0.50
	F	0.18	0.31
Magnesium	M	4.4	8.4
	F	2.3	5.0

From Forbes, G.B.: Nutritional requirements in adolescence. In Suskind, R.M., editor: Textbook of pediatric nutrition, New York, 1981, Raven Press.

*Maintenance needs (2 mg/basal calorie) at age 18 yr are 3500 mg and 2700 mg for males and females, respectively.

growth). Several measurements of the teenager over the period of adolescence are necessary to determine the peak rate of growth. Usually this is impractical since it requires several clinic visits at intervals of about 3 months.

Using the sexual maturity ratings discussed in Chapter 1, it is safe to say that growth is probably at its peak during stage 3 in females and stage 4 in males. A landmark to keep in mind with females is that at menarche most of the growth in height and lean body mass has already occurred. After menarche, nutritional requirements thus are on the decline to adult levels. For the male, however, there is no similar, easily identified developmental milestone. Fortunately, teens' natural appetite is a built-in mechanism for helping them meet their nutritional requirements of growth. The increase in appetite usually parallels the increase in growth rate.

Adolescent boys not only have a longer period of growth than adolescent girls, but their maximal growth rate exceeds that of girls. Their nutritional requirements thus are usually greater for a longer period of time.

Changes in Body Composition

Changes in body composition during this period also influence the need for nutrients. During adolescence, boys gain twice as much lean tissue as girls, and girls deposit proportionately more fat tissue than boys. The result of this phenomenon is that the male as an adolescent and adult has a greater percentage of body weight as lean tissue. He thus has a higher metabolic rate and basal energy expenditure. Fig. 3-1 illustrates the gain in lean body mass and fat mass in adolescent girls and boys.

Both males and females increase the absolute amount of fat in their bodies during adolescence, but the increase in females is much greater. Because of this, although the prepubescent male and female enter puberty with similar body compositions (15% and 19% body fat, respectively), the female exits from adolescence with a greater percentage of body fat (about 23%) than the male (12%).[1,2] This striking difference in adolescence growth between males and females influences nutritional needs. Techniques for assessing body composition are on p. 55.

Because the adolescent male experiences greater gain in bone and lean tissue than the female, he requires more protein, iron, zinc, and calcium than the female for development of these tissues. Another reason for the male's larger requirements for these nutrients is his greater *rate* of growth.

ASSESSMENT OF NUTRITIONAL STATUS

Teenagers are in a fluctuating state of balance between supplying their bodies with needed nutrients and using up the nutrients. At any one time, this flow is the teenager's nutritional status.

Nutritional status is the degree to which the individual's physiological need for nutrients is being met. Nutritional status reflects cellular level me-

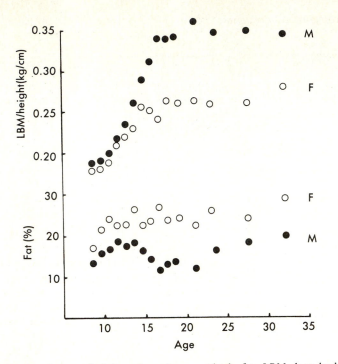

Fig. 3-1. Mean lean body mass/height ratio and percent body fat. *LBM,* lean body mass. (From Forbes, G.B.: Nutritional requirements in adolescence. In Suskind, R.M., editor: Textbook of pediatric nutrition, New York, 1981, Raven Press.)

tabolism, and its measurement is an approximation of the level of cell functioning with regard to availability and use of needed nutrients at a given point in time.

The *nutrition environment* (the factors that influence the nutritional status) is also an important consideration. Such factors as general health history, socioeconomic status, medications, alcohol or tobacco use, family attitudes, and peer group food practices all contribute to the adolescent's diet choices. Table 3-2 summarizes the significance of each of these influences. The health professional should try to understand the effect they have on the adolescent's eating habits.

Nutrition assessment includes study of both the nutritional status and the nutrition environment. Nutrition assessment is the process of gathering information on the nutritional status and nutrient environment of an individual, evaluating this information, and making conclusions both about the type and the amount of nutrients available to the cell and about the factors that affect this availability. Assessment of all the factors in the environment that may influence nutriture is essential if appropriate action to combat problems is going to be initiated as a *nutritional care plan.* The nutritional care plan is dynamic because it allows for processing new information and changing intervention strategies over time.

The extent to which the total nutrition environment is studied depends on the projected use of the nutrition assessment. For example, a great deal of detailed information reflecting nutritional status is needed for a 13-year-old male with Crohn's dis-

Table 3-2. Nutrition environment evaluation guide

Influences	Key Issues	Significance
Likes and dislikes	Does patient dislike any particular food that is a major source of a specific nutrient (for example, milk is a major source of calcium; citrus fruits of vitamin C; meat of high-quality protein)?	Points out need to explore alternative ways to supply nutrients (for example, substitute cheese and yogurt for milk; broccoli and green peppers for citrus fruit; proper combinations of plant foods for meat)
Environment and attitudes Individual	Does patient express interest in his or her diet?	Gives clues to attitude toward role of nutrition in health care
	Are there any behavioral problems that influence patient's food choices?	May indicate need to work with other health team members to resolve problem that temporarily precludes nutrition intervention
	Has patient ever followed a special diet? If so, who prescribed it, what type of diet was it, and when was it prescribed? What instructions did patient receive?	Self-prescribed diet may signal inappropriate or unreliable approach toward control of health by diet; points out medical and educational considerations needed in design of care plan
	Does patient think he or she has been following the diet? Is there evidence to substantiate this?	If discrepancy exists, indicates lack of understanding of diet by patient or unwillingness or inability of patient to make dietary changes
	What difficulties if any does patient see in making dietary changes?	Focuses on issues that need consideration in design of individualized care plan
Family	Who purchases and prepares food in home (that is, partially controls patient's food supply)?	Sets scene for type of action plan suitable to patient and family
	Does patient have adequate cooking facilities and equipment or access to other resources?	May indicate need to provide basic nutrition guidelines, including personalized menu plan
	Are there any cultural, regional, or religious factors that affect patient's food choices?	Requires consideration to tailor care plan to individual needs
Peers	How often does patient eat away from home? Where and with whom does patient eat? Are there specific food intake patterns related to peer influences?	Indicates potential influences of peers on food choices; points out potential efficacy of patient- versus family-oriented care plan

Continued.

Table 3-2. Nutrition environment evaluation guide—cont'd

Influences	Key Issues	Significance
Environment and attitudes—cont'd Schools	Does patient eat at school? Does patient participate in school feeding programs?	School feeding programs with their standardized composition assure minimal nutrient availability and provide reference for accuracy of reported information
	Is there anything about school schedule or cafeteria environment that may discourage appropriate nutrient intake?	"Too little time for lunch" or "no one to eat with" may necessitate consultation with other team members or school to resolve life-style problems
	Is patient in appropriate grade in school? Has patient received food and nutrition information in school courses?	Gives clues to current knowledge of nutrition and level of intellectual functioning; allows practical planning for educational aspects of care plan
Limited food funds	Is patient or family eligible for food stamps; Women, Infants, and Children program (WIC); or reduced-price or free school lunch? Do they participate in programs? Does patient or family receive other social assistance?	Indicates family has limited income and may need assistance with food buying and preparation to assure nutritionally adequate diet; points out need to consider referral to appropriate food program or nutrition education resource
Health-related concerns	Does patient have any food allergies or intolerances (as distinguished from dislikes)?	Excludes foods from diet; indicates need to plan and assure adequacy with alternative food choices
	Are there any physical conditions affecting ability to consume adequate nutrients (for example, mouth sores, swallowing problems, taste abnormalities)?	Indicates need to consider flavor, consistency, and temperature of food in care plan
	Are there any problems in digestion, absorption, or metabolism that will interfere with nutrient utilization? Will any other therapy (drugs, exercise, radiation) affect nutrient needs?	Indicates need to address these problems in diet preparation

Table 3-3. Methods for nutrition assessment

Method	Responsibility	Information
Interview	Professional (with patient participation)	Diet history (24-hour recall, sample intake, and food frequency)
		Medical history
		Psychosocial history
Questionnaire	Client	Food intake records
		Food preference data
		Other data specific to purpose
Direct observation and measurement	Professional (with patient cooperation)	Hospital and school dietary intake
		Clinical data
		Laboratory data
		Behavioral observation data
		Anthropometric data
Other data	Professional	School reports
		Other health professional or agency reports

ease who is scheduled for a course of parenteral nutrition. Information about the nutrition environment would be less vital at this time. However, nutritional care planning for a newly diagnosed 15-year-old diabetic patient would require both nutritional status evaluation and assessment of the nutrition environment. Without both components, the care plan cannot adequately address physiological nutritional needs and the adolescent's ability to meet those needs.

Methods used to obtain needed nutrition information will vary depending on the specific situation. The kind and depth of information needed and the willingness and ability of the adolescent and his or her family to participate will influence the methodologies used. Table 3-3 presents a summary of different methods and the type of information gathering each will facilitate.

There is no single reliable measure of an individual's nutriture. Rather, a combination of dietary, biochemical, and clinical data is collected. As shown in Fig. 3-2, each of these gives a picture of nutritional status at a different point of body

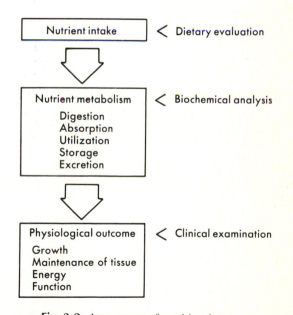

Fig. 3-2. Assessment of nutritional status.

Table 3-4. Progression of nutritional depletion

Stages of Depletion	Examples of Assessment Measures
Inadequate nutrient intake when compared with recommended dietary allowance	Dietary assessment (all nutrients)
Desaturation of tissue levels and stores	Serum ferritin (iron); anthropometric data (energy and protein)
Depletion of circulating nutrient pools	Total serum (iron); plasma vitamin A; serum albumin (protein)
Interference with intermediary metabolism	Hematocrit and hemoglobin (iron); serum alkaline phosphate (vitamin D); erythrocyte transketolase activity (thiamin)
Physiological changes	Irritability (iron); reduced cellular immunity (protein)
Clinical dysfunction	Motor weakness (thiamin); poor dark adaptation (vitamin A)
Structural alterations	Bowed legs (vitamin D); keratomalacia (vitamin A)

(Left margin, spanning rows: "Increasing Depletion"; Right margin, spanning rows: "Increasing Depletion")

functioning. The combination of the three makes up the overall assessment of nutriture.

Nutritional deficiency states are progressive. Table 3-4 summarizes the progression of nutritional depletion and shows how deficiencies of various nutrients may be studied at one or more levels of relative depletion. Coupled with individual variations in nutritional requirements and metabolism, this progression complicates the problem of assessing the teen's nutritional status. Further, the vagueness of "optimal nutrition," the limits of currently available tests, and the lack of appropriate standards necessitate the use of a variety of approaches to study the adolescent.

Dietary Data

Data about the actual nutrient intake of an individual are gathered in a dietary assessment. A number of methods are available, and the choice depends on the specificity desired, the time available, and the cooperation of the adolescent and/or family.

Most of the methods employ an interview between the health professional and adolescent. Good interviewing skills are the basis for acquiring accurate and pertinent information. Teenagers offer a special challenge because they are often suspicious of people they perceive as being in authority. They may be very reluctant to offer information, and probing may be necessary to obtain needed information. Demonstrating a nonjudgmental, caring attitude, explaining why certain information is needed, and allowing verbalization of the teenager's concerns are all practices that will facilitate the development of good rapport and the acquisition of accurate, useful information. This is further discussed in Chapter 10.

The *24-hour recall* is the most commonly used technique for dietary assessment. When used by a skilled interviewer, the technique has the major advantage of giving a qualitative evaluation of a teenager's diet in 15 to 20 minutes.[3] The disadvantages are memory inaccuracies, the difficulty in specifying quantities of foods, and the fact that a single day's food intake may not be representative of the diet.

The accuracy of the 24-hour recall may be increased by taking additional time to go through the entire day's activities. This often jogs the memory as to food intake; allows adolescents to volunteer information they would like known; and gives the interviewer and other health team members much information about the family, peers, and level of activities that will be helpful in planning nutritional care. Alternating between open-ended questions (for example, "What was the first thing you had to eat or drink yesterday?") and more directed questions (for example, "Did you have anything on your toast?") is a good technique to practice. This will aid the interviewer in getting a more accurate and detailed picture of intake without putting words in the mouth of the teenager. The use of food models and measuring devices will assist in estimating quantities of food.

A *usual intake* is very similar to the 24-hour recall in terms of interviewing technique. The focus is simply on a typical day. Rather than asking about what the youth ate yesterday, questions should be directed to what he or she normally eats. This approach *may* give a more representative intake, but it requires more decisions (for example, what is "usual"). The usual intake also invites the adolescent to edit his report and to add nonfood-related information, and although this can be very helpful in terms of gaining broader knowledge about the youth, it generally limits the assessment to only a qualitative evaluation of the diet.

Food frequency questions involve asking how often the teen eats a food or category of foods. The questions usually are asked orally by a trained person but may also be given in a questionnaire format. Fig. 3-3 shows a food frequency form. Food frequency forms can be designed for specific purposes. For example, if there is concern about inadequate iron intake, the foods can be grouped according to their iron contribution to the diet. This tool is very helpful as a check to use with the 24-hour–recall and usual-intake techniques. The use of at least two approaches to evaluating diet

intake increases the validity of the data and allows for more detailed intervention strategies.

Food intake records are written records kept by the individual of all food eaten during a specified period of time. This tool, usually used for 3- to 7-day periods (occasionally longer), gives more valid data if the time is taken to give adequate verbal and written instructions for keeping the records. Food records are a particularly valuable technique to use with adolescents because they allow the health professional to assess not only food intake but also attitude toward nutrition, motivation to change habits, ability to follow directions, and potential ability and willingness to comply with therapeutic plans. In addition to simple records with the type and amount of food eaten, records may also incorporate other life-style factors. These factors may include where the food was eaten, with whom, and how the youth felt at that time. This type of information is essential in planning behavioral modification programs and can contribute much to the health team's overall knowledge of the individual adolescent.

An example of the peripheral knowledge you might gain by using food records is illustrated by a young teenage girl at a clinic who answered questions of all team members with a yes, a no, or a shrug. She had a depressed affect, made little eye contact, and appeared to have little understanding of what was said to her. The health team suspected mild mental retardation until she returned to the nutritionist with a detailed and extensive food record. With this written evidence of the ability to understand and follow directions and of motivation to participate in her own health care, she was reevaluated and found to be above average in intelligence but clinically depressed.

Food preference data can be simple (obtained by asking particular food likes and dislikes as part of a general interview) or detailed (obtained by using a fairly extensive type of checklist questionnaire). Perhaps its greatest asset when dealing with teenagers is in giving adolescents an opportunity to

Name _____

_____

Check below how often patient consumes the following:

	2-3 times/day	1 time/day	2-3 times/week	Seldom	Never
Milk, cheeses, yogurt					
Meat, fish, poultry, eggs, peanut butter, dry beans, nuts					
Citrus fruits, juice					
Orange or dark green leafy vegetables or fruit					
Other fruits, vegetables, potatoes					
Bread, cereal, rice, pasta, crackers					
Cookies, candy, cake, pastries, fruit drinks, soda, shakes, sugar, honey					
Butter, margarine, mayonnaise, salad dressings, gravies, french fries					
Snacks (for example, pretzels, cheese snacks)					
Alcohol, caffeine					
Vitamins, other supplements					
Other (specify)					

Evaluation (refer to Food Intake Evaluation Guide)

1. What would you estimate the calorie consumption to be?

   Appropriate_____ Excessive _____ Inadequate_____

2. Is the patient's typical daily food intake adequate or weak with respect to the following:

	Adequate	Weak
Protein	_____	_____
Calcium	_____	_____
Iron	_____	_____
Vitamin A	_____	_____
Vitamin C	_____	_____

Fig. 3-3. Food frequency form.

Table 3-5. Food intake evaluation guide

Key Information	Possible Indications
Variety of foods eaten	A varied diet is most likely to provide the 40-plus nutrients needed for good health.
Number of servings eaten from each food group	Apparent deficiencies in a food group necessitate a cross-check to determine type, quantity, and frequency of food intake. Less than 3-4 servings of milk, cheese, yogurt, or other milk products may mean insufficient calcium intake. Less than 2 servings of meat, fish, or vegetable protein food may mean insufficient protein and iron intake. Less than 4 servings of fruit and vegetables (1 rich in vitamin A and 1 rich in vitamin C) may mean insufficient vitamin A and vitamin C intake. Less than 4 servings of grain products may mean insufficient vitamin B and protein intake if eaten in combination with less than 2 servings from the meat group.
Time between meals and snacks	Long lapses raise suspicions that a teenager actually did have something to eat. Too short a time lapse may reflect compulsive eating prompted by an emotional problem. Be alert for the "eat/starve" syndrome and possible gorging.
Patient's definition of a serving	What a teen calls a serving may or may not match the "standard" serving. Examples of a single serving in the different food groups follow: Milk and milk products: 1 cup milk or yogurt; 1-inch cube cheese; ½ cup ice cream or custard. Protein foods: 2-3 oz hamburger or steak; 1 whole chicken leg or breast; 2 eggs; 1 cup baked beans; 4 teaspoons peanut butter. Fruits and vegetables: ½ cup or 1 small raw, cooked, or canned. Grain products: 1 slice bread; 1 biscuit, roll, or muffin; ¾-1 cup ready-to-eat cereal; ½-¾ cup cooked cereal or pasta.
Quantity and frequency with which "extras" are consumed (for example, sweets, sauces, gravies, chips, sodas, fried foods, shakes)	Too many extras may indicate that these foods are being eaten in place of more nutrient-dense foods or that too many calories are being consumed.
Beverages consumed (both with and between meals)	Failure to record beverages produces an inaccurate picture of a teen's nutrient intake. Some beverages make a significant contribution to nutritional needs (milk, juices); other beverages (soda, sweetened drinks, alcohol) primarily supply calories.
Dependency on fast foods or quick-fix meals	Excessive use of fast foods or quick-fix meals may indicate a lack of interest in or knowledge of meal planning, cooking, and comparison food costs. Indifference or ignorance toward the value of nutrition signals a particular need to take a close look at the nutritional adequacy of the foods served. Such a dependency could lead to a diet low in fiber and trace elements, possibly low in vitamins and minerals, and high in sodium.

talk about something they feel very sure about. Further, there is an expressed interest in the teen's feelings about food. Often the question, "Are there any foods that you especially like or dislike?" is a good opener with an otherwise nonverbal teenager.

Evaluating the information obtained by one or more of the dietary assessment techniques must precede any recommendations for dietary change. On a qualitative basis, diets can be evaluated using various systems. Using the approach presented in Table 3-5, the diet of a teenager can be rapidly assessed for general adequacy. This assessment should highlight potential weak areas or points that need further investigation and more specific quantitative analysis. The value of the intake record depends on the accuracy of the information obtained and on the factors considered in evaluating that information.

Quantified nutrient intake data are often compared with the recommended dietary allowances (RDA) for age and sex.[4] At best the RDA are general guidelines for populations. They thus must be used with extreme caution when evaluating individual diets. For adolescents they are particularly misleading as to true nutritional needs. In part this is because of the lack of reliable scientific data on which to base the RDA for adolescents. Most of the recommendations are made on data extrapolated from information on the requirements of younger children or adults.[5] Further, the RDA are developed for chronological age groups and not for the physical stages of development that have primary influence on the individual's nutritional needs.

Since there are currently no better guidelines for nutritional needs, the 1980 RDA are used with these reservations in mind. Generally, meeting the RDA for a specific nutrient is considered adequate. When intakes fall below two thirds of the RDA, caution is needed in interpreting the adequacy of the diet. It is possible to make the RDA more specific by taking into account the size of the reference adolescent for whom the requirement is made. This at least will help in evaluating the very small or very large teen's intake. As previously stated, no single index will give definitive information on nutritional status, and if possible a low intake should always be followed by laboratory and clinical measurements to assess potential inadequacy.

ASSESSMENT OF NUTRITIONAL REQUIREMENTS

Energy

The recommended dietary allowances for energy for teenagers of various chronological ages and for each sex are shown in Table 3-6. Although a single number such as 2700 kcal for a male 11 to 14 years of age is stated, a range is also given, in this case 2000 to 3700 kcal. The high figure of the range, 3700 kcal, is almost twice that of the low end, 2000 kcal, thus illustrating the range of energy intakes that exist among teenagers and that probably will meet their needs. It is necessary that energy requirements be stated in this fashion to accommodate the variation in stages of development. For example, some 14-year-old boys are well into their growth spurt, while others have not yet started. The energy allowances thus are proposed as average and approximate.

In determining the energy requirements for an individual teenager, it is useful to adapt the RDA by stating the figures on a per-centimeter-of-height basis using the size of the reference adolescent for each age and sex category. Based on the reference used for the 11- to 14-year-old male, the RDA for calories can be stated as 17.2 kcal/cm height (43.7 kcal/in height), which is 2700 kcal divided by 157 cm (61.8 in) (the height of the reference male). By multiplying the height in cm of the individual teen being assessed or counseled by 17.2 kcal/cm (43.7 kcal/in), the energy requirements for that particular teen can be estimated. However, even when using this technique, the RDA is still only a guide and does not take into account the stage of development of that particular teen. In

Table 3-6. Recommended energy intakes

	Daily Total (kcal)		Daily Total (kcal/cm height)	
Age (yr)	Median*	Range†	Median*	Range†
Children				
7-10	2400	1650-3300	18.2	14.8-22.1
Males				
11-14	2700	2000-3700	17.2	15.1-20.9
15-18	2800	2100-3900	15.9	13.5-20.8
19-22	2900	2500-3300	16.4	15.8-17.1
Females				
11-14	2200	1500-3000	14.0	11.2-17.5
15-18	2100	1200-3000	12.9	7.9-17.3
19-22	2100	1700-2500	12.9	11.6-16.5

From Food and Nutrition Board, National Academy of Sciences–National Research Council: Recommended dietary allowances, ed. 9, Washington, D.C., 1980.
*Median, median energy intake of children followed in longitudinal growth studies.
†Range, 10th and 90th percentiles of the children's energy intake.

addition, it does not account for the tremendous differences in activity that exist between teenagers. The final assessment should be based on the adolescent's present consumption, adequacy of growth, and feelings of health and stamina. Assessment of body composition (p. 55) also helps to define whether energy intake is adequate, too low, or excessive.

Beal[6] looked at the energy intakes of teenagers growing appropriately and found that the 10th to 90th percentiles of the range of intakes was 12.4 to 23 kcal/cm height (31.5 to 58.4 kcal/in height) for males and 6.9 to 19.1 kcal/cm height (17.5 to 48.5 kcal/in height) for females. This illustrates that even when adjusted for size there were some teens whose energy intakes still did not fall within the range of the RDA (Table 3-6).

By perusing these recommendations for energy intake, one can see that when corrected for size the energy recommendations for teenage girls are never as high as those for teenage boys at any age.

Assessment of Adequacy of Energy Intake. The best way to assess the adequacy of the energy intake in the adolescent is to measure growth and body composition. Typical growth measurements are of the height and weight. These are compared to previous height and weight measurements of the teenager and to standard curves derived from data compiled by the National Center for Health Statistics (NCHS).[7] These curves are given in Appendix B. Properly used sequential measurements of the adolescent's height and weight can be very informative. However, because of the unique growth patterns of teenagers, one of the customary uses of the growth grids—determination of "ideal" weight—is inappropriate, a fact that does not appear to be widely appreciated even by those working closely with adolescents.

Typically the height and weight of a teenager are measured and plotted on the NCHS growth curve (the curve contains the heights and weights of children and teenagers 2 to 18 years of age and the percentiles for each age group). Used properly, this clinical practice gives information about whether the teen's growth is staying "in channel" and whether growth is continuing at about the same rate as it has been in the past. This is a good crude measure of energy adequacy.

Used inappropriately, the height and the weight plotted on the charts with the percentile designations are used to determine an "ideal" weight. Although this is a common practice with younger children, for the pubescent child (female taller than 137 cm [54 in] or male taller than 145 cm [57 in]) it is inappropriate to evaluate weight-for-height proportion. Ideal weight should not be defined by recommending that the height and weight should fall on or be close to the same percentile channel. To illustrate the inaccuracy of this practice, consider the 17-year-old female who is 170.1 cm (67 in) tall and is just below the 90th percentile for height for girls of her age. The growth curve charts (Appendix B) are being used improperly when the clinician states that the appropriate weight for this girl should be at the same 90th percentile (about 71.8 kg [158 lb]). This is an incorrect recommendation, as most girls of that height who weigh 71.8 kg (158 lb) will state. Any clinician visually assessing the situation also will verify the error of such a recommendation. These growth curves are not meant to be used in this fashion. The curves merely describe the distribution of heights and weights of a representative sample of teenagers of each age in this country. By the adolescent period, there is a wide distribution of weights at any age. Quite naturally there were overweight teenagers in the population from which the curves were derived because the study was intended to reflect the demographic population distribution in the country, not to measure ideally proportioned teens. This raises the upper percentiles of weight considerably and also skews lower weight percentiles in comparison with shorter heights.

How then *does* the clinician define the appropriate weight-for-height and determine whether there is or has been an excessive or deficient energy intake? It is necessary to turn to the original data from which the percentile charts for height and weight were derived.[8] The important tables from this publication have been included in the appendix of this text (Appendixes C and D).

To use the tables, the clinician locates the height percentile for the age and sex of the individual (Appendix C presents the same percentiles as the NCHS height chart). The 170.1 cm (67 in) 17-year-old female is between the 90th and 95th percentile. By referring to Appendix D, you see that unlike the growth charts there is a range of weights given for both a particular height and a particular age. Unfortunately, there is still no reference to sexual maturity ratings or the stage of physical development. The 50th percentile weight for the height represents the median weight in the sample of teens of that height. The various percentiles above and below also are given.

From our experience in assessing height, weight, and body measurements, it appears that the weight for a teenager of a particular height should be at or between the 25th and 75th percentiles of the weight-for-height as given in these tables. Referring to Table 3-7, you can see that the weight range for the 170.1 cm (67 in) 17-year-old girl is 55.6 to 65.7 kg (122.1 to 144.5 lb), a range of about 10 kg (22 lb). (Appendix D gives weight-for-height percentiles for youths 12 to 17 years of age.)

There still may be teens whose weight is greater than the 75th percentile but who are not overfat. These teens need to be evaluated further with measurement of body fatness. In some situations it is enough to compare a fatfold (also called skinfold) measurement at the single site over the triceps muscles to the triceps-for-weight percentiles in the *National Health Survey*[9] (Appendix E). These NCHS tables give percentiles for triceps fatfold measurements for teens of various weight and age categories.

Teens who are between the 75th and 90th percentiles for weight-for-height but who have fatfolds in lower percentiles according to these NCHS tables usually are an appropriate weight for their height and are very muscular. Adolescents who are above the 75th percentile for weight-for-height and who also have triceps-for-weight percentiles greater than the 75th percentile could be classified as being overweight and overfat. Teens who are below the 25th percentile for weight-for-height and who also have triceps-for-weight percentiles lower than the 25th percentile can be classified as underweight.

Assessment of muscular tissue and body protein stores provides additional useful information in this situation. This can be done by measuring the mid-upper arm circumference, determining the arm muscle area (Appendix F), and comparing it to percentile rankings (Appendix G). Fig. 3-4 provides a guideline for use of these data in evaluating the weight of an adolescent.

In other less obvious situations or in situations needing more precision, it may be necessary to

Table 3-7. Weight in kilograms of girls aged 17 years at last birthday, United States, 1966-70

Height (cm)	Percentile						
	5th	10th	25th	50th	75th	90th	95th
145-149.9	38.6	38.8	40.1	45.1	45.7	51.1	51.2
150-154.9	41.6	42.3	44.6	48.9	53.5	59.2	64.1
155-159.9	44.4	45.5	48.7	53.2	57.7	61.6	76.2
160-164.9	46.8	48.0	50.2	55.4	61.5	72.3	82.3
165-169.9	47.9	50.3	55.1	59.3	65.1	69.4	71.6
170-174.9	50.6	52.9	**55.5**	60.2	**65.7**	76.1	82.7
175-179.9	54.9	56.7	60.1	61.7	75.2	75.9	83.0

Modified from National Center for Health Statistics: Height and weight of youths 12-17 years, United States. In Vital and health statistics, series 11, no. 124, Health Services and Mental Health Administration, Washington, D.C., 1973, U.S. Government Printing Office. Data from The national health survey, U.S. Department of Health, Education, and Welfare, 1973.

calculate the actual percentage of body weight that is made up by fat. A problem arises in finding an indirect method for measuring body fat that is as accurate as the direct measure (cadaver analysis), which of course is impossible. Several techniques of varying accuracy have been developed (Table 3-8). Most are used only in research settings, although some, such as skinfold and girth measurements, can be used clinically.

There has been a great deal of research to determine which body sites for skinfold measurement give the best correlation with body fat. There are differences in the amount of fat located subcutaneously,[1,10] skinfold thickness,[11] and skinfold compressibility[12] that depend on the age, maturation, and sex of the individual. Therefore tables and equations used for body fat percentage determinations must be age-and sex-appropriate for the population or adolescent being evaluated (Table 3-9).[13-17] Ideally the developmental stage of the teen should also be considered, but at this point validated standards specific to maturity ratings do not exist.

Tables for determining body fatness from skinfold measurements in adolescents are scarce. Pařízková[13] measured 10 skinfold sites on 241 Czechoslovakian children 12 to 16 years of age

and developed nomograms for determining body fatness using two skinfold measurements: the subscapular and the triceps skinfolds. Appendix H gives the nomograms. Durnin and Wormersley[14] used British subjects and published tables for determining body fatness using four skinfold site measurements: the subscapular, suprailiac, triceps, and biceps skinfolds. These tables are appropriate to use with teenage girls 16 years of age or older and teenage boys 17 years of age or older (Appendix I). A description of the sites used is given below:

Triceps: midway between the acromial and olecranon processes on the posterior aspect of the arm; the arm held vertically with the fold running parallel to the length of the arm

Suprailiac: vertical fold on the crest of the ilium at the midaxillary line

Subscapular: inferior angle of the scapula with the fold running parallel to the axillary border

Biceps: midway between acromial and olecranon processes on the anterior aspect of the arm; the arm held vertically with the fold running parallel to the length of the arm

In an attempt to develop a clinically useful method for determining body fatness without using any special equipment such as skinfold calipers,

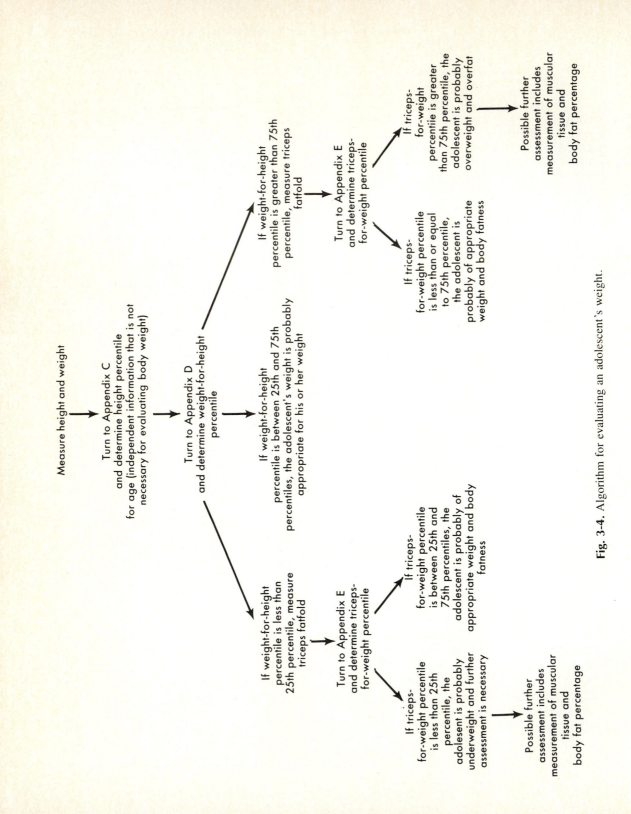

Fig. 3-4. Algorithm for evaluating an adolescent's weight.

Table 3-8. Some techniques for determining body composition

Technique	Procedure	Use
Hydrostatic (underwater) weighing	Subject is weighed in and out of water. Using the difference between these two measurements, it is possible to determine body density and the amount of body fat since muscle is more dense than fat. Formulas are available to make these determinations.	Requires great deal of subject compliance Expensive Cumbersome Accurate Used in some clinical settings
Skinfold (fatfold) measurements	Using a standardized caliper, the thickness of a pinch of skin and underlying fat is measured at various sites on the body. Using age- and sex-appropriate tables, body fat percentage can be determined.	Equipment available Relatively inexpensive Fast Requires little subject compliance Less accurate (depends on technician) Clinically useful
Skeletal diameters	Skeletal diameters are measured at various points on the body (for example, wrist width, knee width). Based on fact that a constant proportion of lean tissue is associated with a given skeletal size, lean body mass can be determined.	Less accurate than hydrostatic weighing or other measurements based on densitometry Time consuming Equipment not readily available Requires little subject compliance Cumbersome formulas
Circumferences (girths)	Circumference measurements are made at various sites on body. Tables and formulas are available to determine body fatness from these measurements.	Easy No elaborate equipment needed Requires little patient compliance
Total body potassium (potassium-40)	Since body naturally emits gamma radiation as potassium-40, this can be counted. Lean tissue containing a standard amount of potassium can thus be measured, and a formula can be used to derive amount of fat tissue.	Accurate Requires little subject compliance Research purposes only Expensive
Total body water	Body water is measured using an isotope dilution technique. Since adipose tissue contains less water than fat tissue, fat tissue can be determined.	Accurate Expensive Research purposes
Soft tissue roentgenography	Using roentgenography or ultrasound techniques, size of subcutaneous fat tissue can be measured since it is of different density than bone or muscle tissue. Using equations that relate size of subcutaneous fat to surface area, the amount of body fat can be determined.	Expensive Research purposes

Table 3-9. Assessment of body fat percentage

Study	Measurements Used	Age and Sex for Standards
Pařízková[13]*	Subscapular and triceps fatfolds	Males and females, 12-16 yr
Durnin and Wormersley[14]*	Subscapular, suprailiac, biceps, and triceps fatfolds	Males 17+ yr; females 16+ yr
Dugdale and Griffiths[15]	Subscapular, suprailiac, biceps, and triceps fatfolds; height and weight	Males 4-12½ yr; females 4-19 yr
Frerichs, Harsha, and Berenson[16]	Height, weight, and triceps fatfold	Males and females, 10-14 yr
Katch, McArdle, and Boylan[17]	Girth measurements	Males and females, 17+ yr

*Tables and nomograms are included in appendixes.

several methods have been proposed using girth or circumference measurements made with a common measuring tape. These methods have been performed on hundreds of people, and the results compared to fatness as determined by hydrostatic weighing or body water measurement. However, these methods are still crude, and at present tables are available only for teenagers 17 years of age and older.[16] The predicted values for body fat using these circumferences, like those from skinfold measurements, come within 2.5% to 4% of the values determined by hydrostatic weighing. In a situation where extreme accuracy is required, these methods therefore would not be appropriate. For those who have spent years in vigorous physical training and who are extremely well muscled, these equations will overestimate body fat. In addition, these measurements are less accurate in obese individuals. The technique is simple, however, and it can be useful clinically, especially when the same method is used over time with a particular individual.

In the future it may be possible to count and measure the size of the fat cells and/or enzymes to determine the level of body fatness.[2] This may give a clearer idea of the metabolic implications and ultimate effect on health of certain levels of fatness.

In the meantime determining body fat percentage is useful for identifying an appropriate weight for an adolescent whose body composition is changing and who also may have an erroneous idea about an appropriate body weight.

Protein

Like the energy recommendation, the RDA for protein for an adolescent can be useful if it is related to the size of the individual rather than to just his chronological age. Table 3-10 gives the RDA for protein based on the height of the reference teenager in each category. This is around 0.3 gm protein/cm height (0.8 gm protein/in height). Beal[6] reported the 10th to 90th percentile of the range of protein intakes among normally growing, healthy teenagers as 0.27 to 0.67 gm/cm height (0.68 to 1.7 gm/in height) for females and 0.42 to 0.86/cm height (1.1 to 2.2 gm/in height) for males.

There are many factors other than the physiological state of the adolescent that affect the amount of protein required. The amino acid composition of the protein, the adequacy of the energy intake, and the overall nutritional status of the adolescent influence the requirement for protein. Other sources offer detailed methods for determining protein requirements for the general population; these requirements therefore will not be discussed here.[4]

Table 3-10. Recommended dietary allowance for protein in adolescence

Age (yr)	Daily Total (gm)	Daily Total (gm/cm height)
Children		
7-10	34	0.26
Males		
11-14	45	0.29
15-18	56	0.32
19-22	56	0.32
Females		
11-14	46	0.29
15-18	46	0.28
19-22	44	0.27

From Food and Nutrition Board, National Academy of Sciences–National Research Council: Recommended dietary allowances, ed. 9, Washington, D.C., 1980.

The RDA for total daily protein intake during adolescence ranges from 44 to 56 gm depending on the sex and age of the teenager. Most teenagers consume this amount of protein and more in a typical day. Even the most rapidly growing large teenager would only require 56 gm of protein. This amount is easily supplied in a day's intake, especially when the adolescent consumes meat and other animal proteins. For example, one pint of milk, a 4-ounce hamburger with bun, and a peanut butter sandwich provide 56 gm of protein.

Based on the RDA, the calories from protein should be about 7% to 8% of the total caloric intake of the teenager. This is low compared to most surveys of adolescents' intakes in this country. The surveys show an intake of 12% to 14% of total calories as protein.[18,19] Thus average intakes of protein among teenagers are above the RDA. However, of all youth adolescents are the least studied in terms of their protein requirements.[20]

Assessment of Adequacy of Protein Intake. As mentioned, the likelihood of a teenager consuming inadequate protein is rare. However, in some cases an adolescent will restrict energy intake for weight reduction or economic reasons. In this case the protein that is consumed will be used to meet energy needs and will not be available for synthesis of new tissue. Another instance of inadequate protein intake might occur in an adolescent with a chronic medical problem such as inflammatory bowel disease that increases protein and energy requirements. In these situations assessment of protein status may be necessary.

An obvious indication of protein inadequacy is a slowing of growth. The problem may be either inadequate protein or inadequate energy to allow the protein to be used for growth. An additional useful measurement is the mid-upper arm circumference, which provides an estimate of the proportion of muscle tissue in the body. The arm muscle area can be calculated and compared to standards for adolescents of various ages.[21] These standards are contained in Appendix G. An arm muscle area at the 5th percentile or lower would indicate severe underweight and malnutrition in the adolescent. Fig. 3-5 illustrates how to determine arm muscle area. Nomograms also are available in Appendix F for determining arm muscle area without the calculations.[22]

Biochemically, a 24-hour urinary creatinine excretion can be used to measure the body muscle mass and protein status in adolescents who are malnourished and underweight. An almost perfect correlation has been shown to exist between creatinine excretion and lean body mass as determined by body potassium measurements.[23] Because of differences in height and percentage of body weight as fat, it is most useful to relate the 24-hour urinary creatinine excretion to body height. A creatinine/height index is derived and compared to the age- and size-appropriate standards in Table 3-11. It is generally assumed that 1 gm of creatinine corresponds to 20 gm of muscle mass. The normal creatinine/height index is not well defined, but it is accepted that a value less than 60% of

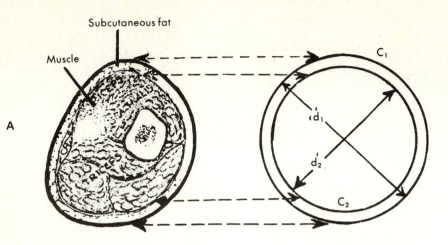

A

1. Measure mid-upper arm circumference in cm and convert it to mm (C_1).

2. Measure triceps skinfold in mm (T).

3. Area $= \pi r^2$ where $r = \dfrac{d_1}{2}$ and $d_1 = \dfrac{C_1}{\pi}$

B

4. Mid-upper arm area in mm^2 (A) $= \dfrac{\pi}{4} \times d_1{}^2$

$$A = \frac{\pi}{4} \times \left(\frac{C_1}{\pi}\right)^2 = \frac{C_1{}^2}{4\pi}$$

5. Mid-upper arm muscle area in mm^2 (M) $= \pi \times \dfrac{d_2{}^2}{4}$ where $d_2 = \dfrac{C_2}{\pi}$ and $C_2 = \pi d_1 - \pi T$

$$M = \frac{(C_1 - \pi T)^2}{4\pi}$$

6. Mid-upper arm fat area in mm^2 (F) $= A - M$

Fig. 3-5. A, Diagram of the cross section of the mid-upper arm. **B,** Calculation of arm area, *A;* arm muscle area, *M;* and arm fat area, *F.* Calculation of arm muscle and fat areas may be avoided by using the nomograms in Appendixes F and G. (Adapted from Krause, M.V., and Mahan, L.K.: Food, nutrition and diet therapy, ed. 6, Philadelphia, 1979, W.B. Saunders Co.)

Table 3-11. Normal values for 24-hr creatinine excretion

Height (cm)	Creatinine Values (mg/24 hr)		
	Both Sexes*	Males†	Females†
55	50.0		
60	65.2		
65	80.5		
70	97.5		
75	118.0		
80	139.6		
85	167.6		
90	199.9		
95	239.8		
100	278.7		
105	305.4		
110	349.8		
115	394.5		
120	456.0		
125	535.1		
130		448.1	525.2
135		480.1	589.2
140		556.3	653.1
145		684.3	717.2
150		812.3	780.9
155		940.3	844.8
160		1068.3	908.8
165		1196.3	
170		1324.3	
175		1452.3	
180		1580.3	

From Merritt, R.J., and Blackburn, G.L.: Nutritional assessment and metabolic response to illness of the hospitalized child. In Suskind, R.M., editor: Textbook of pediatric nutrition, New York, 1981, Raven Press.
*Data from Viteri, F.E., and Alvarado, J.: Pediatrics **46**:696, 1970.
†Data from Cheek, D.B., editor: Human growth: body composition, cell growth, energy and intelligence, Philadelphia, 1968, Lea & Febiger.

standard indicates severe tissue and protein depletion and that a value less than 80% of standard indicates moderate depletion.[24] The intake of meat that contains creatine has some effect on the creatinine levels, so it is wise to get at least three values and to have the adolescent avoid a high meat intake on the days of testing.

Other measures of protein status that are useful for the chronically ill or very malnourished teen are measures of the visceral protein status. These include measurement of serum concentrations of liver secretory proteins (for example, albumin, transferrin, prealbumin, and retinol-binding protein). Low levels of these proteins indicate decreased availability of amino acids for protein synthesis. Albumin is a less sensitive indicator of protein malnutrition than some of the other proteins. Immunocompetence (the ability of the body to generate an immune response to a foreign protein) also can be assessed as a measure of protein nurture. This is easily measured using lymphocyte count and intradermal skin testing.[24]

Minerals

The maximal growth rate of males exceeds the maximal growth rate of females. Because of this difference and the male's eventual greater body size, the adolescent male has greater mineral needs than the female. During the growth spurt, the need for all minerals increases, but three are particularly important: calcium (for increased skeletal mass), iron (for the expansion of blood volume), and zinc (for the generation of new skeletal and muscular tissue). Dietary surveys have consistently shown iron and calcium to be of concern in the teenager's diet.[25-31] More recently, there has been increasing emphasis on the role of zinc.[32]

Calcium. Calcium requirements increase with the growth of lean body mass and the skeleton. About 99% of the body's calcium is in the bone, so the increase in calcium requirements depends on the skeletal growth rate and the rate of ossification of the bone. Forty-five percent of the total adult skeleton is laid down during adolescence, but growth in skeletal mass continues past the adolescent period into the third decade.[33]

The peak daily increments of calcium are greater, last longer, and occur later in males than in females. At the peak of their growth spurt, the daily accumulation of calcium is as much as 400 mg in boys and 240 mg in girls. The average daily increment is 180 to 210 mg in boys and 90 to 110 mg in girls during the period from 10 to 20 years of age.[34] Body calcium is a function of stature, and calcium content increases by 20 gm/cm final height (50.8 gm/in final height). Therefore the difference between the calcium in a tall man's body (95th percentile) can be 36% greater than in a small man's body (5th percentile). The difference between a tall woman and a short woman is about 20%. Although data are not available, the same differences probably exist for adolescent bodies.[34,36]

The RDA for calcium in the United States is currently 1200 mg for both sexes until 18 years of age and 800 mg thereafter. This recommendation is 500 to 600 mg higher than the recommendations in other countries. This discrepancy results from the United States' emphasis on peak retention values for individuals in the growth spurt. These values are high so that all adolescents' needs will be covered even though the values may be much more than required for some. The customary high calcium intake, which means that the body is accustomed to absorbing less calcium, and the high protein intake, which leads to poorer calcium retention, are additional reasons for the high U.S. calcium recommendation.[37,38] About 20% to 30% of the ingested calcium is absorbed depending on the needs and the usual intake of the teen.[39] Calcium absorption can vary widely: from 53% when the intake is 190 mg/day to 17% when the intake is 3000 mg/day.[40]

There has been discussion about the calcium/phosphorus ratio and opinions differ as to how important this is in the diet. It appears that the calcium/phosphorus ratio in the diet affects the homeostasis of calcium and phosphorus in the body and thus the integrity of the skeleton. Since the RDA for calcium and phosphorus are both 1200 mg, the recommended calcium/phosphorus ratio is 1:1.[4,41] It has been shown, however, that the human can tolerate a wider range of ratios—between 2:1 and 1:2. Some speculate that if the diet contains sufficient calcium, calcium absorption may not be affected by the calcium/phosphorus ratio.[39] Much more research needs to be done in this area, especially since calcium has been found to be one of the nutrients consistently low in the diets of teenagers[25-31] and since recent estimates indicate that the calcium/phosphorus ratio in the U.S. diet as available for consumption is approximately 1:1.7.[43] This seems to be a trend in the wrong direction.

Since 1967, there has been a 6% decrease in estimated available calcium and an unchanged phosphorus level in the average American diet.[43] During the same period, there has also been a 4% increase in protein in the diet.[43] Sources of dietary phosphorus that lower the calcium/phosphorus ratio are carbonated beverages (of which teens drink a great deal), processed meats and cheeses, refrigerated bakery products, and several food additives that contain phosphates. From 1960 to 1973, there was a 22% decrease in milk consumption and an 11% increase in soft drink consumption in the United States.[44]

The concern over the calcium/phosphorus ratio is due to the desire to prevent osteoporosis. The present consensus seems to be that the development of osteoporosis is not so much related to calcium intake in old age but to the amount of bone present in early adult life. In other words, the natural process of demineralization has more bone to work on when the individual reaches adulthood with the maximal amount of bone mineralization.[4] This seems to be even more reason to assess the calcium/phosphorus ratio in the diet of the teenager and to recommend good sources of calcium in the diet.

Assessment of Adequacy of Calcium Intake. The best way to assess the adequacy of the calcium intake in the adolescent is to measure the mineralization of the bone. Most frequently this is done with a roentgenogram of the metacarpal bones of the hand. However, a more accurate assessment is achieved using the photon activation technique, which is available in some medical centers.[45] In general the serum calcium concentration is useless because it does not vary in normal individuals. Despite widely varying calcium intakes, serum calcium concentration will not vary because the various regulatory mechanisms such as vitamin D and parathyroid hormone are so efficient at maintaining the proper calcium concentration.

In adults an elevated serum alkaline phosphatase would indicate abnormal calcium status, but in growing youngsters and teens an elevated serum alkaline phosphatase is normal. In practical terms the best way to assess calcium adequacy is through assessment of the diet for calcium, protein, and the presence of items such as oxalate and phytate, which decrease calcium absorption, and vitamin D, which promotes calcium absorption. The reader should consult a basic nutrition text for a discussion of the factors that affect calcium absorption.

Iron. For both the male and female, the need for iron increases with rapid growth and the increase in muscle mass, blood volume, and respiratory enzymes. In the female, there is the additional need with menarche because of iron loss during menstruation. The iron losses from menstruation in adolescents vary widely, but it appears that the losses are correlated with absorption of iron.[46]

The adolescent male during the peak of his adolescent growth needs even more iron than the menstruating adolescent female. Since the iron required for growth is partially dependent on the blood volume increase caused by growth of lean body mass, the adolescent male requires more iron because he is gaining more lean body mass at a faster rate than the female.

In addition, the iron need depends on the size of the adolescent. The large, fast-growing boy will require more iron than the small adolescent of the same age. Table 3-12 shows that a boy growing at the 3rd percentile for weight who is not in the peak of his growth spurt requires only 6.6 mg iron/day. On the other hand, a male growing at the 97th percentile for weight who is in the peak of his growth spurt would require 25.8 mg iron/day or almost four times as much.[47] In girls the difference is only about twice as much.

The same iron intake thus could be more than adequate during one phase of adolescence and less than adequate during another. Iron deficiency anemia, which is discussed in Chapter 7, may result if iron intake is not increased. In a group of over 14,000 subjects who had a constant iron intake of 6 to 9.5 mg/day after infancy, the rate of anemia increased from 2% in the 11-year-old male to 30% in the 15-year-old male, largely because of growth in lean body mass.[47] In girls the rate of anemia is not as great but is almost twofold higher in the 15-year-old female than in the 11-year-old female.

The RDA for iron for female teenagers is 18 mg/day. The RDA is the same for males until 19 years of age when it decreases to 10 mg/day. The females's RDA remains high at 18 mg/day since her increased requirement is long-term because of the continuation of menstruation after adolescence and throughout the child-bearing years. Table 3-12 indicates that this RDA of 18 mg/day for the male will not meet the requirements for his fast-growing body during the peak of growth. Ideally his body stores will help meet these requirements. Each kilogram of lean body mass gained requires 46 mg of iron. Hepner[47] has calculated that the adolescent boy growing at the 50th percentile would require

Table 3-12. Calculated iron requirements for males and females at the 3rd, 25th, 75th, and 97th percentile for body weight (from 10-16 years of age)

Percentile Rating	Calculated Iron Requirements (mg)					
	Daily Dietary Need*		Peak Daily Dietary Need*		Cumulative Need†	
	Male	Female	Male	Female	Male	Female
3rd	6.6	5.1	13.2	10.3	966	751
25th	9.3	5.2	18.6	10.4	1360	772
75th	11.0	5.5	21.9	11.0	1610	794
97th	12.9	5.7	25.8	11.9	1885	836

From McKigney, J.I., and Munro, H.N., editors: Nutrient requirements in adolescence, Cambridge, Mass., 1978, The MIT Press. Copyright © 1978 The Massachusetts Institute of Technology.
*Period of adolescent growth spurt.
÷Total body iron increment represented by muscle tissue increase during 10-16 year interval.

42 mg of iron/kg gained (19 mg iron/lb gained) as compared to 31 mg iron/kg gained (14.1 mg iron/lb gained) for the adolescent girl growing at the 50th percentile. Gaines and Daniel[48] found that intakes of iron in both females and males increased as physiological age increased. However, there was still no correlation between the amount of intake and transferrin saturation. This was probably related to the difference in iron absorption caused by the composition of the diet and the peculiarities of the individual. Iron absorption is estimated to be between 5% and 10% in adolescence,[49] and rapid growth can increase it.

The average concentration of iron in the American diet is 6 mg/1000 kcal.[50] Meeting the 18 mg RDA can be a problem, especially for the adolescent female who has an iron requirement similar to the adolescent male but a smaller energy requirement. For the female it is almost impossible to meet the RDA without an iron supplement.

Assessment of Adequacy of Iron Intake. In addition to the functional forms of iron—hemoglobin, myoglobin, and iron in enzymes—there are storage forms of iron that can amount to 30% of the total body iron content. Iron deficiency is seen first in these iron stores. Only after these stores are depleted is there a reduction in the functional forms of iron such as hemoglobin. Neither the measurement of hemoglobin nor the presence of anemia is a very sensitive measure of iron status. Assessment of the storage and transport forms of iron (serum ferritin), transferrin saturation percentage, and total iron-binding capacity (TIBC) are much better early indexes of iron deficiency. Other measures are total serum iron, mean corpuscular volume (MCV), and mean corpuscular hemoglobin concentration (MCHC).

In addition, taking into account the developmental stages or sexual maturity stages is useful because iron requirements are so dependent on growth in lean body mass. Table 3-13 presents the hematocrits for adolescents in various stages of sexual maturity below which anemia is assumed to be present. For teenagers the use of chronological standards for anemia rather than standards based on sexual maturity stages might result in deceptive interpretations of test results.

Iron deficiency has been found in teenagers of all races, in both sexes, and at all levels of economic status.[29,51,52] However, as can be seen in Table 3-13, the standards below which anemia is considered present are lower for blacks than for

Table 3-13. 15th Percentile of hematocrits below which anemia is assumed to be present

Sexual Maturity Stage	Black Males	White Males	Black Females	White Females
1	34.9	35.6	34.0	35.8
2	36.0	36.9	35.3	36.6
3	37.1	38.2	36.0	37.0
4	38.2	39.6	36.2	36.7
5	39.3	40.6	35.8	35.9

Modified from Daniel, W.A.: Dietetic Currents **3**(4):15, 1976. Courtesy of Ross Laboratories, Columbus, Ohio.

whites. Girls between 12 and 16 years of age were found to consume 9 to 13 mg iron/day, and boys the same age consumed 10 to 16 mg iron/day.[53]

Zinc. The need for zinc in adolescence is of particular importance because of the rapid growth rate and sexual maturation. Zinc is also an integral part of 40 metalloenzymes. With the onset of puberty, there is a striking increase in the retention of zinc in both males and females that is closely related to the increase in lean body mass. For each kilogram gained in lean body mass, 28 mg of zinc is required.[54] Between the ages of 11 and 17, the average retention exceeds 0.4 mg/day.[55] Table 3-1 indicates how much greater the retention of zinc is during the peak of the growth spurt than during the rest of adolescence.

It is now known that zinc is essential for the growth and sexual maturation of the adolescent. This vital role is explained in part by zinc's central role in nucleic acid metabolism. Severe zinc deficiency in groups of adolescent boys in Iran and Egypt caused a syndrome of dwarfism, hypogonadism, anemia, and hepatosplenomegaly.[56,57] However, even milder deficiencies seem to cause some growth retardation and a delay in sexual maturity in otherwise healthy adolescents. Zinc supplementation in these adolescents resulted in increased growth and sexual maturation.[58] Hambidge and co-workers[59] measured hair zinc in nor-

mal, healthy individuals of middle and upper income 4 to 40 years of age. Five percent had hair zinc levels of 70 μg/gm. These levels were comparable to those found in the Middle Eastern adolescents with zinc deficiency.[59] After zinc supplementation, appetite, dietary intake, taste acuity, linear growth rate, and hair zinc levels improved.[59] Hambidge and co-workers[59] concluded that marginal zinc status could be a clinically relevant problem in a normal population.

As with iron, the percentage of dietary zinc that is absorbed is variable but is usually in the range of 20% to 30%. Also like iron, zinc from animal protein is more available for absorption, and factors such as phytate and fiber decrease zinc absorption. The percentage of zinc absorbed is also dependent on the quantity in the diet and the present zinc status of the adolescent.[60]

Assessment of Adequacy of Zinc Intake. When assessing zinc deficiency in the adolescent, the following clinical features are important: growth retardation, delayed closure of the epiphyses, delayed sexual maturation, hypogeusia (decrease in taste sensation), dysgeusia (abnormal taste sensation), and chronic skin problems (including parakeratosis and possibly acne, which is discussed in Chapter 7).

Any adolescent in whom there is a falling-off of growth should have zinc status evaluated. Laboratory support for the clinical diagnosis of zinc deficiency is provided by a low plasma zinc level. However, low plasma zinc levels can occur without zinc depletion in certain circumstances (for example, during acute infections and hypoproteinemic states, or when circulating levels of estrogen are high).[60] Levels of erythrocyte zinc, urinary zinc excretion, and parotid saliva zinc may also be useful, although the standards for these tests are just beginning to be determined. Serum alkaline phosphatase activity is frequently depressed in zinc-deficient states, so this may be an indicator of zinc deficiency.[60]

One study suggests that adolescents are at a high

Table 3-14. Recommended daily dietary allowances[a]

	Age (yr)	Weight		Height		Protein (gm)	Fat-Soluble Vitamins		
		(kg)	(lb)	(cm)	(in)		Vitamin A (μg RE)[b]	Vitamin D (μg)[c]	Vitamin E (mg α-TE)[d]
Females	11-14	46	101	157	62	46	800	10	8
	15-18	55	120	163	64	46	800	10	8
	19-22	55	120	163	64	44	800	7.5	8
Males	11-14	45	99	157	62	45	1000	10	8
	15-18	66	145	176	69	56	1000	10	10
	19-22	70	154	177	70	56	1000	7.5	10

Modified from Food and Nutrition Board, National Academy of Sciences–National Research Council: Recommended dietary al-

[a] The allowances are intended to provide for individual variations among most normal persons as they live in the United States which human requirements have been less well defined.

[b] Retinol equivalents. 1 retinol equivalent equals 1 μg retinol or 6 μg β-carotene.

[c] As cholecalciferol. 10 μg cholecalciferol equals 400 IU of vitamin D.

[d] α-Tocopherol equivalents. 1 mg d-α tocopherol equals 1 α-TE.

[e] 1 NE (niacin equivalent) is equal to 1 mg of niacin or 60 mg of dietary tryptophan.

[f] The folacin allowances refer to dietary sources as determined by *Lactobacillus casei* assay after treatment with enzymes (con-

risk for zinc deficiency during periods of rapid growth. The lowest concentrations of plasma zinc occurred during infancy and puberty. The steepest decline occurred in females at the age of 10.8 years and in males at 12.9 years. Plasma zinc levels appeared to be lowest at the times of the greatest growth.[61]

Twelve youths, 5 to 17 years of age, who had short stature were assessed for their zinc status. Compared to 40 control children, their plasma zinc levels did not differ, but the hair zinc levels were significantly lower in the experimental group.[62] Five adolescents with Crohn's disease who had arrested linear growth were also studied, and four were found to have plasma zinc levels significantly lower than those of the control group.[62] This appears to be evidence verifying zinc's role as a contributing factor in abnormal growth in some populations of adolescents.

Hair Analysis. Hair zinc also can be used as a measure of zinc status. Measurement of hair zinc is an example of a chemical analysis of tissue that can be used for assessing nutritional status, particularly the long-term intake of a nutrient. Hair analysis for zinc is probably the most tested hair mineral analysis and may prove to be a very good technique for determining zinc nutriture. However, hair analysis should only be used in conjunction with other data such as plasma zinc when determining the zinc status of individuals.[63]

A careful examination of the use of hair analysis reveals some problems that must be kept in mind:

1. Concentrations of metals in the hair can be correlated with the amount of exposure of that individual to that metal. For example, the concentration of lead in hair has been found to be lowest in rural populations groups, higher in urban groups, and highest in individuals who live close to lead smelters.[64] Air, tobacco smoke, water, sweat, shampoos, and hair sprays can deposit trace elements on the surface of the hair.

2. Although measurements made in any laboratory today generally can be assumed to be accurate, comparisons of data obtained from different

Water-Soluble Vitamins							Minerals					
Vita-min C (mg)	Thia-min (mg)	Ribo-flavin (mg)	Niacin (mg NE)[e]	Vita-min B6 (mg)	Fola-cin[f] (μg)	Vita-min B12 (μg)	Cal-cium (mg)	Phos-phorus (mg)	Mag-nesium (mg)	Iron (mg)	Zinc (mg)	Iodine (μg)
50	1.1	1.3	15	1.8	400	3.0	1200	1200	300	18	15	150
60	1.1	1.3	14	2.0	400	3.0	1200	1200	300	18	15	150
60	1.1	1.3	14	2.0	400	3.0	800	800	300	18	15	150
50	1.4	1.6	18	1.8	400	3.0	1200	1200	350	18	15	150
60	1.4	1.7	18	2.0	400	3.0	1200	1200	400	18	15	150
60	1.5	1.7	19	2.2	400	3.0	800	800	350	10	15	150

lowances, ed. 9, Washington, D.C., 1980.
under usual environmental stresses. Diets should be based on a variety of common foods in order to provide other nutrients for

jugases) to make polyglutamyl forms of the vitamin available to the test organism.

laboratories often show large variations in absolute values.

3. There is little agreement about precisely what constitutes normal concentrations of trace elements in hair. Until there is more information, any hair analysis must be looked at with a very critical eye.

4. Different laboratories use different procedures to remove contaminants and analyze different proportions of trace elements. These differences are major sources of inconsistency.

5. The actual techniques of analysis vary between the laboratories, and at present there are no standard reference materials with which to calibrate instruments. Fortunately, the International Atomic Energy Agency is particularly interested in nuclear techniques for hair analysis and is attempting to develop standards.

As a result of the interest in hair analysis, many laboratories have sprung up across the country, particularly on the West Coast. These laboratories often produce elaborate and impressive computer printouts that presume to evaluate the nutriture for dozens of minerals despite lack of evidence supporting the technique's effectiveness for this purpose. Proposed therapy using nutritional supplements to the diet is not potentially as dangerous as chelation therapy, which is also often suggested. Chelation therapy, which binds metal ions to hasten their removal from the body, can also remove essential metals. Educating the public about the limitations and dangers of such techniques is very important. Adolescents especially will need the information, as they belong to a generation trained to trust such technology.

Other Minerals. Recommended allowances for other minerals such as magnesium, phosphorus, and iodine are given in Table 3-14. The daily increments for magnesium are given in Table 3-1. The magnesium needs for growth are relatively small, but the maintenance needs during adolescence are not known.[35]

Phosphorus does not appear to be a problem since the total body phosphorus in the adult is

Table 3-15. Estimated safe and adequate daily dietary intakes of selected vitamins and minerals*

	Vitamins			Trace Elements†						Electrolytes		
Age (yr)	Vita- min K (µg)	Biotin (µg)	Panto- thenic Acid (mg)	Copper (mg)	Man- ganese (mg)	Fluo- ride (mg)	Chro- mium (mg)	Selenium (mg)	Molyb- denum (mg)	Sodium (mg)	Potassium (mg)	Chloride (mg)
Infants												
0-0.5	12	35	2	0.5-0.7	0.5-0.7	0.1-0.5	0.01-0.04	0.01-0.04	0.03-0.06	115-350	350-925	275-700
0.5-1	10-20	50	3	0.7-1.0	0.7-1.0	0.2-1.0	0.02-0.06	0.02-0.06	0.04-0.08	250-750	425-1275	400-1200
Children												
and 1-3	15-30	65	3	1.0-1.5	1.0-1.5	0.5-1.5	0.02-0.08	0.02-0.08	0.05-0.1	325-975	550-1650	500-1500
4-6	20-40	85	3-4	1.5-2.0	1.5-2.0	1.0-2.5	0.03-0.12	0.03-0.12	0.06-0.15	450-1350	775-2325	700-2100
Adolescents 7-10	30-60	120	4-5	2.0-2.5	2.0-3.0	1.5-2.5	0.05-0.2	0.05-0.2	0.10-0.3	600-1800	1000-3000	925-2775
11+	50-100	100-200	4-7	2.0-3.0	2.5-5.0	1.5-2.5	0.05-0.2	0.05-0.2	0.15-0.5	900-2700	1525-4575	1400-4200
Adults	70-140	100-200	4-7	2.0-3.0	2.5-5.0	1.5-4.0	0.05-0.2	0.05-0.2	0.15-0.5	1100-3300	1875-5625	1700-5100

Modified from Food and Nutrition Board, National Academy of Sciences–National Research Council: Recommended dietary allowances, ed. 9, Washington, D.C., 1980.

*Because there is less information on which to base allowances, these figures are not given in the main table of RDA and are provided here in the form of ranges of recommended intakes.

†Since the toxic levels for many trace elements may be only several times usual intakes, the upper levels for the trace elements given in this table should not be habitually exceeded.

about one half that of calcium. In addition, the absorption rate of phosphorus is higher than of calcium, about 50%, and the usual American diet provides more phosphorus than calcium.[35]

Of the trace minerals, many such as copper, chromium, cobalt, and iodine are known to be essential. The estimated safe intakes are given in Table 3-15. Iodine nutriture was assessed in the *Ten State Nutrition Survey,* and there was no evidence of iodine deficiency in the adolescent population surveyed.[29]

Fluoride has been shown to be important at a level of 1.5 mg/day, and ranges of 1.5 to 2.5 mg/day have been proven safe in many studies.[65] These levels confer some caries prevention protection. Dental caries were shown to be an extensive problem among adolescents surveyed in the *Ten State Nutrition Survey.*[29] Chapter 7 contains further discussion of dental caries in adolescence.

When looking at trace mineral status, it is important to examine interactions between nutrients. For example, it is postulated that the ratio of zinc to copper in the diet is related to the incidence of cardiovascular disease and that a lower zinc/copper ratio is better.[66] It is also important to remember that since many trace minerals have not been adequately studied in adolescents, many possible interactions are unknown.

VITAMINS

The requirements for vitamins during adolescence increase with the growth rate. Thiamin, riboflavin, and niacin requirements are dependent on the energy (especially carbohydrate) intake. Thus with the increased energy intake during adolescence, there is an increase in the RDA for these vitamins. In the case of vitamins A, E, C, B_6, and folic acid, the RDA during adolescence are the same as those for adulthood. An exception is vitamin D. Because of the rapid rate of skeletal growth, the requirement for vitamin D in adolescence is 10 μg cholecalciferol (400 IU); this requirement is lowered to 7.5 μg in adulthood. However, the RDA for all vitamins except vitamin D are greater during adolescence than during childhood. For most of the vitamins, the requirements during adolescence have been determined from interpolation of nutritional requirements determined for adults or for younger children.[5]

Vitamin A is one vitamin shown to be low in the diets of over one third of the adolescents 10 to 16 years of age surveyed in the *Texas Nutrition Survey.*[31] Similar numbers of children were found to have low serum vitamin A concentrations. A clinical manifestation of vitamin A deficiency (follicular hyperkeratosis) was found in about 7% to 9% of the adolescent age group.[31]

In another study, liver vitamin A values collected during autopsy showed that liver stores of vitamin A appeared to be much lower among people 11 to 20 years of age than in either young children or adults. The physiological significance of this observation is unknown.[67] Maturation and growth appear to influence plasma levels of vitamin A in normal children, and the levels are largely independent of the size of the liver reserves. A relatively large amount of vitamin A can be stored in the liver, and plasma vitamin A levels appear only to reflect nutritional status when liver reserves have been almost completely exhausted. A more useful index of vitamin A status appears to be the retinol-binding protein, a transport protein for vitamin A.

Low intakes of vitamin C have also been reported.[28] McGanity[31] reported that the incidence of clinical manifestations of vitamin C deficiency may be as high as 9% in the adolescent population. Vitamin C intake does not seem to be a problem for most adolescents, but it might be for those who absolutely avoid all fresh fruits and vegetables and/or smoke cigarettes. In addition, vitamin C intake should be kept as high as possible to enhance the iron absorption that is so important during the adolescent years.

Intake of folic acid has been frequently found to be low in the diets of American teenagers.[68] In

Table 3-16. Biochemical measurements of nutritional status

Nutrient	More Sensitive	Less Sensitive
Protein	Plasma amino acids	Total serum protein
	Hair root morphology	
	Serum albumin	
	Urinary creatinine/height index	
	Urinary hydroxyproline	
	Serum retinol-binding protein	
	Serum transferrin	
Lipids	Serum cholesterol (high density lipoprotein and low density lipoprotein)	
	Serum triglycerides	
	Lipoproteins	
Vitamin A	Serum vitamin A	Blood leukocytes
	Serum carotene	
	Serum retinol	
	Liver retinol stores	
	Retinol-binding protein	
Vitamin D	Serum 25-hydroxy-vitamin D_3	Urinary calcium
	Serum alkaline phosphatase	Serum phosphorus
		Serum parathormone
Vitamin E	Hydrogen peroxide erythrocyte hemolysis test	Platelet assessment
	Serum or plasma tocopherol	
Vitamin K	Plasma factors II, VII, IX, X	Prothrombin time
Thiamin	Urinary thiamin	Blood pyruvate
	Erythrocyte transketolase activity	
	Thiamin pyrophosphate effect	

Modified from Krause, M.V., and Mahan, L.K.: Food, nutrition and diet therapy, ed. 6, Philadelphia, 1979, W.B. Saunders Co.

addition, vitamin B_6 intake has been found to be low when compared to the RDA.[28,69] The tests presently used to assess vitamin nutriture are given in Table 3-16.

In summary, because of the paucity of information available about the vitamin requirements during adolescence, it is difficult to make recommendations for intake. As we learn more about the functions of vitamins, our biochemical tests for assessing their nutriture will improve. We may be able to define vitamin deficiency states before they reach the functional or clinical stage.

CLINICAL ASSESSMENT

Physical *signs* and *symptoms* of malnutrition occur in the later stages in the progression of a deficiency state and are found in only a small number of cases. Further, the signs and symptoms are nonspecific, as seen in Table 3-17. They may represent nonnutritional causes or multiple nutritional deficiencies. Nevertheless, a careful physical examination with attention to possible physical signs of malnutrition is very important to enable correlation with laboratory and dietary data.

Table 3-16. Biochemical measurements of nutritional status—cont'd

Nutrient	More Sensitive	Less Sensitive
Riboflavin	Urinary riboflavin Erythrocyte glutathione reductase	
Nicotinic acid	N^1-methyl-2-pyridone-5-carboxylamide (2-pyridone)/N^1-methylnicotinamide urinary excretion ratio	Urinary N^1-methyl nicotinamide
Vitamin B_6	Tryptophan load test (mg xanthurenic and kynurenic acids excreted in urine) Plasma pyridoxal phosphate	Urinary pyridoxine excretion (μg/gm creatinine) Blood transaminase (serum glutamic-pyruvic transaminase and serum glutamic-oxalo-acetic transaminase)
Folic acid	Red cell folate	Serum folate Bone marrow film Thin blood film Urinary formiminoglutamic acid excretion
Vitamin B_{12}	Serum B_{12} Serum thimidylate synthetase Urine methylmalonic acid	Bone marrow film Thin blood film Schilling test
Vitamin C	Serum ascorbic acid Leukocyte ascorbic acid	Urinary ascorbic acid
Iron	Iron deposits in bone marrow Serum iron Transferrin saturation percentage Serum ferritin	Hemoglobin Hematocrit Thin blood film
Iodine		Urinary iodine Thyroid function tests
Zinc	Serum and plasma zinc	Hair zinc
Magnesium	Serum magnesium	

Functional tests such as dark adaptation for vitamin A status and taste thresholds for zinc status may also be incorporated into the clinical evaluation. Although these measures also are generally nonspecific and should be used in conjunction with other findings, they have the advantage of greater sensitivity than some of the physical signs of malnutrition. Functional problems clearly indicate a need for aggressive therapeutic nutritional intervention. Thus as more objective functional tests become available, they should be included in the assessment of nutritional status.

NUTRITIONAL CARE PLAN AND EDUCATIONAL GOALS

Following a comprehensive nutrition assessment, the health professional proceeds with a nutritional care plan. The plan should consider all significant data and be directed toward alleviating any nutritional problem.

Problem Areas

Studies consistently have shown that nutrients can be lacking in teens' diets. Most frequently,

Table 3-17. Physical and functional signs indicative or suggestive of malnutrition

	Normal Appearance	Signs Associated with Malnutrition	Possible Disorder or Nutrient Deficiency	Possible Nonnutritional Problem
Hair	Shiny; firm; not easily plucked	Lack of natural shine; dull and dry Thin and sparse Silky and straight; fine Dyspigmented Flag sign Easily plucked (no pain)	Kwashiorkor and, less commonly, marasmus	Excessive bleaching of hair Alopecia
Face	Skin color uniform; smooth, pink, healthy appearance; not swollen	Nasolabial seborrhea (scaling of skin around nostrils) Swollen face (moon face) Paleness	Riboflavin Kwashiorkor Iron	Acne vulgaris
Eyes	Bright, clear, shiny; no sores at corners of eyelids; membranes a healthy pink and moist; no prominent blood vessels, mound of tissue or sclera; normal dark adaptation	Pale conjunctiva Red membranes Bitot's spots Xerophthalmia (conjunctival dryness) Corneal xerosis (dullness) Nyctalopia (night blindness) Keratomalacia (softening of cornea) Redness and fissuring of eyelid corners Arcus cornealis (white ring around eye) Xanthoma palpebrarum (small yellowish lumps around eyes)	Anemia (iron) Vitamin A Riboflavin; pyridoxine Hyperlipidemia Vitamin A	Bloodshot eyes from exposure to weather, lack of sleep, smoke, or alcohol
Lips	Smooth; not chapped or swollen	Angular stomatitis (white or pink lesions at corners of mouth) Angular scars Cheilosis (redness or swelling of lips and mouth)	Riboflavin	Exposure to weather

Modified from Jelliffe, D.B.: The assessment of the nutritional status of the community, World Health Organization Monograph, no. 53, Geneva, 1966; McLaren, D.S.: Nutritional assessment. In McLaren, D.S., and Burman, D., editors: Textbook of pediatric nutrition, Edinburgh, 1976, Churchill Livingstone; Christakis, G., editor: Nutritional assessment in health programs, Washington, D.C., 1973, American Public Health Association, Inc.; and Krause, M.V., and Mahan, L.K.: Food, nutrition and diet therapy, ed. 6, Philadelphia, 1979, W.B. Saunders Co.

Table 3-17. Physical and functional signs indicative or suggestive of malnutrition—cont'd

	Normal Appearance	Signs Associated with Malnutrition	Possible Disorder or Nutrient Deficiency	Possible Nonnutritional Problem
Tongue	Deep red in appearance; not swollen or smooth	Scarlet and raw tongue Magenta tongue (purplish) Swollen tongue Filiform papillae atrophy or hypertrophy Taste alterations; increased taste thresholds	Nicotinic acid Riboflavin Niacin Folic acid Vitamin B_{12} Zinc	Leukoplakia
Teeth	No cavities; no pain; bright	Mottled enamel Caries (cavities) Missing teeth	Fluorosis Excessive sugar	Periodontal disease Poor health habits
Gums	Healthy; red; do not bleed; not swollen	Spongy; bleeding Receding gums	Vitamin C Calcium	Periodontal disease Malocclusion
Glands	Face not swollen	Thyroid enlargement (front of neck swollen) Parotid enlargement (cheeks become swollen)	Iodine Starvation	Inflammatory enlargement of thyroid
Skin	No signs of rashes, swellings, dark or light spots	Xerosis (dryness) Follicular hyperkeratosis (sandpaper feel to skin) Petechiae (small skin hemorrhages) Pellagrous dermatosis (red swollen pigmentation of areas exposed to sunlight) Excessive bruising Flaky paint dermatosis Scrotal and vulval dermatosis Xanthomas (fat deposits under skin around joints)	Vitamin A Vitamin C Nicotinic acid Vitamin K Kwashiorkor Riboflavin Hyperlipidemia	Environmental exposure Physical abuse
Nails	Firm; pink	Koilonychia (spoonshaped) Brittle; ridged	Iron	
Subcutaneous tissue	Normal amount of fat	Edema Fat below standard Fat above standard	Kwashiorkor Starvation; marasmus Obesity	

Continued.

Table 3-17. Physical and functional signs indicative or suggestive of malnutrition—cont'd

	Normal Appearance	Signs Associated with Malnutrition	Possible Disorder or Nutrient Deficiency	Possible Nonnutritional Problem
Muscular and skeletal systems	Good muscle tone; some fat under skin; can walk or run without pain	Muscle wasting	Starvation; marasmus; kwashiorkor	
		Craniotabes (thin, soft skull bones in infant)		
		Frontal and parietal bossing (round swelling of front and side of head)		
		Epiphysial enlargement (swelling of ends of bones)	Vitamin D	
		Persistently open anterior fontanel (soft area on head closes late)		
		Knock knees or bow legs		
		Musculoskeletal hemorrhages	Vitamin C	
		Calf muscle tenderness	Thiamin	
		Thoracic rosary	Vitamin D; vitamin C	
		Fractures in elderly	Osteoporosis	
Cardiovascular system	Normal heart rate and rhythm; no murmurs or abnormal rhythms; normal blood pressure for age	Cardiac enlargement	Thiamin	Anxiety
		Tachycardia		
		Elevated blood pressure	Sodium	
Gastrointestinal system	No palpable organs or masses (in children, however, liver edge may be palpable)	Hepatosplenomegaly	Kwashiorkor	
Nervous system	Psychological stability; normal reflexes	Psychomotor changes	Kwashiorkor	Depression
		Mental confusion	Nicotinic acid	Psychiatric disorder
		Depression	Thiamin	
		Sensory loss	Pyridoxine	
		Motor weakness	Vitamin B_{12}	
		Loss of position sense		
		Loss of vibration		
		Loss of ankle and knee jerks		
		Burning and tingling of hands and feet (paresthesia)		
Total body	Strength and energy sufficient for daily functioning	Extremely and easily fatigued	Iron; protein-energy malnutrition	
		Motor weakness	Thiamin	

these nutrients are iron, calcium, riboflavin, and vitamin A.[28,29,70] In addition, other surveys have shown that dietary intakes of folic acid, vitamin B[6], and zinc are often below the recommended levels for teens.[68,69,71]

On the other hand, there is the problem of excessive intakes. Preliminary estimates from the *Health and Nutrition Examination Survey* data indicate that intakes for total fat, saturated fats, added sugar, protein, and sodium were higher than levels specified in the dietary goals.[72]

Dietary guidelines or dietary goals developed by the U.S. Departments of Agriculture and Health, Education, and Welfare for health promotion and nutritional well-being are listed below:

DIETARY GUIDELINES FOR AMERICANS*

Eat a variety of foods
Maintain ideal weight
Avoid too much fat, saturated fat and cholesterol
Eat foods with adequate starch and fiber
Avoid too much sugar
Avoid too much sodium
Drink alcohol only in moderation

Many of these recommendations run counter to the eating habits of adolescents. The relationship between dietary factors and major health problems is not entirely clear, and the dietary goals therefore are very controversial. Most of the controversy relates to the recommendation to reduce dietary fat and cholesterol. Many scientists feel that it is not prudent to recommend such dietary changes for the entire population. However, there is enough preliminary evidence to suggest that many major health problems of America's adults and many potential health problems of America's adolescents are linked to diet.

*From U.S. Department of Agriculture and U.S. Department of Health, Education, and Welfare: Nutrition and your health: dietary guidelines for Americans, Washington, D.C., 1979, U.S. Government Printing Office.

Intervention strategies for nutrition improvement may include education regarding specific nutritional needs and food sources; counseling; behavior modification approaches to altering eating habits; referral to other resources such as the local food stamp program; or recommendation of appropriate supplements. In all cases, the plan should be individualized and, to the extent possible, should include suggestions for the adolescent and his or her family. Further, each care plan should have a follow-up and reassessment component.

Responsibility for nutritional care in today's health care system can fall on almost any health professional. All health professionals should be aware of common nutritional problems of adolescents and make appropriate referrals to nutritionists for in-depth assessments and development of individualized nutritional care plans in cooperation with other team members. A team approach allows teenagers to select the individual with whom they can develop the best rapport and facilitates reinforcement of care plan components from different points of view. In this manner, today's adolescent will have an opportunity to receive high-quality nutritional care.

SUMMARY

Because of differences in rates of growth and changes in body composition, the nutritional needs of adolescent boys are greater than those of adolescent girls. Many of these requirements are not adequately met by teens because of life-style factors and available choices from the food supply. Intakes most likely to be inadequate are iron, calcium, zinc, vitamin B[6], folic acid, vitamin A, and riboflavin. Nutrition assessment should involve close scrutiny of the status of these nutrients. A more likely finding in adolescents, however, is an excessive consumption of fat, sodium, and sugar. This should be appraised and addressed in the adolescents' total health care.

REFERENCES

1. Pařízková, J.: Body fat and physical fitness, The Hague, 1977, Martinus Nijhoff Publishers.
2. Chumlea, W.C., and others: Size and number of adipocytes and measures of body fat in boys and girls 10 to 18 years of age, Am. J. Clin. Nutr. **34:**1791, 1981.
3. Gregor, J.L., and Etnyre, G.M.: Validity of 24-hour dietary recalls by adolescent females, Am. J. Public Health **68:**70, 1978.
4. Food and Nutrition Board, National Academy of Sciences–National Research Council: Recommended dietary allowances, ed. 9, Washington, D.C., 1980.
5. Dwyer, J.: Nutritional requirements of adolescence, Nutr. Rev. **39:**56, 1981.
6. Beal, V.A.: Nutritional intake. In McCammon, R.W., editor: Human growth and development, Springfield, Ill., 1970, Charles C Thomas, Publisher.
7. National Center for Health Statistics: National Center for Health Statistics growth charts, 1976. In Monthly vital statistics report **25**(3), Supplement (HRA) 76-1120, Rockville, Md., June, 1976, Health Resources Administration.
8. National Center for Health Statistics: Height and weight of youths 12-17 years, United States. In Vital and health statistics, series 11, no. 124, Health Services and Mental Health Administration, Washington, D.C., 1973, U.S. Government Printing Office.
9. National Center for Health Statistics: Skinfold thickness of youths 12-17 years, United States. In Vital health and statistics, series 11, no. 132, Health Services and Mental Health Administration, Washington, D.C., 1974, U.S. Government Printing Office.
10. Forbes, G.B., and Amirhakimi, G.H.: Skinfold thickness and body fat in children, Hum. Biol. **42:**401, 1970.
11. Lee, M.M.C., and Ng, C.K.: Post mortem studies of skinfold caliper measurement and actual thickness of skin and subcutaneous tissue, Hum. Biol. **37:**91, 1965.
12. Hammond, W.H.: Measurement and interpretation of subcutaneous fat: with norms for children and young adult males, Br. J. Prev. Soc. Med. **9:**201, 1955.
13. Pařízková, J.: Total body fat and skinfold thickness in children, Metabolism **10:**794, 1961.
14. Durnin, J.V.G.A., and Wormersley, J.: Body fat assessed from total body density and its estimation from skinfold thickness: measurements on 481 men and women aged from 16-72 years, Br. J. Nutr. **32:**77, 1974.
15. Dugdale, A.E., and Griffiths, M.: Estimating body fat mass from anthropometric data, Am. J. Clin. Nutr. **32:**2400, 1979.
16. Frerichs, R.R., Harsha, D.W., and Berenson, G.S.: Equations for estimating percentage of body fat in children 10-14 years old, Pediatr. Res. **13:**170, 1979.
17. Katch, F.I., McArdle, W.D., and Boylan, R.B.: Getting in shape, Boston, 1979, Houghton Mifflin Co.
18. Heald, F.P., Remmell, P.S., and Mayer, J.: Caloric, protein and fat intake in children and adolescents. In Heald, F.P., editor: Adolescent nutrition and growth, New York, 1969, Appleton-Century-Crofts.
19. Frank, G.C., and others: Dietary studies of rural school children in a cardiovascular survey, J. Am. Diet. Assoc. **71:**31, 1977.
20. Irwin, M.I., and Hegsted, D.M.: A conspectus of research. In Nutritional requirements of man, New York, 1980, The Nutrition Foundation.
21. Frisancho, A.R.: New norms of upper limb fat and muscle areas for assessment of nutritional status, Am. J. Clin. Nutr. **34:**2540, 1981.
22. Gurney, J.M., and Jelliffe, D.G.: Arm anthropometry in nutritional assessment: nomogram for rapid calculation of muscle circumference and cross-sectional muscle fat areas, Am. J. Clin. Nutr. **26:**912, 1973.
23. Forbes, G.B., and Bruining, G.J.: Urinary creatinine excretion and lean body mass, Am. J. Clin. Nutr. **29:**1359, 1976.
24. Merritt, R.J., and Blackburn, G.L.: Nutritional assessment and metabolic response to illness of the hospitalized child. In Suskind, R.M., editor: Textbook of pediatric nutrition, New York, 1981, Raven Press.
25. Wharton, M.A.: Nutritive intake of adolescents, J. Am. Diet. Assoc. **42:**306, 1963.
26. Hodges, R.E., and Krehl, W.A.: Nutritional status of teenagers in Iowa, Am. J. Clin. Nutr. **17:**200, 1965.
27. Hampton, M.C., and others: Caloric and nutrient intakes of teenagers, J. Am. Diet. Assoc. **50:**385, 1967.
28. Schorr, B.C., Sanjur, D., and Erickson, E.C.: Teenage food habits: a multidimensional analysis, J. Am. Diet. Assoc. **61:**415, 1972.
29. U.S. Department of Health, Education, and Welfare: Ten state nutrition survey, 1968-1970, Department of Health, Education, and Welfare Publication (HSM) 73-8133, Atlanta, 1973, Health Services and Mental Health Administration, Centers for Disease Control.
30. Hodges, R.E.: Vitamin and mineral requirements in adolescence. In McKigney, J.I., and Munro, H.N., editors: Nutrient requirements in adolescence, Cambridge, Mass., 1976, The MIT Press.
31. McGanity, W.J.: Problems of nutritional evaluation of the adolescent. In McKigney, J.I., and Munroe, H.N., editors: Nutrient requirements in adolescence, Cambridge, Mass., 1976, The MIT Press.
32. Sandstead, H.H.: Zinc nutrition in the United States, Am. J. Clin. Nutr. **26:**1251, 1973.

33. Garn, S.M., and Wagner, B.: The adolescent growth of the skeletal mass and its implication to mineral requirements. In Heald, F.P., editor: Adolescent nutrition and growth, New York, 1969, Appleton-Century-Crofts.

34. Committee on Nutrition, American Academy of Pediatrics: Calcium requirements in infancy and childhood, Pediatrics 62:826, 1978.

35. Forbes, G.B.: Nutritional requirements in adolescence. In Suskind, R.M., editor: Textbook of pediatric nutrition, New York, 1981, Raven Press.

36. Cohn, S.H., and others: Changes in body chemical composition with age measured by total body neutron activation, Metabolism 25:85, 1976.

37. Johnson, N.E., Alcantara, E.N., and Linkswiler, H.: Effect of level of protein intake on urinary and fecal calcium and calcium retention of young adult males, J. Nutr. 100:1425, 1970.

38. Margen, S., and others: Studies in calcium metabolism. I. The calciuretic effect of dietary protein, Am. J. Clin. Nutr. 27:584, 1974.

39. Wilkinson, R.: Absorption of calcium, phosphorus and magnesium. In Nordin, B.E.C., editor: Calcium, phosphate and magnesium metabolism, New York, 1976, Churchill Livingstone, Inc.

40. Heany, R.P., Saville, P.D., and Recker, R.R.: Calcium absorption as a function of calcium intake, J. Lab. Clin. Med. 85:881, 1975.

41. Life Sciences Research Office: Evaluation of the health aspects of phosphates as food ingredients, SCOGS-32, Bethesda, Md., 1975, Federation of American Society for Experimental Biology.

42. Cheek, D.B., editor: Human growth: body composition, cell growth, energy and intelligence, Philadelphia, 1968, Lea & Febiger.

43. Marston, R.M., and Welsh, S.O.: Nutrient content of the national food supply, Natl. Food Rev. p. 19, Winter 1981.

44. Phillips, M.C., and Briggs, G.M.: Milk and its role in the American diet, J. Dairy Sci. 58:1751, 1975.

45. Russell, W., and others: Bone mineral status measured by direct photon absorptiometry in childhood renal disease, Pediatrics 60:864, 1977.

46. Greger, J.L., and Buckley, S.: Menstrual loss of zinc, copper, magnesium and iron by adolescent girls, Nutr. Rep. Int. 16:639, 1977.

47. Hepner, R.: In McKigney, J.I., and Munro, H.D., editors: Nutrient requirements in adolescence, Cambridge, Mass., 1976, The MIT Press.

48. Gaines, E.G., and Daniel, W.A.: Dietary iron intakes of adolescents, J. Am. Diet Assoc. 65:275, 1974.

49. Sjolin, S.: Anemia in adolescence, Nutr. Rev. 39:96, 1981.

50. Finch, C.A.: Iron nutrition, Ann. N.Y. Acad. Sci. 300:221, 1977.

51. Shank, R.E., and others: Evaluation of iron deficiency as a cause of mild anemia in adolescent girls, Enzyme 18:240, 1974.

52. Daniel, W.A., Jr., Gaines, E.G., and Bennett, D.L.: Iron intake and transferrin saturation in adolescents, J. Pediatr. 86:288, 1975.

53. U.S. Department of Health, Education, and Welfare and Food and Nutrition Board, National Academy of Sciences–National Research Council: Iron nutriture in adolescence. Department of Health, Education and Welfare Publication (HSA) 77-5100, Washington, D.C., 1976.

54. Widdowson, E.M., McCance, R.A., and Spray, C.M.: The chemical composition of the human body, Clin. Sci. 10:113, 1951.

55. Forbes, G.B., and Hursh, J.B.: Age and sex trends in lean body mass calculated from K40 measurements: with a note on the theoretical basis for this procedure, Ann. N.Y. Acad. Sci. 110:255, 1963.

56. Prasad, A.S., Halsted, J.A., and Nadimi, M.: Syndrome of iron deficiency anemia, hepatosplenomegaly, hypogonadism, dwarfism, and geophagia, Am. J. Med. 31:352, 1961.

57. Sandstead, H.H., and others: Human zinc deficiency, endocrine manifestations and response to treatment, Am. J. Clin. Nutr. 20:422, 1967.

58. Ronoghy, H., and others: Controlled zinc supplementation for malnourished school boys: a pilot experiment, Am. J. Clin. Nutr. 22:1279, 1969.

59. Hambidge, K.M., and others: Low levels of zinc in hair, anorexia, poor growth, and hypogeusia in children, Pediatr. Res. 6:868, 1974.

60. Hambidge, K.M.: Trace elements in pediatric nutrition, Adv. Pediatr. 24:191, 1977.

61. Butrimovitz, G.P., and Purdy, C.: Zinc nutrition and growth in a childhood population, Am. J. Clin. Nutr. 31:1409, 1978.

62. Solomons, N.W., and Rosenfield, R.L.: Growth retardation and zinc nutrition, Pediatr. Res. 10:923, 1976.

63. Solomons, N.W.: On the assessment of zinc and copper nutriture in man, Am. J. Clin. Nutr. 32:856, 1979.

64. Maugh, T.H.: Hair: a diagnostic tool to complement blood serum and urine, Science 202:1271, 1978.

65. Committee on Biologic Effects of Atmospheric Pollutants, National Academy of Sciences–National Research Council: Fluorides, Washington, D.C., 1971.

66. Klevay, L.M.: Hypercholesterolemia in rats produced by an increase in the ratio of zinc to copper ingested, Am. J. Clin. Nutr. 26:1060, 1973.

67. Raica, N., Jr., and others: Vitamin A concentration in human tissues collected from five areas in the United States, Am. J. Clin. Nutr. 25:291, 1972.

68. Daniel, W.A., Jr., Gaines, E.G., and Bennett, D.L.: Dietary intakes and plasma concentration of folate in healthy adolescents, Am. J. Clin. Nutr. **28:**363, 1975.
69. Kirksey, A., and others: Vitamin B_6 nutritional status of a group of female adolescents, Am. J. Clin. Nutr. **31:**946, 1978.
70. Huenemann, R.L., and others: Teenage nutrition and physique, Springfield, Ill., 1974, Charles C Thomas, Publisher.
71. Gregor, J.L., and others: Nutritional status of adolescent girls in regard to zinc, copper and iron, Am. J. Clin. Nutr. **31:**269, 1978.
72. Dwyer, J.: Diets for children and adolescents that meet the dietary goals, Am. J. Dis. Child. **134:**1073, 1980.

Chapter 4

Adolescent Life-Style and Eating Behavior

MARY STORY

Biological, psychological, cognitive, social, and developmental changes have a dynamic effect on the eating behavior of adolescents. The adolescent's search for independence and identity, active life-style, and concern for appearance may result in missed meals, eating away from home, increased snacking, and adoption of fad diets and nontraditional eating patterns. This chapter will look at adolescent eating behavior within its larger developmental and social context and will explore factors influencing adolescent food behavior and dietary practices.

FACTORS INFLUENCING EATING BEHAVIOR

Food behavior is an individual's response to stimuli related to the selection, procurement, distribution, manipulation, storage, consumption, and disposal of food.[1] An individual's food behavior is part of an intricate habit system embedded in psychological makeup, social and physical environments, and total life-style.[2] To understand food behavior in an individual or a cultural group, there must be an awareness of the factors influencing food selection. An inadequate knowledge of the variables influencing food behavior is a major obstacle in food-habit modification.

To improve the eating habits and nutritional sta-
tus of teenagers one must understand the adolescent subculture and the multiple variables, both external and internal, that affect it (Chapter 2). An adolescent's food habits are influenced by many sources: family and peers, emotional environment, and psychological and social development.

Fig. 4-1 depicts several influences on adolescent food behavior. The internal and external factors do not act directly on food behavior, but because they are integrated by the individual and incorporated into the life-style, they thus affect food behavior.[3]

Family

The family unit is recognized as the predominant influence on the individual's food behavior. The family mediates the child's dietary intake in two distinct ways: (1) the family is the provider of food, and (2) the family transmits food attitudes, preferences, and values that affect lifetime eating habits.

As adolescents move toward independence and autonomy, family influence changes. Indeed, food habits of adolescents reflect the weakening of parental influence. During these years, family commensalism may decline as newly acquired independence results in adolescents spending more time away from home and eating more meals outside the home.

Even when family commensalism is valued and

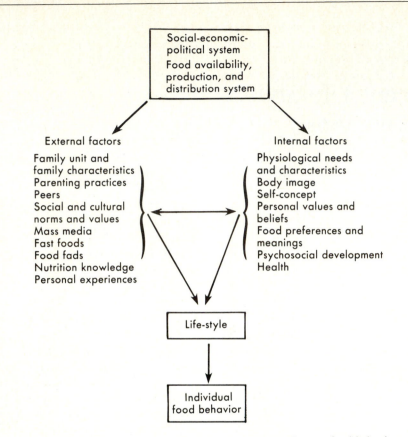

Fig. 4-1. Schematic diagram of factors influencing adolescent food behavior.

family relationships are strong, changes in adolescent food habits, although sometimes minor, may still be evident. Food habits developed earlier in life may undergo temporary changes. Before adolescence, it is relatively simple for parents to set rules and for the preadolescent to abide by them without question. For example, parents may tell children that they have to clean their plates before eating dessert or that they have to drink milk and not soda pop with their dinners. Around puberty, however, children begin to develop more abstract thought processes (Chapter 2). At this stage the adolescent begins to perceive the world in more abstract and logical ways and to think in terms of

possibilities and hypothetical situations. Developing formal operational skills enables adolescents to "read" other people, including parents, in more sophisticated and complex ways. This new skill can be annoying to parents when their teen points out inconsistencies between the parents' stated principles and their behavior.[4] The adolescent may become unwilling to accept the parents' word as a given, particularly if the parents' ideas are not logically founded. Parents may be in for a challenge and an argument if they insist that their children need to eat breakfast daily if the parents themselves do not.

Contrary to popular thinking, however, researchers have found that most adolescents and their parents enjoy positive family relations and generally are satisfied with the way they get along.[5] A minority of parents, however, are unable or unwilling to adapt to the maturational process of adolescence, and disequilibrium ensues (Chapter 2). Adolescents whose family relationships are dysfunctional and whose parents are authoritarian and rigid often use food as a vehicle to express rebellion against parental authority. This parental style may foster erratic and bizarre food practices such as wild binges, strong food aversions, food refusals, crazy diets, fasting regimens, and missed meals. A propensity toward this type of food behavior may also be found in teens with very permissive parents. In this case the behavior is an attempt to force the parents to set some limits on the teen's behavior. Likewise, parents who nag, scold, or pressure their children into eating as they should may find that this approach yields negative consequences and that the teen invariably becomes upset, angry, and rebellious. Parents should be advised to make an effort to allow their teens independence but also to provide a physical environment that facilitates healthy adolescent development and an emotional climate that encourages adaptive choices.[6] Parents can stock the kitchen with nutritious snack foods (for example, cooked chicken, raw vegetables, milk, cheese, fruit, nuts, raisins, and popcorn) and encourage their teenagers to help themselves.

In the past the majority of American families were composed of two parents with one or more children all living together. In most of these families the father was employed outside of the home, but the mother was not. No longer are the majority of adolescents exposed to this traditional family structure. The two changes in family structure that have had the most profound impact on family commensalism are the significant increase in single-parent families and the return to the work force of many mothers.[7] Such changes in the nuclear family and in the mother's work role can have pro-

found effects on the family's eating practices. These changes are partially responsible for the belief that the time-honored family meal is becoming less and less important to the American family. In fact, however, this popular view may be a myth.

In a report in which 1254 heads of households were interviewed, 70% felt that there was too little emphasis on the family eating together.[8] Youth also valued family commensalism: one recent study found that of 194 adolescents, 77% believed that eating at least one meal a day with family members is important.[9] The teens most frequently gave these reasons: (1) it was a time to communicate with the family, and (2) it made them feel a part of the family. Not surprisingly, 90% stated that their parents placed more importance on the family meal than they did.

Family meals were unimportant to about one fourth of the students. These students gave a variety of reasons, including apathy and indifference ("It just doesn't matter") and lack of time ("Everyone is coming and going at different times"; "Everyone has their own thing to do"). Family conflict also contributed to this negative attitude. Incessant arguing and fighting at the dinner table is stressful and is not conducive to positive family interactions and a sense of unity.

It should not be assumed, however, that lack of conflict around the dinner table will automatically provide a medium for family discussion, transmission and promotion of values, and enhancement of family togetherness. A Minnesota study found that a television was on most of the time during the evening meal in one third of the households surveyed. This was especially true in rural homes (47%) as compared with urban (30%) or suburban (21%) homes.[9] If a television is on during the meal, family interaction may decrease.

In short, family eating practices are among the most important influences, both positive and negative, on the food habits of adolescents. Family disorganization that leaves teens on their own with respect to eating fosters poor eating habits. In my experience adolescents whose diets are the poorest are those who eat alone or with their friends; those who eat with their families on a regular basis usually eat better and have more adequate diets. In general, families eat best when they eat together in a relaxed and loving atmosphere and when mealtime conversation is pleasant.

Peers

During the early teen years, as the dependent relationship with parents begins to loosen, the peer group plays an increasingly larger role in the life of the adolescent. Although the family continues to have an impact during adolescence, there is a shift in orientation and identification from parents to peers, and peers become a pivotal force that may exert even more influence over behavior than parents. It appears, however, that the greater the antagonism toward and the emotional distance from the parents, the greater the need to be part of the peer group. Thus adolescents with poor parental relationships will be more susceptible to peer group control and influence over behavior.[10] Regardless of the extent of influence, peers clearly play a role of fundamental importance in shaping and modifying adolescent behavior, beliefs, attitudes, and values. The peer group defines what is socially acceptable and dictates conformity to group values regarding school and learning, dress, language, entertainment idols and music preferences, and food and beverage choices.

The role of the peer group in influencing food behavior has rarely been explored. However, it seems logical that peers would have considerable influence over food choices considering the large amounts of time that adolescents spend with each other. Adolescents often spend more time with peers than with parents. In one investigation of 766 young adolescents, it was found that the youth spent more than twice as much time with peers than with parents over the course of a weekend.[7] Adolescents desperately want approval, particularly by their peers, and peer pressure and group con-

formity thus can be important determinants in food acceptability and selection. Eating is an important form of recreation and socialization among friends. In this group context, foods selected and consumed usually need to meet the approval of the peer group.

Teenagers, especially those just entering adolescence, who have a chronic illness (for example, diabetes) that necessitates adherence to a dietary regimen different from their peers may be teased. They face considerable social pressures and risk alienation and social isolation when adhering to their prescribed diet (Chapter 7). Likewise, an adolescent who is overweight and trying to lose weight may find it exceedingly difficult to comply with a diet plan and still feel part of the group when everyone goes out for hot fudge sundaes. These individuals may require counseling to help them cope and deal with social and peer group pressures to conform.

Nutrition-conscious parents tend to believe that they have 10 or 12 years during which to influence and establish a child's good eating habits—long enough to make the adolescents fairly impervious to other external influences. Although it is true that eating habits are formed in infancy and may have lasting effects, children who have nutritionally sound dietary habits throughout childhood may experience marked changes during adolescence for several reasons, one of which is the desire to fit in with their friends. A study of adolescents found that adolescents gave these major reasons for not drinking milk: (1) it is a food for babies and children; (2) it makes them (especially girls) fat; and (3) their peers do not drink it (soft drinks were considered the appropriate social drink with their peers).[11] This last reason is influenced by the marketing messages and ads that soft drink producers use to promote and sell their products to young people: fun parties on the beach with Coca-Cola. Madison Avenue succeeds again.

Symbolic meanings that are attributed to food in general or to specific foods are numerous. Meanings can connote either strong or weak, positive or negative, values and attitudes. To be accepted into an eating pattern, a food must possess a positive value or at least not a negative one. The stronger the positive value, the greater the chance that the food will be considered acceptable. These implied meanings are learned.[12] Various studies have measured the implied meanings of selected foods among high school students in the Southeast.[13,14] Spinach and most meats were associated with male images, which supports the belief that meats symbolize masculinity and manhood. Among the foods associated with feminine images were hot tea, jello salad, and cottage cheese. Foods associated with the words "teenager" and "young" were preferred, and less-preferred foods were associated with the words "baby," "adult," and "old." Applesauce, pudding, and carrot strips were foods associated more with a sick person than a well person. The implied symbolic meanings of various foods may determine whether they will be eaten by teens in a social setting. In speaking with a 15-year-old male who attended an all-boys school and was bored with bringing the same lunch to school everyday, I suggested that he add variety by bringing a tossed salad. He looked at me in horror and commented that although he liked salads and ate them frequently at home, he would never bring one to school because the other boys would think he was a sissy. It was acceptable to eat salads at home but not in the presence of friends.

Media

Mass media as a means of communication consist of two forms: the print media (newspapers, magazines, and books) and the audiovisual media (radio, television, and film). Through media adolescents are exposed to a wide variety of views, ideas, and attitudes. The omnipresence of the media makes it virtually impossible to ignore or to escape its role in influencing attitudes and behavior.

In addition to the basic information provided, most media carry advertising. Advertising is a powerful form of communication in that its sole purpose is to entice, grab attention, make an impression, and persuade consumers to buy things. Advertisers and industry are keenly aware of the important role adolescents have as consumers. Adolescents are a unique group from an economic standpoint. Although adults unquestionably have greater earning power and higher incomes, a large part of their income goes for fixed expenses such as housing, food, utilities, and health care. Adolescents, on the other hand, generally do not have to contribute to these costs and as a result often have more discretionary money to spend. The adolescent age group thus is a coveted market.

Advertisers selling appearance-related products take advantage of the adolescent's need for self-esteem, their desire to be attractive, popular, and sexually appealing, and their need to be accepted. A vast array of beauty treatments, cosmetics, acne medications, shampoos, toothpastes, clothing, athletic and physique development equipment, dietary aids and treatments, and foods and beverages (for example, candy, gum, soda pop, and snacks) are targeted toward the youth market. One manipulative technique for selling products is to have sport heroes, fashion models, popular actors and actresses, or those who possess a certain "in" look endorse the item. These ads also reinforce society's desired body images: thin and svelte for females and strong and athletic looking for males.

The power of the mass media in influencing food beliefs, food attitudes, and eating patterns is well acknowledged.[15] However, the degree of the media's impact is difficult to quantify or measure. This difficulty accounts for the lack of scientific research in this area. In the last 15 years media, especially advertising, have been lambasted by concerned-citizen groups for having a detrimental effect on the eating habits of American children. Of the various forms of media, television has had the greatest impact on children's eating habits. It is estimated that children between the ages of 6 and

16 watch approximately 24½ hours of television per week or an average of 3½ hours every day. Even when they reach 17 to 18 years of age, adolescents still watch approximately 17½ hours per week or an average of 2½ hours every day.[7,16,17] During this time, they are exposed to both implicit and explicit messages related to food, eating behavior, and ideal body image through not only television commercials but also program content.

Gussow has pointed out the powerful implicit messages of television commercials:

The heavy advertising of beer and soft drinks, for example, delivers a message far more potent than the urging to buy any single product. In terms of this message it doesn't really matter whether someone going to the refrigerator gets out a Pepsi or a Coke, a 7-Up or a Budweiser. What matters is that a thirsty American goes to the refrigerator to open up a container rather than to the sink to open the tap. That behavior has been sold to us.[18]

Other advertising messages associate foods of dubious nutritional value with emotions of love, romance, peer popularity, and success. For example, the concept behind many of the soda pop commercials oriented to youth is that a life of fun, popularity, and success comes with drinking that particular soda. Advertisers strive to inextricably link their product with a certain desired image. The image sells the product.

Life-style behaviors that foster poor eating habits are also repeatedly portrayed on television commercials. People in successful occupations are shown as eating on-the-run or being too busy to eat nutritiously. Commercials also encourage snacking between meals, usually on high-calorie, low-nutrient snacks. These advertisements are frequently filled with attractive, healthy-looking, slender people living energetic lives. The commercials thus present a dichotomous situation in which individuals are able to remain slim and full of energy and yet have eating habits that may be counter to this. As Kaufman aptly summarized it, "Television presents viewers with two sets of conflicting messages. One suggests that we eat in ways almost guaranteed to make us fat; the other suggests that we strive to remain slim."[19]

Because commercial advertising has carried the brunt of the blame in the eyes of nutritionists and concerned-citizen groups for negatively influencing the eating patterns of children and youth, the effects of television programming have been largely ignored. Although the messages related to food and eating behavior on network television programs are certainly more subtle and less direct than commercials, they nonetheless may have a strong impact on attitudes and preferences toward food. Not only does observational learning take place during program watching, but adolescents may attempt to emulate the behavior of their favorite stars and may pick up cues regarding foods, beverages, and eating.

Kaufman[19] recently identified and analyzed food-related messages on 10 top-ranking prime-time television programs. Results showed that 65% of the references to food in programs were to beverages (particularly alcoholic beverages) and to sweets. The analysis indicated that television program characters frequently snacked on foods of low-nutrient density, rarely ate a balanced meal, ate on-the-go, and used food primarily for the satisfaction of social and emotional needs. The majority (88%) of the program characters were thin or average in body type, and only 12% were overweight or obese. The thin or average body types were more often associated with positive personal and social characteristics such as intelligence, popularity, and attractiveness.

Magazine reading also increases during adolescence.[20] As would be expected, boys prefer sports and men's magazines (for example, *Sports Illustrated* and *Playboy*), and girls choose young people's, women's, and fashion magazines (for example, *Seventeen, Redbook,* and *McCall's*). Undoubtedly, these newspapers and magazines become a source of information on food and nutrition. Printed materials have been found to be a

Table 4-1. Ratings of diet and nutrition information in popular magazines

Magazine	Circulation	Nutrition Articles Reviewed			Percent Accurate
		Accurate	Inaccurate	Total	
Generally Reliable					
Redbook	4,200,000	28	1	29	97
Reader's Digest	18,000,000	20	1	21	95
Good Housekeeping	5,400,000	37	3	40	93
Inconsistent					
Glamour	1,800,000	41	10	51	80
Vogue	1,100,000	19	5	24	79
Woman's Day	7,500,000	35	12	47	74
Ms.	490,000	8	3	11	73
Seventeen	1,500,000	15	6	21	71
Family Circle	7,400,000	24	17	41	59
McCall's	6,300,000	17	13	30	57
Ladies' Home Journal	5,400,000	14	14	28	50
Unreliable					
Mademoiselle	920,000	17	20	37	46
Essence	600,000	10	17	27	37
Cosmopolitan	2,800,000	14	24	38	37
Harper's Bazaar	630,000	12	29	41	29
Organic Gardening	1,300,000	2	6	8	25
Prevention	2,000,000	3	28	31	10

From Hudnall, M.: American Council on Science and Health News & Views **3**(1):1, 1982.

main source of nutritional information among a wide range of consumers.[21,22] The nutritional information presented in the popular press varies widely in validity and accuracy. Unfortunately, information that is erroneous and deceiving may be published and is protected under the First Amendment to the Constitution, which guarantees freedom of the press.

Recently, diet and nutrition articles from selected popular magazines were reviewed.[23] The magazines were rated according to the following criteria: (1) scientific soundness and accuracy of the information; (2) credentials of the authors or consultant experts; and (3) safety, sensibility, and effectiveness of the weight-loss diets. Table 4-1

summarizes the results of these findings. Less than one fourth of the sample magazines were rated as "generally reliable." Unfortunately, a large proportion of the articles in popular magazines do not present accurate and reliable nutritional information and thus help to disseminate and perpetuate nutritional myths and invalid claims. This is of serious concern since adolescents as a rule do not possess the necessary skills to distinguish facts from fallacies.

TYPICAL EATING BEHAVIOR

To modify and improve the dietary habits and nutritional status of teenagers, health-care providers and nutrition educators must recognize and be aware of teenagers' typical eating behaviors.

Food Preferences

Food preferences are formed as a result of the complex interaction of many factors in an individual's environment. These preferences play a critical role in influencing food choices and consumption.

Food-preference studies conducted in the United States among the adolescent population indicate strong homogeneous trends that cut across regional lines, ethnic backgrounds, and urban, suburban, and rural areas. Various studies[13,14,24-26] have shown that the most popular food items among adolescents are soda pop, milk, steak, hamburgers, pizza, spaghetti, chicken, french fries, ice cream, oranges, orange juice, apples, and bread. The least-preferred foods are liver and vegetables (especially green leafy vegetables).

The uniformity of these food preferences is not influenced, at least to any significant extent, by differences between regions or between urban and rural areas. In addition, there appears to be conformity among a variety of diverse groups. The above-mentioned food items, for example, were popular with black and white adolescents living in the Southeast[13,25] and with Cherokee teenagers in North Carolina.[26] Garton and Bass[27] found foods preferred by deaf adolescents to be similar to those preferred by hearing adolescents. This conformity reflects the influence of the mass media on food habits. The national media's role in shaping and reinforcing the uniformity of food preferences in our nation's youth should not be underestimated.

A poll recently was conducted in Minnesota to provide insight into how teens perceive food and the meanings it has in their everyday lives.[28] Several of the questions were designed to ascertain adolescents' food preferences. The students' responses showed little variation when asked to respond to the question, "Suppose that you have just spent the last year traveling through the galaxy on a space shuttle. You've had nothing to eat but food capsules and water and now it is your first day back on Earth. What would you want to eat and why?" Overall, the responses were beef and potatoes, the stereotypical standard American fare. The answers also reflected the influence of fast foods on the teenage diet. The following responses illustrate this influence:

"Steak, french fries, pop, milk shake, or beer."
"A steakburger, fries, malt, and salad with pop."
"Steak or prime rib, baked potato, Texas toast, and a salad."
"Pizza with extra cheese and beer."
"A double cheeseburger, heavy on everything, fries, shake, hot apple pie."
"Taco John's, McDonald's, or Arby's."

High school students were also asked, "If someone from another planet asked you what kinds of foods American teenagers eat, what would you say?" The nearly unanimous response from urban, suburban, and rural adolescents was fast food. The answers included the following responses: "junk food," "burgers, pizza, fries, fast foods," "fast foods that don't take time to prepare or buy," "sweets," and "greasy, hot, junky foods."

The question also asked, "If your visitor asks what kind of foods teenagers tend not to eat, what would you tell him?" Again, the unanimous responses were liver, spinach, and vegetables.

Not surprisingly, vegetables (excluding potatoes) have a low acceptance among adolescents. Adolescents accept raw vegetables more readily than cooked ones and sweet-tasting vegetables (such as corn) over bland or bitter ones.[13,25,26,29] Walker, Hill, and Milman[29] found that children's and adolescents' rejection of certain vegetables appeared to be based on such factors and prejudices as (1) early negative conditioning, (2) rejection of "baby foods," and (3) faulty generalization from attributes such as color, shape, or odor.

Fast Foods

The number of fast-food restaurants has mushroomed in the last decade. Ten years ago there were approximately 30,000 fast-food outlets in the United States; today there are almost five times as many.[30] In 1978 fast-food sales amounted to over $19 billion.[31] The advent of fast-food restaurants and their rapidly continuing growth undoubtedly has had not only a great impact on the American diet as a whole but also on the teenager's diet.

In their quest for independence, adolescents spend more time away from the home and consume more of their meals and snacks outside the home. Fast-food restaurants thus hold great appeal for the adolescent population. Not only are they a prime employer of adolescents, but they also provide a socially acceptable and casual place to hang out and "make the scene." The food is inexpensive and priced within an adolescent's budget. Convenience adds to the popularity because there is no preparation or cleanup time. Ordering requires a minimum of decision making, service is fast, and the food is filling. Food can either be eaten on the premises or taken out, and it can be eaten informally without utensils or plates. Another key to the fast-food chains' success among adolescents is that the food served is the type of food teenagers like: hamburgers, french fries, soft drinks, shakes, and pizza. All of these features that contribute to the desirability of fast foods are heavily promoted by the industry's advertising campaigns. In 1977 McDonald's spent $120 million for advertising; Burger King spent $40.5 million; and Kentucky Fried Chicken spent $32.3 million.[32]

The influence of the fast-food concept on school-lunch programs throughout the country is becoming widespread, with the schools adopting fast-food meal patterns. Clark County Schools of Las Vegas, Nevada, first initiated this idea by having the school food service provide a wide variety of fast-food items such as pizza, hamburgers, burritos, and tacos.[33] Student response to this trend has been very positive, with improved lunch participation and reduced plate waste. Pulaski County, Arkansas, experimented with the fast-food route for 2 months in one high school. Participation jumped from 280 to 1350 students daily, and the program's $11,000 deficit become an $878 profit.[34] Despite this success, fast-food lunches in the schools remain controversial. Many critics believe that this approach emphasizes and reinforces the least healthful features of the American diet: foods that are high in calories, fat, salt, and sugar. This does not foster the eating of a variety of foods to ensure an adequate diet.

As fast foods have assumed an ever-expanding role in the American diet, several researchers have analyzed the nutritional value of these foods. Speculation has centered on the nutritional impact fast foods have on the American diet. Shannon and Parks[33] have noted that the nutritional impact of fast foods is dependent on (1) the frequency and extent to which consumers use fast foods, (2) the nutritional value of fast foods, and (3) the selection consumers make from fast foods. Occasional visits to fast-food restaurants will have little impact on the nutritional value of a week's diet. However, for some adolescents the mainstay of the diet may be fast foods. Depending on which fast foods are chosen, the quality of other foods being consumed, and the person's nutritional and energy needs, nutritional deficits may occur in these individuals.

One of the criticisms of fast-food restaurants has been the limited number of food choices that are available to consumers. However, a recent trend among fast-food chains has been increased menu diversification. Some chains now feature an open salad bar that provides a wider range of food choices.

Table 4-2 shows the nutritional values of five meals that are typically served at fast-food restaurants and compares them to the RDA for adolescents. The table shows that significant quantities of

Table 4-2. Nutritional values of meal combinations from fast-food restaurants

	RDA (11-18 yr)		McDonald's		Burger King	
	Female	Male	Hamburger, Fries, Coke	Big Mac, Fries, Vanilla Shake	Hamburger, Fries, Coke	Whopper, Fries, Vanilla Shake
Calories	2200 (2100)*	2700 (2800)*	571	1135	562	1152
Fat (gm)	—	—	22	53	19	53
Protein (gm)	46	45 (56)*	15	38	14	43
Vitamin A (retinol equivalents)	800	1000	19.8	179.2	4.2	129.8
Vitamin C (mg)	50 (60)*	50 (60)*	14.2	17.9	2.1	29
Riboflavin (mg)	1.3	1.6 (1.7)*	0.20	1.1	0.02	0.08
Thiamin (mg)	1.1	1.4	0.37	0.63	0.02	0.05
Calcium (mg)	1200	1200	60	495	57	439
Phosphorus (mg)	1200	1200	187	729	246	595
Iron (mg)	18	18	2.9	4.8	3	7.2
Sodium (mg)	—	—	649	1320	426	1073

Modified from Young, E.A., Brennan, E.H., and Irving, G.L.: Update: nutritional analysis of fast foods, Dietetic Currents **8**(2):6, 1981 (Ross Laboratories, Columbus, Ohio).
*Values in parentheses represent the RDA for the 15- to 18-year-old age group.

some nutrients can be supplied from these meals. A McDonald's hamburger, fries, and 8-ounce Coke provide roughly one third of the RDA for adolescents for energy, protein, and thiamin. However, this meal contributes only 16% of the RDA for iron, 5% of the RDA for calcium, and 2% of the RDA for vitamin A. When a Big Mac and shake is substituted for a regular hamburger and Coke, the nutritional value for this meal is substantially increased. Although this latter meal would provide 41% of the RDA for calcium (because of the shake) and from 20% to 25% of the RDA for iron and vitamin A, it also provides more calories: 54% of the RDA for teenage girls and 40% for teenage boys.

Although typical fast-food meals generally are high in calories, with a range of 900 to 1300 calories/meal, they fall short on certain nutrients. Adolescents who are in their growth period need the excess calories. They have an advantage over adults because they can consume foods that have a high-calorie/low-nutrient ratio and still meet their nutritional needs. A teenage boy who requires 3700 calories/day; frequently eats a Big Mac, fries, and a shake; and also consumes other high-quality nutritious foods throughout the day would have no problem meeting his nutritional requirements. On the other hand, a teenage girl who has completed her growth and requires only 1700 calories/day would have a difficult time incorporating the above meal into her diet. She could not meet all of her nutritional needs without exceeding her energy allowance. The teenage girl who is dieting has an even greater problem.

The following appear to be the major limitations of fast-food meals[32,35]:

1. Iron density is often low compared with the iron requirements of teenagers.
2. Calcium, riboflavin, and vitamin A are low unless milk or a shake is ordered.

3. Vitamin C is low if french fries or fruit juice are not included.
4. There are few sources of folic acid or fiber.
5. The percent of energy from fat is high in certain meal combinations.
6. Sodium content of fast-food meals is high.
7. Certain meal combinations are excessive in energy when compared with the amounts of nutrients provided.

Whatever their limitations, fast foods are an integral component of many adolescents' diets. Although fast foods can contribute nutrients to the diet, they cannot completely meet the nutritional needs of teens. Both adolescents and health professionals should be aware that fast foods are acceptable nutritionally when consumed judiciously and as part of a well-balanced diet. When they become the mainstay of the diet, however, there is cause for concern.

Nutrition education of adolescents should address and identify the limitations and potential problems of fast foods. It should suggest how, with proper selection, these foods can be combined and incorporated with other foods into an overall nutritionally adequate food plan. In addition, adolescents need to be taught the skills with which to make wise food choices from available menu items. Nutrition educators must help teens to become informed decision makers about their diets.

Irregular Meals

Meal skipping and eating irregularly are common during adolescence and are especially prevalent during middle and late adolescence. Parents lament, "I can't get my teenagers to sit down long enough to eat. They are always on the go." Numerous studies have documented the fact that adolescents are chronic meal skippers.[36-41] The number of meals teens miss and eat away from home increases from early adolescence to late adolescence. One study that investigated food patterns of 6200 youth found that the percentage of one or more missed meals per day increased from 10% in the seventh grade to 25% in the twelfth grade.[41] This steady increase reflects the growing need for independence and time away from the home. According to studies, the evening meal appears to be the most regularly eaten meal of the day.[9,26,40] In assessing meal patterns of 194 high school students in Minnesota, it was found that 82% of the youth ate an evening meal 5 to 7 days a week. Females were found to skip the evening meal, as well as breakfast and lunch, more often than males.[9]

Busy schedules may cause many teens to miss meals. Part-time jobs, athletics, and social activities may interfere with regular meal times, and unless the meal is made up, the day's energy and nutrient intake may be inadequate. Adolescents have stressed that the pressure for time and their commitments to activities affect their eating habits. Students commonly view themselves as being too busy to worry about food and proper eating.

Hinton and co-workers[39] looked at psychological, sociological, and physiological factors that influenced eating behavior in 140 adolescent girls. Girls who scored high on personal adjustment, emotional stability, family relations, and conformity missed fewer meals and had better diets than other girls. Girls whose families criticized their eating habits tended to skip more meals. The researchers also found that when health was considered an important factor in selecting food, diets tended to be adequate. However, when status, sociability, independence, and enjoyment had high value, poor food practices resulted.

The meals missed most often by adolescents are breakfast and lunch. Breakfast is frequently neglected and is omitted more by teens and young adults (under 25 years of age) than by any other age group in the population.[42] According to the *1977-78 Nationwide Food Consumption Survey* (NFCS),[42] 19% of teenage girls (12 to 18 years of age) and 11% of teenage boys of the same age missed this meal. A study of 288 Cherokee teenagers found that 38% of the females and 28% of the males missed this meal.[26] These and other findings indicate that females are more likely to miss breakfast (along with other meals) than males. A likely explanation is the pursuit of thinness and frequent attempts at dieting. Many teenage girls believe that they can either lose or control their weight by omitting breakfast (or lunch) and therefore cutting out calories. Girls who are dieting should be counseled that this approach is likely to accomplish just the opposite: by midmorning or lunch they may be so hungry they may overcompensate for the "saved calories."

Age also plays a role in breakfast eating, and younger adolescents eat breakfast more frequently than older adolescents.[41,43,44] The NFCS data reported that although 15% of teenagers skipped this meal, only 5% of the younger children did so.[42]

It is well known that nutrition knowledge and positive attitudes toward nutrition are not necessarily applied to everyday food practices. Seventy-five teens (males and females) were asked whether they felt it was important to eat breakfast every day. Eighty-nine percent answered affirmatively and gave reasons such as, "it keeps you going," "gives you vim and vigor," "without it you'd slow way down during the day," and "you feel better during the morning—more awake." Although a high value was placed on the importance of breakfast, only 60% ate breakfast on a regular basis (more than 4 days a week).[45]

The majority of foods eaten by these adolescents were traditional American breakfast foods such as eggs, toast, cereals, milk, and juice. These culturally appropriate breakfast foods represent a very narrow range of foods given our food supply. We have been inculcated to have a very myopic view of what constitutes acceptable breakfast foods. These definitions and attitudes become so firmly ingrained that breakfast food choices become severely limited. Breakfast might become more popular among teenagers if they realized that their choices were not limited to cereals and eggs. Since adolescents may not be as firmly grounded as their parents in what is appropriate food for breakfast, parents must be challenged and educated to overcome and reformulate their ideas about appropriate and acceptable foods for breakfast. Parents must be made to understand that there are no nutritional dictates specifically defining which foods are acceptable for breakfast. Sandwiches, soup, hamburgers, or leftovers from dinner the night before are all acceptable options that could get teens off to a good day's start. A good breakfast should provide at least 300 calories, contribute toward meeting the day's nutritional needs, and provide sufficient protein and fat to give a sense of satiety until the next meal. Omission of breakfast can adversely affect the nutrient intake for the day if there is no "catch up" on food intake later.

The influence of breakfast on learning and productivity is discussed further in Chapter 8.

Snacking

There have been several noticeable changes in the food consumption, eating behaviors, and meal patterns of Americans since the beginning of the twentieth century. One such pattern change that is characteristic of a different life-style and reflects a more casual eating pattern is increased snacking.[12] Despite its reputation (which is well deserved) as being closely linked with the adolescent life-style, this trend is not limited to this age group. Although teens have been found to eat more frequently than adults, the disparity between these two groups is not as great as some would like to believe. According to the NFCS, 56% of teenagers (12 to 18 years of age) ate four or more times in one day as compared with 46% of the adults (19+ years of age).[42] Despite the prevalence of snacking in America, many still consider it to be unhealthy. Indeed, the belief that food should be eaten three times a day is still a deeply entrenched concept and persists despite an altered life-style. One report found that 41% of family members felt that more emphasis should be placed on the importance of not snacking between meals. Furthermore, 59% of parents considered snacking a serious health threat.[8]

These beliefs are often based on the notion that between-meal snacks spoil your appetite for standard meals and are high in calories and low in nutrients. Whether between-meal snacking warrants its reputation for interfering with the nutrient intake of adolescents depends on the quality and quantity of foods consumed as snacks. Snacking may make a significant contribution to the total nutrient intake of a teen and, depending on the food choice, can provide an adequate balance of nutrients. The *Ten State Nutrition Survey* (TSNS) showed that snacks eaten by teens were not just empty calories as had been believed.[38] Both males and females obtained a substantial proportion of their recommended caloric intake—about 23%—from between-meal snacks. The mean nutrient intake per 100 calories from between-meal snacks met or exceeded the RDA for protein, riboflavin, and ascorbic acid, although the intake of thiamin was slightly below standard. Nutrients most limited in snacks were vitamin A, calcium, and iron. Thus, although the nutrient density of snacks was less than that consumed as meals, snacks made a significant contribution to meeting total daily nutritional needs, especially for vitamin C.[35]

For the adolescent who is either physically active or in a growth period, between-meal snacking may be essential for meeting daily energy and nutritional needs. For example, teenagers who require 3500 or more kcal/day would have a difficult time meeting their need for energy by relying solely on three meals a day. Studies have also shown that adolescents who do not snack between meals or who eat less than three times a day have poorer diets than those eating more frequently.[44]

Parents need to understand that adolescents have greater energy needs than adults. It is not uncommon to hear parents say exasperatingly, "My teenage son eats all the time. I don't know where the food goes. He's like a bottomless pit. For a snack he used to eat two or three cookies and a glass of milk, and now he'll eat the whole cookie jar and drink a quart of milk. He's eating us out of house and home." It is important for parents to realize that this increase in appetite is normal and that as growth ceases the appetite will diminish. Food costs will rise for the household with a teenager, so the food buyer, especially if on a limited food budget, may need counseling and assistance on how to maximize food buys and provide nutritious, inexpensive snacks.

There is little doubt that snacking is a way of life for many teens. The NFCS data showed that two thirds of the 1424 teenagers surveyed snacked during a 1-day period. Almost half of the snacking occurred in the evening, with less in the afternoon and the smallest proportion in the morning. The peak periods for snacks were in the afternoon from 2 to 4 PM (20% of snacking occasions) and in the evening from 8 to 10 PM (27%).[46]

The most frequently reported snack item for teenagers was soft drinks. Among teenage boys the most popular snacks were (in descending order or popularity) soft drinks, milk, bakery products, bread, milk desserts, salty snacks, meats, and fruits. Favorite snacks of teenage girls appeared to be soft drinks, bakery products, milk desserts, salty snacks, fruit, milk, candy, bread, and meat. Vegetables and, to a lesser extent, fruits were seldom mentioned as snacks. Peanut butter and nuts also played an insignificant role as snack choices.[46]

The NFCS results indicated that sugar-containing snacks were among the most frequently consumed food items.[46] This is of serious concern considering the relationship between sugar intake and the development of dental caries.[47,48] Tooth decay is very prevalent during the adolescent years and is one of the major public health problems for this age group. Chapter 7 discusses dental caries in adolescence.

Since between-meal snacking can have a positive relationship to the overall nutritional status of

Table 4-3. Selected snack foods and their nutritional contribution

Food	Amount	Calories	Vitamin A (IU)	Vitamin C (µg)	Calcium (mg)	Iron (mg)
Fresh orange	1	65	260	66	54	0.5
Low-fat yogurt (fruit flavored)	1 cup	230	120	1	343	0.2
Dried apricots	½ cup	220	7085	8	43	3.6
Tomato juice	1 cup	45	1940	39	17	2.2
Low-fat milk (2%)	1 cup	120	500	2	297	0.1
Bran muffin	1	105	90	—	57	1.5
Canned tuna	3 oz	170	70	—	7	1.6
Strawberries	1 cup	55	90	88	31	1.5
Cheddar cheese	1 oz	115	300	—	204	0.2
Whole wheat crackers	2	45	—	—	7	0.5
Orange juice	1 cup	110	500	124	27	0.5
Raw cauliflower	½ cup	16	35	45	15	0.65
Raw broccoli	½ cup	20	1940	70	68	0.6
Grapefruit	½	50	540	44	20	0.5
Blueberries	½ cup	45	75	10	11	0.75
Raw carrots	1	30	7930	6	27	0.5
Pumpkin (dried kernels)	½ cup	387	100	—	35	7.8
Peanut butter	1 tablespoon	95	—	—	4	0.3
Sunflower seeds	½ cup	405	35	—	87	5.1
Ice cream	1 cup	270	540	1	176	0.1
Fresh peach	1	40	1330	7	9	0.5

Modified from U.S. Department of Agriculture: Home and Garden Bulletin, no. 72, Washington, D.C., 1977, Agricultural Research Service.

the teen, this practice should not be discouraged. However, adolescents should be taught to select foods that provide the essential nutrients and to limit their consumption of cariogenic foods. Teens tend to eat what is convenient and on-hand in the kitchen. Parents therefore can make sure nutritious, low-cariogenic snack foods are available. Nutritious and easy-to-prepare snack foods to keep on hand are fresh fruits, milk, bread and sandwich fillings, cheeses, fruit juices, raw vegetables, peanut butter, nuts, seeds, popcorn, and whole grain crackers. Studies have indicated that adolescent diets are lowest or deficient in calcium, iron, vitamin A, and ascorbic acid.[24,42,44,49] Foods that are good sources of these nutrients should be encour-

aged and made available for snack consumption. Table 4-3 shows foods that are good sources of some of these nutrients.

ALTERNATIVE LIFE-STYLES AND DIET EXPERIMENTATION

A central issue in adolescence is the establishment of identity, a sense of yourself as a unique person (Chapter 2). Because food is charged with emotional connotations and symbolic meanings, it may be used as a means of establishing independence and of expressing an adolescent's identity and uniqueness. Food choices convey strong messages about the individual to both the family and the outside world. Eating patterns such as vegetarian diets or food fads may be adopted as a way of testing adult restrictions, exploring new roles and life-styles, and attempting to assert and gain control over your life.

According to Hill,[4] some adolescents may define themselves almost totally in terms of what parents are not and value least. This "negative identity" appears to occur among adolescents who live in conflict-filled family settings. Disturbed parent-child relationships and the adoption of a negative identity may be expressed through food habits. For example, the son of a beef farmer may choose a vegetarian regimen, or the daughter of a dedicated health food advocate may indulge in a diet primarily consisting of junk foods. The adolescents thereby reject the kind of identity formation their parents represent.

Even if teenagers are in stable family settings and have acquired nutritionally sound eating habits before adolescence, they still are vulnerable to idiosyncratic and faddish eating behaviors. Pressures to conform and fit a cultural ideal, combined with their search for independence and identity, place adolescents at a high risk for food fads and deviant food behaviors. The adoption of faddish or bizarre diets is generally a transient experience and in most cases will pass in a short time. Although certain beliefs may be harmless (for example, the athlete who believes that wheat germ possesses magical powers and will give a winning edge to a performance), other practices such as excessive intake of minerals or vitamins may compromise the health of the individual.

During adolescence, both males and females become extremely preoccupied and sensitive about their size and physical appearance. A high value is placed on physical attractiveness. Adolescents critically and harshly compare themselves with an imagined or socially determined standard, and body dissatisfaction becomes inevitable. Studies indicate that teenage males wish to have larger biceps, shoulders, chest, and forearms, and females desire smaller hips, thighs, and waist. One study showed typical dissatisfaction with body images: 70% of adolescent females wanted to lose weight, but not more than approximately 15% were actually obese; on the other hand, 59% of the males wanted to gain weight, but only 25% were lower than average weight.[44] Diet is often used as an attempt to manipulate physical appearance. For males this may mean using protein supplements in the hopes of building a well-muscled body. For females it may mean attempting an endless stream of quick-loss diets in the pursuit of thinness. Adolescents who are dissatisfied with their bodies or athletes who desperately want to be champions are yearning for miraculous transformations. They thus are attracted to diet products and dietary schemes that promise instant and magical results. Adolescents' vulnerability and anxiety about physical appearance make them easy prey for purveyors of and advertisements for nutritional supplements, special food products, and books and gadgets for weight reduction. As shown in Fig. 4-2, these advertisements rely heavily on strong emotional appeal and exaggerated claims. Teens are inundated with confusing and conflicting information via beauty magazines, television, newspapers, friends, family, and teachers and often have difficulty sorting out fact from fiction.

Fad Diets and Weight-Reduction Schemes

Weight reduction can be expensive. In 1980 $105 million was spent in the United States for weight-loss schemes alone.[50] Newspapers and magazines abound with ads for weight-reducing aids and diets, and best-seller book lists usually have at least one diet book that is a current hit. The gimmicks vary but most bear the same message: "quick, safe, and painless weight reduction—without hunger." Indeed, ads for many of these gimmicks make dieting sound like more fun than eating.[49] Adolescent girls who are striving to con-

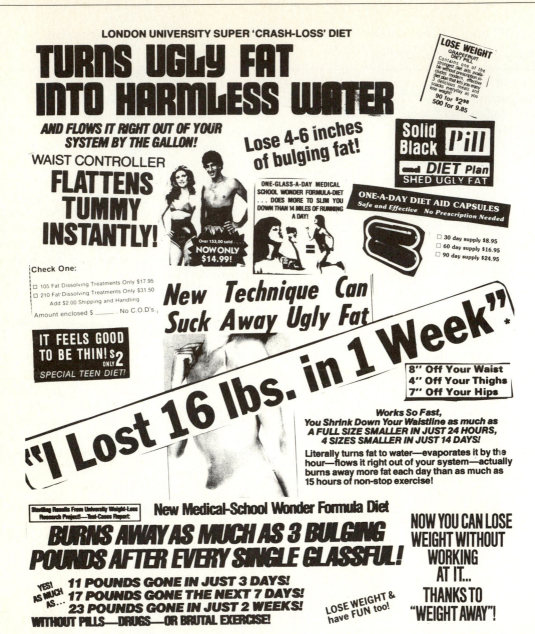

Fig. 4-2. Examples of enticements and advertisements for weight-loss products featured in popular magazines.

Table 4-4. Nonprescription diet aids

Product	Example	Action	Comment
Candies to curb appetite	Ayds Fructose tablets	Suppress appetite by raising blood glucose levels	Harmless; candies usually contain carbohydrate, fat, vitamins, and minerals Expensive; fruit juice before meal could have similar effect[51]
Over-the-counter appetite suppressants	Appendrine Control Dexatrim Prolamine Dietac Dex-A-Diet II Anorexin	Most contain phenylpropanolamine (PPA) that reduces appetite temporarily Many also contain caffeine	PPA and caffeine are mild stimulants PPA can be dangerous to those with heart disease, high blood pressure, diabetes, or hyperthyroidism[50,52,53] Center for Science in the Public Interest, a public interest group, has proposed banning PPA in diet aids[54]
Local anesthetics	Reducets Spantrol Diet-trim	Benzocaine, a local anesthetic, is the active ingredient Anesthetics presumably deaden taste buds	No controlled studies demonstrate efficacy[53]
Bulking agents	Pretts Taper	Contain methylcellulose, which has affinity for water Increase in volume supposedly tricks stomach into feeling full	Because methylcellulose swells in intestine, not in stomach, it has limited effectiveness[50,52]
Diuretics	Diurex	Cause body to lose water and thus reducing body weight Weight loss short lived	No loss of body fat Can be dangerous because of dehydration and loss of potassium Should only be used under direction of physician
Exotic and secret cures	Spirulina Kelp Soolim (100% herbal extract)	Questionable action	Not shown to be effective in controlled studies
Amylase inhibitors	Calorex	In vitro amylase inhibitors inhibit action of pancreatic enzyme amylase and thus are thought to prevent digestion and absorption of starch In vivo they cause diarrhea and gastrointestinal distress	Not shown to be effective[53] Banned from marketplace by FDA in 1982

form to the cultural ideal of beauty and the social norms of thinness are likely to experiment with crash diets and other quick weight-loss regimens. Fig. 4-2 shows the myriad of diet aids that are being promoted, and Table 4-4 depicts some of the nonprescription diet aids now available.[49]

Health professionals who work with adolescents and their families should keep abreast of these current popular diets and fads since questions are commonly asked about their effectiveness. There is a critical teaching moment when an adolescent says, ''My friend just lost 10 pounds on the La Costa Spa diet. Is that a good diet?'' The health professional should use this opportunity to educate and discuss the advantages and disadvantages of the diet. New fad diets crop up continually, and although many appear ludicrous to health-care providers, these diets capture the public's attention and interest many adolescents who lack the necessary skills to evaluate the diets.

Nontraditional Diet Patterns

Many older adolescents and young adults motivated by ecological or environmental concerns, philosophical or religious convictions, or health interests adopt a wide variety of nonstandard eating patterns. The most common diets followed are vegetarian or semivegetarian regimens and diets that emphasize natural or organically grown foods.

Although vegetarian diets are composed of diverse dietary patterns, they generally fall into four main subgroups. Lacto-ovo-vegetarians consume plant foods, dairy products, and eggs; lacto-vegetarians consume plant foods and dairy products but no eggs; pure vegetarians reject any food of animal origin including milk and eggs; and fruitarians eat only raw or dried fruits, nuts, honey, and olive oil. Individual vegetarians frequently do not fall conveniently into any one category. For example, some lacto-vegetarians or pure vegetarians may eat fish. It is not uncommon for an adolescent or young adult to describe themself as being vegetarian but to exclude only red meat from their diet.

Vegetarianism has existed for thousands of years and is a basic religious tenet among Hindu sects, Buddhists, Zorastrians, and other groups. In more modern times vegetarianism is practiced by Trappist monks and Seventh-Day Adventists.[55] Vegetarianism, however, is in no way limited to religious orders or philosophical cults. Historically, many individuals and communities have resorted to vegetarian diets out of necessity because of shortages of animal foods.

During the nineteenth century, a major health reform movement led by Sylvester Graham that emphasized vegetarian regimens and whole grain foods became popular in the United States. Grahamism flourished throughout the United States, and several colleges offered Graham diets for their students.

In the late 1960s there was once again a major vegetarian and natural food movement in the United States. The adherents were primarily adolescents and young adults, many of whom identified with the ''counterculture.'' Like Grahamism, the movement prompted several American colleges and universities to begin to offer vegetarian and natural food menus in their cafeterias.[56]

A wide variety of reasons motivated young people to adopt the newer vegetarian diets. Diet justifications included spiritual purification, awakening, and rebirth; mind expansion; health ''maximization''; ecological law; gluttony avoidance; and opposition to killing and aggressive behavior.[57,58] Although this was by no means a homogeneous group, many of the ''new vegetarians'' joined the new religious cults that were largely based on Oriental thought systems and that addressed man in his total physical, mental, and spiritual self. Each cult has its own dietary patterns and proscriptions, and risks of dietary inadequacy therefore vary considerably.

One cult that advocated extremely stringent and rigid dietary proscriptions was the Zen macrobiotic movement based on Zen Buddhism and the ancient Chinese dualism of yin and yang. It should be noted that several deaths and cases of vitamin deficiences were reported in individuals who attempted to practice the most extreme aspect of the Zen macrobiotic regimen.[59] As a result, the original dietary proscriptions were liberalized. In general, as many of the cults have matured, their diet practices have become more liberal and sensible.

Many individuals and population groups have adhered to vegetarian diets over a lifetime and have demonstrated excellent health and well-being. Lacto-ovo-vegetarian diets tend to be nutritionally similar to diets containing meats. Vegetarians who do not include eggs and/or milk products present a more difficult problem. However, the National Academy of Sciences' Food and Nutrition Board has stressed that pure vegetarian diets can be nutritionally adequate. These diets can meet the nutritional needs of all ages if careful attention is paid to selecting a diet that has sufficient calories; a good balance of essential amino acids; and adequate sources of protein, calcium, riboflavin, iron, vitamin A, vitamin D, and vitamin B_{12}.[60]

However, potential problems can arise with the adoption of a vegetarian diet. Adequately meeting the energy needs of growing adolescents who are vegetarians may be difficult for three reasons: (1) the bulkiness of most staple foods, (2) the poor energy digestibility of some plant foods, and (3) the fact that vegetarian diets are often much lower in fat content.[61] Some of the inadequacy of energy intake can be overcome if fats are consumed in sufficient quantities. If caloric needs are not met, protein is used as an energy source rather than for tissue growth, maintenance, and repair. It is necessary therefore to assess the protein/calorie ratio of the diet. Both the quantity and the quality of the protein in the diet must be considered. High-quality protein refers to a protein that not only contains all the essential amino acids but has these amino acids in amounts proportional to the body's need for them. Although animal foods provide high-quality protein, plant foods do not contain all the essential amino acids in the quantities and propor-

tions needed. The protein quality of plant foods can be increased by combining two plant foods, each lacking a different essential amino acid, at the same meal. This process is called mutual supplementation. A recent discussion on this topic with practical application is available.[62]

Other nutritional concerns with a strict vegetarian or ''vegan'' diet are inadequate intakes of calcium, iron, zinc, and vitamins D and B_{12}. Bioavailability of calcium and zinc are negatively affected by diets high in fiber or phytate.[61] Without an adequate calcium intake, growing adolescents would be at high nutritional risk. Because vitamin B_{12} is found almost exclusively in foods of animal origin, a strict vegetarian diet would be lacking in vitamin B_{12} unless supplements or fortified foods are ingested. It becomes obvious that the level of nutritional risk involved is dependent on the food choices made. To minimize or eliminate the risk of nutritional inadequacy, vegetarian diets should contain a variety of foods.[63]

Management of Dietary Fads and Unconventional Diets

Although many of the dietary patterns that teens adopt may appear aberrant and bizarre, it is important to keep in mind that the food habits of others can differ from your own without representing cultism, faddism, or quackery.[64] Teens can meet their nutrient needs in a variety of ways.

When encountering adolescents on fad or atypical diets, several aspects need to be taken into account.[65] It is first necessary to determine why the particular diet has been adopted. What are the underlying reasons and motivating factors? You must next determine what constitutes the diet and how long it has been followed. On what basis are food choices made? What is the nutrient content of the diet? Are the dietary practices beneficial, neutral, or harmful? Are there nutritional and health risks involved?

A thorough dietary assessment as discussed in Chapter 3 is essential. In addition, a physical examination may indicate the need for biochemical tests to substantiate high or low nutrient levels or nutritional disorders. When food faddism occurs in young adolescents, serial anthropometric data are critical.[65]

The health implications of the fad or cult should be made clear to the adolescent and the parents. An unconventional diet pattern or food fad can cause considerable conflict between adolescents and their parents and may aggravate and exacerbate the existing relationship. If the food pattern chosen is nutritionally adequate, parents need to be reassured that this may only be a transient experience and encouraged to try to remain flexible and tolerant of the situation.

The best way to attempt to bring about change is to work within the teens' ideological framework and system of beliefs. Chapter 10 further discusses counseling methods.

SUBSTANCE USE AND ABUSE

Substance use and abuse in adolescence is a public health problem of major significance and concern. The substances most widely abused by adolescents are tobacco, alcohol, and marijuana.[66]

Cigarette smoking continues to be popular despite firm evidence of its deleterious physical effects. Although a recent nationwide survey found that cigarette smoking among high school seniors had declined since 1977, it also found that about 15% of the seniors smoked half a pack or more each day, with females smoking more than males.[66]

For several years it has been hypothesized that cigarette smoking diminishes body stores of vitamin C. It has been repeatedly observed that cigarette smokers have lower plasma vitamin C levels than nonsmokers.[67-71] Pelletier[72] reported an average 25% reduction in serum vitamin C levels for those who smoked less than 20 cigarettes a day and an approximately 40% reduction for those who smoked more than 20 cigarettes a day.

Although there is general agreement in the literature that smokers do have lowered plasma levels of vitamin C, the significance of this effect in terms of vitamin C requirements has not been elucidated.[70]

Extent of Use

Alcohol is widely abused by adolescents. A recent study estimated that 1.3 million Americans between 12 and 17 years of age have a serious drinking problem.[73] In 1979 a survey of high school seniors showed that 52% of the males and 31% of the females reported having taken five or more drinks in a row at least once during the 2 weeks preceding the survey; 26% of the males and 12% of the females did so three or more times. Both sets of figures have risen 3% to 4% since 1976. Only a small portion (about 6%) reported daily or near daily use of alcohol during the previous 30 days.[66]

Although marijuana smoking increased rapidly during the 1970s, use among high school seniors now has leveled off. In 1979 35% of the students reported some use during the past month, with more males smoking marijuana than females. About 10% of high school seniors reported daily use.[66] These survey findings do not include high school dropouts. As a group, dropouts use drugs more and are more apt to abuse chemicals. If this population group were added to the sample, drug-use rates would probably be even higher.[66]

Combining alcohol with other drugs (primarily marijuana) is a common occurrence among adolescents. Teens who drink heavily are also likely to use and abuse other drugs. One study found that among adolescents who had tried or used four or more illicit drugs, 80% were also heavy drinkers.[74] Use of drugs in combination with alcohol may potentiate the overall chemical effect. Moreover, the effects of polychemical use on the adolescent body are as yet unknown.

Nutritional Implications

Extensive literature addresses the interrelationship between chronic alcohol consumption and nutritional status. Malnutrition has been found to be a common sequela among adult alcoholics. Alcoholics are most prone to nutritional deficiencies of protein, the water-soluble vitamins (particularly thiamin, niacin, riboflavin, and pyridoxine), and the minerals magnesium, potassium, and zinc.[75-79] Unfortunately, there has been little research that looks at the nutritional status of the adolescent alcohol abuser or the physiological effects of alcohol on the growth process.

Adolescents who chronically abuse alcohol or drugs are extremely vulnerable to nutritional disorders. If heavy chemical intake begins in the prepubertal child and continues into puberty, the increased nutrient needs for growth and development may not be met and nutritional deficiencies and compromised growth may ensue. Even if chronic alcohol use begins after the growth spurt, the adolescent is still at considerable risk for deficiencies because the body may be left with little or no nutrient reserves. Malnutrition may result from inadequate food intake or from maldigestion and malabsorption caused by alcohol. Furthermore, chronic long-term alcohol consumption may result in damage to the organs such as the liver. This damage in turn can alter the metabolism and storage of several nutrients.[75,76]

Chronic medical complications of alcoholism such as cirrhosis, portal hypertension, and cerebellar degeneration are manifested after several years of heavy drinking and therefore are distinctly uncommon in adolescents.[80] Gastritis (inflammation of the stomach lining) and, to a lesser extent, pancreatitis and toxic hepatitis are signs of heavy alcohol intake in adolescents.[80]

Iron deficiency is a common finding among adolescents of both sexes (Chapter 7). Curiously, in a study of 68 black adolescent chemical abusers, iron deficiency anemia was nonexistent. In fact,

hematocrit and hemoglobin values were all in the acceptable range.[81] It has been postulated that acute alcohol ingestion increases iron absorption, possibly through stimulation of gastric acid secretion. This results in increased solubility of ferric iron in the small intestine.[75]

As with alcohol, there is little study of the nutritional status of adolescent drug users. Marijuana is the most common illicit drug being used by adolescents, and it is being used increasingly by young children.[82] Marijuana has short-term effects on reflexes, behavior, vision, learning, memory, and the cardiopulmonary system. In addition, it alters perceptions of time and space and affects sensory perceptions. Long-term effects on health are unknown, and the relation of marijuana to maturational changes has not been determined.

Marijuana reportedly stimulates the appetite and causes a transient increase in the amount of food consumed.[83-85] The pharmacological basis of the effect of tetrahydrocannabinol (THC), the active ingredient in marijuana, on eating behavior is unclear. Studies have found no association between THC and alterations in blood glucose or insulin.[82,86,87] Because moderate doses of THC influence central nervous system functions, it has been suggested that THC may alter normal feeding behavior by interacting with hypothalamic feeding mechanisms.[88] Other investigators speculate that the so-called hunger induced by marijuana is actually a social effect caused by the suggestibility of the group in which it is smoked.[81]

Whatever the cause, a common result of marijuana smoking is an increased appetite known as "the munchies." Brown[89] looked at food habits and preferences of college students (17 to 21 years of age) using chemicals. Sixty-nine percent indicated that marijuana increased their appetite. Another study found that of 68 black adolescent chemical users, 86% who smoked marijuana reported they got "the munchies." The types of food preferred when "stoned" were (in decreasing order of preference) sweets, beverages (mainly soda pop), meat, fruits, vegetables, salty snacks, bread, and crackers.[81]

Only a very small percentage of adolescents who abuse drugs are hard drug addicts. Since food is not usually a primary concern for these narcotic-dependent persons, nutritional problems may be expected. General malnutrition, anemia, decreased appetite, gastrointestinal distress, and emaciation have been reported.[90,91] Anorexia, nausea, vomiting, and constipation are common side effects of narcotics.[92]

In addition to the physiological effects of opiates, food intake may be compromised by the fact that the limited money available is often used for purchasing drugs rather than food. Inadequate dietary intakes and vitamin deficiencies have been observed in drug-dependent individuals.[90,93]

The effect of chemicals on nutritional status is dependent on serveral factors: type of drug, dose, duration and frequency of use, prior health and nutritional status, stage of physical growth, and nutritional adequacy of the diet consumed. The abuse of drugs and alcohol may have a deleterious effect on the nutritional health of adolescents. Therefore it is important that nutrition evaluation be an essential component in the comprehensive care of adolescents who are chronically abusing chemicals. Nutrition intervention and counseling should play a major role in the physical rehabilitation process.

IMPROVING NUTRITION OF ADOLESCENTS

It is a commonly held notion that adolescents have atrocious eating habits. Despite this popular notion, U.S. adolescents in general are not suffering from marked signs of malnutrition or nutritional deficiency diseases. In fact, as a group they are relatively well nourished and in good nutritional health. However, growth demands, life-style, and psychosocial characteristics of teens do make them potentially vulnerable to nutritional problems, and a small but significant percentage of them do have nutritional disorders. Certain physiological or environmental stresses in adolescence (for example, poverty, chronic substance abuse, pregnancy, chronic illness, or an intensely rapid growth spurt) may precipitate nutritional deficiencies (Chapter 3).

When discussing the eating habits of adolescents, it must be remembered that many of the eating practices that are considered characteristic of this age group actually reflect the eating practices of the rest of the American population (for example, frequent snacking, missed meals, eating on-the-run, being too busy to eat, reliance on convenience foods, eating at fast-food places, going on fad diets, and eating too many "junk foods"). Although these practices are not endemic to adolescents, they are accentuated during this time. Many of these particular dietary practices run counter to the dietary guidelines given on p. 73. The following are potential areas of concern for this age group: low consumption of fruits, vegetables, and dairy products; low intake of dietary fiber; dietary excess of sugars and sweets; and high intakes of total fat, saturated fat, and cholesterol.

Many researchers believe that the adolescent period is a time particularly vulnerable to the initiation of nutrition-related health problems that occur in later life.[94] It becomes a challenge for nutrition educators to work with youth and their families to bring about prudent dietary modifications.

Roles of Parents and Teens

Parents have instrumental and critical roles to play in guaranteeing the nutritional adequacy of their teens' diet. Although it is true that parents may have little control over what their teens are eating outside the home, they can control what is brought into the home. It is my experience that most of the teens' food intake occurs in the home. (Many teens do not want to spend their money on food when they can get it at home free.) Those who are not home for the evening meal will generally come home and "catch up" later in the evening. They tend to eat what is available and convenient. Parents can capitalize on this. They can help the adolescent maintain nutritional health and promote good nutrition by stocking the kitchen with a variety of nourishing ready-to-eat foods that comply with the dietary guidelines. Fresh fruits and juices, low-fat yogurt, cheese and milk, nuts or sunflower seeds, raw vegetables, whole grain or enriched crackers (unsalted) are all examples of nutritional foods. Since adolescents are partial to soda pop, salty snack foods (for example, chips and pretzels), and sweets, it is wise to limit the availability of these foods in the home. Although parents can play a facilitative role by having a variety of food on hand, they need to respect the emerging independence of their children and allow them to make their own food choices as much as

possible. Parents also should be encouraged to alter their own diets to serve as positive role models for their children.

Although parents should not be expected to drastically alter their family schedule to fit their teenagers' schedule, they should be encouraged to try to work out a family arrangement so that mealtimes will not conflict with outside activities (for example, work or sports) that are important to the teen. Both male and female adolescents should be encouraged to assume food-related responsibilities such as meal planning and preparation, gardening, or food processing. Acquiring food-related skills and responsibilities is essential for both sexes. Adolescents who are interested in cooking and experimenting with foods should be encouraged to do so as illustrated in Fig. 4-3. Cooking can increase self-esteem and can be a creative outlet. The

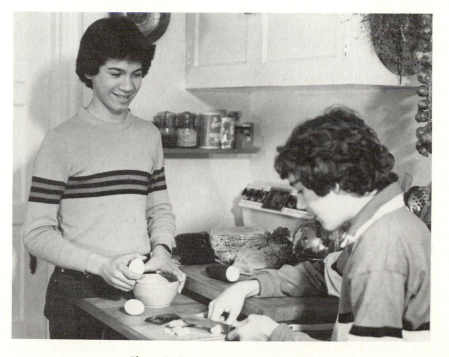

Fig. 4-3. Two friends making a meal.

novice cook is bound to have failures in the kitchen. The family needs to be sensitive to this and remember that this is part of the learning process. Overly criticizing the food or becoming irate if a dish is ruined can have disastrous and long-lasting effects on the adolescent's interest in cooking. Despite hectic family schedules, family meals should be encouraged. The aim should be for an enjoyable experience free from family friction and volatile topics. Everyone will eat better.

Parents often assume that they have no influence over what their children eat outside the home. However, in many settings such as schools and food stands at recreational and sporting events, parents can urge that alternative choices be provided and that vending machines offer more nutritious selections.

Roles of Health Professionals and Nutrition Educators

When helping adolescents adopt more healthful and nutritious food practices and choices, their life-style must be considered. Adolescents lead busy lives, and food usually receives only a fraction of their attention. Food is often viewed with a catch-as-catch-can attitude. As anyone working with adolescents knows, to be effective dietary changes and improvements must fit into their life-style. It is necessary to find more opportunities to provide adolescents with the food they need and like. These foods in turn will contribute to meeting their physical and social needs.

Becoming judgmental and expressing negative biases will only serve to alienate adolescents and may cause them to reject all counseling. What is needed is effective communication between the adolescent and the health professional and the establishment of trust and rapport. Every attempt must be made to understand teens' way of thinking and to listen to their point of view. Young people need to be taken seriously and respected for their system of beliefs.

If the diet pattern is nutritionally inadequate, nutritional counseling is warranted as discussed in Chapter 10. Adolescents generally have many questions about their particular diet and how it affects them. They want information about nutrition. These questions should be answered in a straightforward manner. Adolescents do not want to be lectured, talked down to, or ridiculed. They want to share information, have their ideas listened to, and be involved in exploring possible alternatives. In a counseling session, adolescents should be helped (1) to appreciate their nutritional needs, (2) to understand how well or how poorly their choices are satisfying those needs, and (3) to make selections that will improve the situation.

Adolescents should be taught that they have the responsibility for the nutriture of their own body. Nutrition educators can play a facilitative role in teaching them the skills that will enable them to make informed decisions regarding their food choices.

SUMMARY

An adolescent's food habits are reflective of many and diverse influences, such as the family, peers, and media, and are influenced by the adolescent's own psychosocial development. Because of great indifference and autonomy, adolescents become increasingly responsible for making their own food choices. Simultaneously, adolescent life-styles may result in erratic eating patterns and food choices that are nutritionally less than optimal. It then becomes a challenge for the health professional to work with teens and their families to teach them the skills necessary for the development of nutritious and health-promoting food habits.

REFERENCES

1. Bass, M.A., Wakefield, L.M., and Kolasa, K.M.: Community nutrition and individual food behavior, Minneapolis, 1979, Burgess Publishing Co.
2. Hochbaum, G.M.: Human behavior and nutrition education, Nutr. News **40**(1):1, 1977.

3. Schafer, R., and Yetley, E.A.: Social psychology of food faddism, J. Am. Diet. Assoc. **66:**129, 1975.

4. Hill, J.P.: Understanding early adolescence: a framework, Chapel Hill, 1980, Center for Early Adolescence, University of North Carolina.

5. Steinberg, L.D.: Understanding families with young adolescents, Chapel Hill, 1980, Center for Early Adolescence, University of North Carolina.

6. Hamilton, E.M., and Whitney, E.: Nutrition: concepts and controversies, St. Paul, 1979, West Publishing Co.

7. Santrock, J.W.: Adolescence, Dubuque, Iowa, 1981, Wm. C. Brown Group.

8. The General Mills American family report, 1978-79: Family health in an era of stress, Minneapolis, 1979, General Mills. (Conducted by Yankelovich, Skelly and White, Inc.)

9. Haugen, D.L.: The relationship of family meals to food habits and attitudes of youth in Minnesota, plan B master's paper, Minneapolis, 1981, University of Minnesota.

10. Muuss, R.E., editor: Adolescent behavior and society: a book of readings, ed. 3, New York, 1980, Random House, Inc.

11. John, M.E., and Price, H.: The story of adolescents and milk, Progress Report 204, University Park, Pa., 1959, Agricultural Experiment Station.

12. Gifft, H.H., Washbon, M.B., and Harrison, G.G.: Nutrition, behavior and change, Englewood Cliffs, N.J., 1972, Prentice-Hall, Inc.

13. Carlisle, J.C., Bass, M.A., and Owsley, D.W.: Food preferences and connotative meaning of foods of Alabama teenagers, School Food Serv. Res. Rev. **4**(1):19, 1980.

14. McConnell, S.: Selected food preferences and some connotative meanings of foods by high school students in Hancock County, Tennessee, master's thesis, Knoxville, 1974, University of Tennessee.

15. Manoff, R.K.: Potential uses of mass media in nutrition programs, J. Nutr. Ed. **5:**125, 1973.

16. Schramm, W., Lyle, J., and Parker, E.B.: Television in the lives of children, Stanford, Calif., 1961, Stanford University Press.

17. Ruben, A.M.: Television usage, attitudes, and viewing behaviors of children and adolescents, J. Commun. **21:**355, 1977.

18. Gussow, J.: Counternutritional messages of TV ads aimed at children, J. Nutr. Ed. **4:**48, 1972.

19. Kaufman, L.: Prime-time nutrition, J. Commun. **30**(3):37, 1980.

20. Avery, R.K.: Adolescents' use of the mass media, Am. Behav. Sci. **23:**53, 1979.

21. Jalso, S.B., Burns, M.M., and Rivers, J.M.: Nutritional beliefs and practices, J. Am. Diet. Assoc. **47:**263, 1965.

22. Walker, M.A., and Hill, M.M.: Homemakers' food and nutrition knowledge, practice, and opinions, Home economic research report, no. 39., Washington, D.C., Nov. 1975, U.S. Department of Agriculture, Agricultural Research Service.

23. Hudnall, M.: American Council on Science and Health survey: how popular magazines rate on nutrition. ACSH News and Views **3**(1):1, 1982.

24. Schorr, B.C., Sanjur, D., and Erickson, E.C.: Teenager food habits: a multidimensional analysis, J. Am. Diet. Assoc. **61:**415, 1972.

25. Coffey, K.A.: Food behaviors of adolescents relative to adiposity, doctoral thesis, Knoxville, 1977, University of Tennessee.

26. Story, M.: Food and nutrition practices and anthropometric data of Cherokee Indian high school students in Cherokee, North Carolina, doctoral thesis, Tallahassee, 1980, Florida State University.

27. Garton, N.B., and Bass, M.A.: Food preferences and nutrition knowledge of deaf children, J. Nutr. Ed. **6:**60, 1974.

28. Resnick, M., Hedin, D., and Simon, P.: Youths' views on food and nutrition: the Minnesota youth poll, St. Paul, Center for Youth Development and Research, University of Minnesota, Agricultural Experiment Station. (In press.)

29. Walker, M.A., Hill, M.M., and Milman, F.D.: Fruit and vegetable acceptance by students, J. Am. Diet. Assoc. **62:**268, 1973.

30. Fast-food chains, Consumer Reports **44:**508, 1979.

31. Van Dress, M.G.: Fast-food industry growth, Natl. Food Rev., p. 35, Winter 1980.

32. Young, E.A., Brennan, E.H., and Irving, G.I.: Update: nutritional analysis of fast-foods, Dietetic Currents **8**(2):6, 1981.

33. Shannon, B.M., and Parks, S.C.: Fast-foods: their nutritional impact, J. Am. Diet. Assoc. **76:**242, 1980.

34. Little Rock schools seek food stamps for school lunch, Community Nutrition Institute Weekly Rep., vol. 2, no. 28, 1981.

35. McNutt, K.W., and McNutt, D.R.: Nutrition and food choices, Chicago, 1978, Science Research Associates, Inc.

36. Macdonald, L.A., Wearring, G.A., and Moase, O.: Factors affecting the dietary quality of adolescent girls, J. Am. Diet. Assoc. **82:**260, 1983.

37. Greger, J.L., Divibliss, L., and Aschenbeck, S.K.: Dietary habits of adolescent females, Ecol. Food Nutr. **7:**213, 1979.

38. Thomas, J.A., and Call, D.L.: Eating between meals: a nutrition problem among teenagers? Nutr. Rev. **31:**137, 1973.

39. Hinton, M.A., and others: Eating behavior and dietary intake of girls 12 to 14 years old, J. Am. Diet. Assoc. **43:**223, 1963.

40. Huenemann, R.L. and others: Food and eating practices of teenagers, J. Am. Diet. Assoc. **53:**17, 1968.

41. Edwards, C.H., and others: Nutrition survey of 6,200 teenage youths, J. Am. Diet. Assoc. **45:**543, 1964.

42. Science and Education Administration: Nationwide food consumption survey, 1977-78, Preliminary Report 2, Hyattsville, Md., Sept. 1980, U.S. Department of Agriculture.

43. Minnesota Department of Education: 1977 Minnesota student breakfast survey, St. Paul, 1978, Minnesota Department of Education. (Prepared by L. Kreisman.)

44. Huenemann, R.L. and others: Teenage nutrition and physique, Springfield, Ill. 1974, Charles C Thomas, Publisher.

45. Story, M., Coachman, V., and Van Zyl York, P.: Eating practices and beliefs of black adolescents, Unpublished research, Minneapolis, 1982, Adolescent Health Program, University of Minnesota.

46. Pao, E.M.: Eating patterns and food frequencies of children in the United States, Hyattsville, Md., Oct. 1980, U.S. Department of Agriculture, Human Nutrition, Science, and Education Administration, Consumer Nutrition Center.

47. Pipes, P.L.: Nutrition in infancy and childhood. ed. 2, St. Louis, 1981, The C.V. Mosby Co.

48. Edgar, W., and others: Acid production in plaques after eating snacks, J. Am. Dent. Assoc. **90:**418, 1975.

49. Barrett, S.: Diet facts and fads. In Barret, S., editor: The health robbers, ed. 2, Philadelphia, 1980, George F. Stickley Co.

50. Economics of food faddism, Nutr. and M.D. **7:**4, April 1981.

51. Guthrie, H.A.: Introductory nutrition, ed. 5, St. Louis, 1983, The C.V. Mosby Co.

52. CSPI asks control of reducing drugs, CNI Weekly Rep. **2:**42, 1981.

53. White, P.L., and Selvey, N.: Nutrition and the new health awareness, JAMA **247:**2914, 1982.

54. A nasal decongestant and a local anesthetic for weight control, Med. Lett. Drugs Ther. **21**(16):65, 1979.

55. Todhunter, E.N.: Food habits, food faddism, and nutrition, World Rev. Nutr. Diet. **16:**286, 1973.

56. Deutsch, R.M.: The new nuts among the berries, Palo Alto, Calif. 1977, Bull Publishing Co.

57. Erhard, D.: The new vegetarians. I. Vegetarianism and its medical consequences, Nutr. Today **8**(6):4, 1973.

58. Erhard, D.: The new vegetarians. II. The Zen macrobiotic movement and other cults based on vegetarianism, Nutr. Today **9**(1):20, 1974.

59. White, P.L., and Mondeika, T.D.: Foods, fads and faddism. In Goodhart, R.S., and Shils, M.E., editors: Modern nutrition in health and disease, ed. 6, Philadelphia, 1980, Lea & Febiger.

60. Committee on Nutrition, Academy of Pediatrics: Nutritional aspects of vegetarianism, health foods and fad diets, Pediatrics, **59:**361, 1977.

61. MacLean, W.C., and Graham, G.G.: Vegetarianism in children, Am. J. Dis. Child. **134:**513, 1980.

62. Trahms, C.M.: Vegetarianism as a way of life. In Worthington-Roberts, B.S., editor: Contemporary developments in nutrition, St. Louis, 1981, The C.V. Mosby Co.

63. Nutrition and vegetarianism, Dairy Council Digest **50**(1): 1, 1979.

64. Pfeffer, K.H.: The sociology of nutrition, malnutrition and hunger in developing countries. In Blix, G., editor: Food cultism and nutrition quackery, VIII Symposium of the Swedish Nutrition Foundation, Stockholm, 1972, Almquist & Wiksells International.

65. Robson, J.R.K.: Food faddism, Pediatr. Clin. North Am. **24**(1):189, 1977.

66. Bachman, J.G., Johnston, L.D., and O'Malley, P.M.: Smoking, drinking, and drug use among American high school students: correlates and trends, 1975-1979, Am. J. Public Health **71:**59, 1981.

67. Brook, M., and Grimshaw, J.J.: Vitamin C concentration of plasma and leukocytes as related to smoking habit, age and sex of humans, Am. J. Clin. Nutr. **21:**1254, 1968.

68. Pelletier, O.: Smoking and vitamin C levels in humans, Am. J. Clin. Nutr. **21:**1259, 1968.

69. Pelletier, O.: Vitamin C status of cigarette smokers and nonsmokers, Am. J. Clin. Nutr. **23:**520, 1970.

70. Callabrese, E.J.: Nutrition and environmental health: the influence of nutritional status on pollutant toxicity and carcinogenicity, vol. 1, The vitamins, New York, 1980, John Wiley & Sons, Inc.

71. Calder, J.H., Curtis, R.C., and Fore, H.: Comparison of vitamin C in plasma and leucocytes of smokers and non-smokers, Lancet **1:**556, 1963.

72. Pelletier, O.: Vitamin C and cigarette smokers, Ann. N.Y. Acad. Sci. **258:**156, 1975.

73. National Institute of Alcohol Abuse and Alcoholism: Young people and alcohol, Alcohol Health & Research World, p. 2, Summer 1975.

74. Morrissey, E.R.: Alcohol-related problems in adolescents and women, Postgrad. Med. **64**(6):111, 1978.

75. Shaw, S., and Lieber, C.S.: Nutrition and alcoholism. In Goodhart, R.S., and Shils, M.E., editors: Modern nutrition in health and disease, ed. 6, Philadelphia, 1980, Lea & Febiger.

76. Iber, F.L.: In alcoholism the liver sets the pace, Nutr. Today. **6:**2, 1977.

77. Li, T.K., Schenker, S., and Lumeng, L., editors: Alcohol and nutrition, Research Monograph, no. 2, Washington, D.C., 1979, U.S. Department of Health, Education, and Welfare.

78. Becker, C.E.: Medical consequences of alcohol abuse, Postgrad. Med. **64**(6):88, 1978.

79. Vitale, J.J., and Coffey, J.: Alcohol and vitamin metabolism. In Kissin, B., and Begleiter, A., editors: The biology of alcoholism, vol. 1, Biochemistry, New York, 1971, Plenum Press.

80. Farrow, J.A.: Considerations in the evaluation and management of adolescent alcohol abuser, J. Curr. Adol. Med. **2**(9):9, 1980.

81. Story, M., Coachman, V., and Van Zyl York, P.: Nutritional status of black adolescent with chemical abuse problems, Unpublished research, Minneapolis, 1982, Adolescent Health Program, University of Minnesota.

82. American Academy of Pediatrics, Committee on Drugs: Marijuana, Pediatrics **65**:652, 1980.

83. Hollister, L.E.: Hunger and appetite after single doses of marijuana, alcohol and dextroamphetamine, Clin. Pharmacol. Ther. **12**:44, 1970.

84. Abel, E.L.: Effects of marijuanna on the solution of anagrams, memory and appetite, Nature **231**:260, 1971.

85. Gluck, J.P., and Ferraro, D.P.: Effects of Δ^9-THC on food and water intake of deprived and experienced rats, Behav. Biol. **11**:395, 1974.

86. Hollister, L.E., Richards, R.K., and Gillespie, H.K.: Comparison of tetrahydrocannabinol and synhexyl in man, Clin. Pharmacol. Ther. **9**:783, 1968.

87. Podolsky, S., Paffavina, C.G., and Amaral, M.A.: Effects of marijuana on the glucose tolerance test, Ann. N.Y. Acad. Sci. **191**:54, 1971.

88. Life Science Division, Army Research Office: A review of the biomedical effects of marijuana on man in the military environment. Bethesda, Md., 1970, Federation of American Societies for Experimental Biology.

89. Brown, J.: Diet and the new drugs: eating habits of some drug users, Ecol. Food Nutr. **2**:21, 1973.

90. Gambera, S.E., and Krohn-Clark, J.A.: Comments on dietary intake of drug-dependent persons, J. Am. Diet. Assoc. **68**:155, 1976.

91. Aylett, P.: Some aspects of nutritional state in "hard" addicts, Br. J. Addict. **73**:77, 1978.

92. Brecher, E.M.: Licit and illicit drugs, Boston, 1972, Little, Brown & Co.

93. Nakah, A.E., and others: A vitamin profile of heroin addiction, Am. J. Public Health **69**:1058, 1979.

94. Greenwood, C.T., and Richardson, D.P.: Nutrition during adolescence, World Rev. Nutr. Diet. **33**:1, 1979.

Chapter 5

Eating Disorders

JANE MITCHELL REES

Although recent and precise figures are not available, as many as 30% of U.S. teens are said to be obese.[1,2] The number of teens with diagnosed anorexia nervosa is growing,[3-6] and many anorexic teens remain undiagnosed and untreated.[2,6-8] In addition, many teenagers who fall between these two extremes in physical appearance have eating disorders that are as yet unlabeled and untreated. Because these disorders are so common among adolescents, professionals interested in adolescent nutrition must understand them completely.

SPECTRUM OF EATING DISORDERS IN ADOLESCENTS

Eating disorders can best be studied when the physical symptoms are viewed as a spectrum with developmental obesity at one end and anorexia nervosa at the other (Fig. 5-1). Between are people at normal and abnormal weights. All along the spectrum people hold in common basic underlying psychological problems. These problems interfere to varying degrees with the normal functioning of the affected people.[2,9,10] In developing responses to life these people often use food inappropriately. Food-related behaviors and the resulting deviation in weight, the most observable aspects of these disorders, are usually the focus of attention of the

affected person, the lay public, and often the health professional. It is the underlying neurophysical and psychodevelopmental mechanisms, however, that are the essential focuses of more fundamental study needed by clinicians who are treating the disorders.[2,10]

Because of rapid physical growth and body-image development in the adolescent period, eating disorders are of special concern at this time. These changes intensify associated self-esteem problems. Anorexia nervosa, for example, is a disorder so tied to body-image distortion that it is most commonly seen in adolescence, the period when a person is most vulnerable to body-image problems.[6]

Body image refers to the mental picture a person has of him- or herself and includes thoughts and feelings about the physical self.[11-13] The body image has its developmental origins in children's first perceptions of themselves as separate beings in space. Thereafter body image develops with the child's changing concept of self. Because of rapid physical changes in adolescence, body-image development advances rapidly during this period. During adolescence, teens begin to conceive of themselves as having adult rather than children's bodies. Just as a person may experience confusion about other aspects of life in adolescence, there

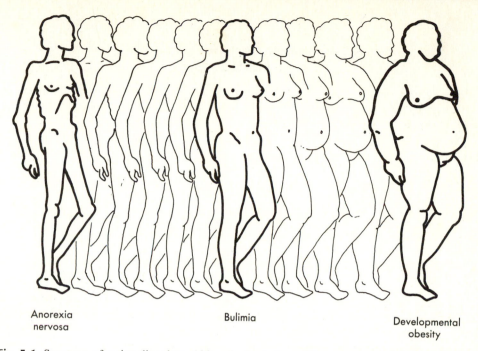

Anorexia
nervosa   Bulimia   Developmental
                                                                obesity

Fig. 5-1. Spectrum of eating disorders. Although physical conditions vary, underlying psychological characteristics are held in common across the spectrum.

may be confusion with regard to body image. In a classic study Dwyer and co-workers[14] showed that not one of 500 high school subjects felt satisfied with all body parts. As might be expected, the adolescents expressed dissatisfaction with parts that most characterize physical attractiveness to teens. In other cases, however, they were uncomfortable with their head, feet, and hand size. The overall lack of adjustment to their physical being that they expressed demonstrates the confused body-image ideas teens often hold.

In the Dwyer study young women generally wanted smaller body parts and young men larger body parts. These feelings are responsible for both the great number of teenage females who diet whether or not they are actually overweight[6,15] and the number of teenage males who spend money for "muscle-building" kits and dietary supplements.

The great need to conform at this stage further complicates the teenager's body-image development. Bodily overconcern leads teens to spend a great deal of energy in contemplation of the physical aspects of their being. Messages about bodies from the media, family, and friends and comparisons with peers are incorporated into feelings about their own bodies.

Progress in adopting a normal adult body image will be interrupted for the teen with an eating disorder. Bruch[10] and others[6,13,14,16-24] described distortions of body image in both anorexic and obese teens.

Teens with severe eating disorders fail in varying degrees to carry out the developmental tasks of adolescence described in Chapter 2.[10] The developmental problems of these teens are summarized in the box on p. 106. The most striking of their

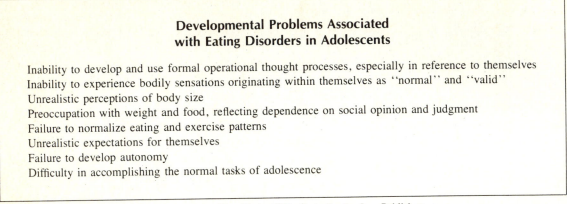

Developmental Problems Associated with Eating Disorders in Adolescents

Inability to develop and use formal operational thought processes, especially in reference to themselves
Inability to experience bodily sensations originating within themselves as "normal" and "valid"
Unrealistic perceptions of body size
Preoccupation with weight and food, reflecting dependence on social opinion and judgment
Failure to normalize eating and exercise patterns
Unrealistic expectations for themselves
Failure to develop autonomy
Difficulty in accomplishing the normal tasks of adolescence

Data modified from Bruch, H.: Eating disorders, New York, 1973, Basic Books, Inc. Publishers.

problems is a failure to develop autonomy.[9,10] The result is that these young people feel ineffective and out-of-control. They fail to establish significant friendships and opposite-sex relationships outside their families.[12] This leads to a continuing cycle of dependence on inappropriate habits related to food and exercise in an attempt to derive gratification from life.[10] These teens fail to experience bodily sensations originating in themselves as "normal" and "valid." Instead, they respond excessively to external cues and social opinions and judgments.[9,16]

Teens with eating disorders are perfectionists,[16] and they often misinterpret their roles in light of other's (most often their family's) expectations.[10] For example, anorexic teens struggle with all human energy to live up to their narrowed perceptions of success.[16] By contrast, developmentally obese teens sense their inability to be perfect and often resign themselves to failure without making an effort to reach goals.[2,10]

In recent years theories about the origin of such problems have turned to the structure and interaction of the teens' families. Although obese teens are a much less homogeneous group than anorexic teens, the family patterns of teens with various eating disorders have much in common.[2,10,25]

Minuchin[25] has described such families as being psychosomatic. They are enmeshed, overprotective, and rigid and have a low tolerance for conflict.

The study of eating disorders to date has focused on three recognizable syndromes: anorexia nervosa, obesity, and bulimia.[26] Because subgroups are being studied in current research,[16] it is expected that advanced diagnostic classifications with specific etiological features will be isolated from the general categories in the future. Knowledge of the disorders will be greatly enhanced when these subgroups are more well defined.

ANOREXIA NERVOSA

The term *anorexia nervosa* is actually a misnomer. The implication that affected persons have a lack of appetite has been shown to be invalid.* Superficially, the motivation to be thin keeps anorexic persons from eating.[6,10] In over 100 years of description in the literature,[6,16] a combination of symptoms has come to be recognized as characteristic of the disorder. Although certain of these symptoms may be seen in other disorders, the

*References 3, 8, 10, 16, 25, 27, 28.

combination is unique in anorexia nervosa. They are collected in the Feighner criteria* as cited in Vigersky and others[8]:

A. Age of onset prior to 25.
B. Anorexia with accompanying weight loss of at least 25 per cent of original body weight.
C. A distorted, implacable attitude toward eating, food, or weight that overrides hunger, admonitions, reassurance, and threats: e.g. (1) Denial of illness with a failure to recognize nutritional needs, (2) apparent enjoyment in losing weight with overt manifestations that food refusal is a pleasurable indulgence, (3) a desired body image of extreme thinness with overt evidence that it is rewarding to the patient to achieve and maintain this state, and (4) unusual hoarding or handling of food.
D. No known medical illness that could account for the anorexia and weight loss.
E. No other known psychiatric disorder with particular reference to primary affective disorders, schizophrenia, obsessive-compulsive and phobic neuroses.
F. At least two of the following manifestations: (1) amenorrhea; (2) lanugo; (3) bradycardia (persistent resting pulse of 60 beats per minute or less); (4) periods of overactivity; (5) episodes of bulimia; (6) vomiting (may be self-induced).

These criteria can be used as a basis for making a diagnosis, although in many cases there will be variations in the symptoms manifested by any individual. Despite these variations, anorexia nervosa can still be recognized by the experienced clinician.[16,29] For example, if all other symptoms correspond to the criteria but the amount of weight has not yet reached 25%, it definitely would be necessary to institute treatment and to make the diagnosis without reservation. One source of variation is that patients may be seen at different stages in the disorder as outlined on p. 108.

The Feighner criteria focus more on physical symptoms at the crisis stage than on the underlying psychological symptoms. Recognition of the psychological symptoms, however, is of equal importance. In Bruch's terms[9] the principle psychological features of anorexia nervosa are "a relentless pursuit of thinness" and "a misuse of the eating function in efforts to solve or camouflage problems that otherwise appear insolvable," that is, problems resulting from arrested development.

The majority of anorexic patients are adolescents, although anorexia nervosa has been seen in other age groups.[3] The disorder is not commonly seen in males,[3,6,10] and only 8%[30] and 11%[31] of anorexic teens were male in two groups studied. Males, however, appear to experience anorexia nervosa in essentially the same form as females.[7,10,31,32]

The disorder occurs predominantly in affluent classes[6] and nations[2,10] and is supported by a cultural paradox in which food is abundant and used lavishly for purposes other than survival on the one hand, and slimness is highly valued on the other.[2,9,16,33] These cultural values are strong internal messages that have great impact on a teen who has not developed autonomy. Crisp[30] speculates that the lack of a similar value on slimness in males accounts for the small number of males seen with the disorder.

Theories about Etiology of Anorexia Nervosa

Theories about the etiology of anorexia nervosa have evolved from the initial psychoanalytic idea that alleged the disease stemmed from an inability to deal with innate sexual drives, through a period where it was ascribed to endocrinological deficits,[16] to the more recent notion that contends the disorder grows out of disturbed patterns of interaction with family members or the family as a whole.[25] Bruch's work[10] was the first to incorporate a broader focus than simply the patient and her symptoms. Bruch described an interaction pattern in which the mother misperceives the needs of her child from infancy on and/or the child fails to express her needs clearly. In any case the child

*From Feighner, J.P., and others: Diagnostic criteria for use in psychiatric research, Arch. Gen. Psychiatry **26**:57-63, 1972. Copyright 1972, American Medical Association.

acquiesces to the mother's misguided ministrations. During the period of infancy and childhood, the daughter is so controlled by her mother that she does not develop a true sense of self as distinguished from the mother.

As adolescence approaches, the body develops, and demands for decisions and performance in many areas increase, the teenager panics at her lack of ability to cope independently. She develops rituals related to eating in an effort to be thin and "good."[6] To gain her "independence," the teen regresses[32] to the period where independence ordinarily begins.[34] In this early stage the principal manner to demonstrate growing independence open to the child is eating behavior.[35] This image of the child striving for autonomy provides a framework for more complex psychiatric conceptualizations and places the nutritional component of the eating disorder in theoretical perspective.

Minuchin's more recent approach[25] describes how not only the relationship with the mother but interrelationships within the family system foster the anorexic state. If family members are enmeshed in a system that does not allow development of appropriate roles, the system can produce a variety of psychomatic problems. The particular direction toward anorexia nervosa may be determined when the main themes of family interaction are related to food, fitness, and appearance.[3,9,25] It has also been speculated that children are vulnerable to anorexia nervosa when interpersonal relationships are more crucial to their sense of worth than accomplishments based on activity.[32] Minuchin and co-workers[25] postulate that this trait in itself grows out of family behavior patterns. However, certain individuals may have more innate characteristics leading them, as opposed to their siblings, to develop anorexia nervosa within "anorexogenic" families.[25]

The possibility that a biochemical mechanism may be responsible for the development of anorexia nervosa continues to be investigated.[8,36] Although various mechanisms have been proposed, none so far has been demonstrated to be primary or causative. These mechanisms appear to be the result of the psychological stress, malnutrition, and starvation.[37] The fact that patients and their families fit such characteristic and complex patterns would cast doubt on the existence of a primary physiological cause in most cases.[3,6,7,10,25] However, it may yet be found that biochemical factors contribute to the development of the disorder.

One of the reasons anorexia nervosa has been so puzzling is that clinicians have observed it in various stages.[3,9] Most writings and the Feighner criteria are concerned with the disease at the time when starvation has brought the patient near death. However, experience with the disorder shows that patients typically can be seen in three stages: (1) physical manifestation, (2) crisis, and (3) long-term recovery.

An arbitrary division of anorexia nervosa into progressive stages, which actually range on a continuum, reduces the confusion over the differences seen in individual patients at any given time. Studying the disorder in stages can enhance the recognition of the initial problems and point out the need to sustain therapy through the years necessary to facilitate development of full adult potential. A protocol for assessment of eating disorders is provided in Fig. 5-2.

Physical Manifestation

Psychological State. From the family's point of view, the anorexic teen usually is a "model child" until she begins to develop a compulsive attitude about her weight.[6,10,32] She has fit into the family unit and met their high expectations.[32] She has worked extremely hard at school, being satisfied with nothing less than excellent grades.[6,9,25]

Suddenly, the whole family erupts in conflict over her eating behavior. The teen herself has become more troubled about her role in life. She is unable to sustain peer friendships and she is very anxious about relationships with males.[25] She is confused by the need to establish more adult be-

Patient name _____
Birth date   _____
Number   _____

	Date	Date	Date

Motivation
  Desire to lose weight
  Goals
  Insight			

Family characteristics
  Eating disorders
  Other diseases
  Natural or other parent			

Parental attitude toward weight problem
  Role of food in family
  Perceptions of weight problem
  Attempts to intervene			

Social relationships
  Friends
  School
  Social life and activities
  Social skills
  Teasing			

Physical activity
  Exercise and frequency
  Family activity patterns
  Hobbies and interests
  Personal feeling about activity			

Mental function
  Intellectual achievement
  School performance			

Emotional-psychological status
  Depression
  Locus of control
  Body image
  Self-esteem
  Oral expression
  Coping skills
  Compulsiveness			

Eating behavior
  Control over food intake
  Meal pattern
  Bizarre eating habits
  Knowledge of nutrition
  Nutritional adequacy			

Medical data
  Clinical findings
  Thyroid status			

Growth and adiposity
  Weight history
  Maturation stage
  Menses
  Body fatness
  Growth velocity
  Age			

Plan			

Fig. 5-2. Clinical assessment of eating disorder. (Developed by Mahan, K., and Rees, J., Adolescent Clinic and Child Development and Mental Retardation Center, University of Washington, Seattle, Wash.)

havior patterns and clings to the rigid standards of childhood.[3,6] She isolates herself. Life appears to be out of her control. She has conflicting feelings about living as her parents direct, is hurt by their critical comments, and begins to realize that she must assert herself.[3] She takes a stand and will not compromise on her eating and exercise habits.[3,6,12,16] She feels that she is too fat and must be slim to prove that she is a worthy person.[10,32] She is increasingly preoccupied with her rituals and is hostile and angry when her family interferes. She denies her illness.[10,38,39]

A wide range of distorted perceptions has been noted by those describing the psychological aspects of anorexia nervosa. These distorted perceptions are related specifically to body size, sex, hunger, rest, satiety, temperature, pleasure, and control and to "feeling states" in general.[2,3,6,10,28] In looking for underlying mechanisms, the question has been raised whether the abnormal reactions to physiological needs by anorexic teens are the result of distorted perceptions or of an "anhedonic" orientation.[32] In other words, do anorexic teens perceive these aspects of life differently, or do they ignore such sensations to deny themselves the pleasure of resolving these feelings by gratifying experiences? To date this question has not been conclusively answered. However, these distorted perceptions appear to result from the psychological development peculiar to the anorexic teen, which leads to failure to develop ability in formal operations.[9] Without formal operations, the individual is dependent on a narrow range of more stereotypical responses to psychological and physical needs.

The inability to conceptualize leads to confusion over the intellectual capacity of these teens since they usually maintain high academic standards. It needs to be pointed out that high marks in secondary and certain college courses can be achieved by rote learning that does not demand the ability to link independent ideas into an integrated whole. Further, the high academic achievements of an-

orexic teens may represent an overachievement as a result of obsessive study rather than intellectual ability.[6,38,40] Such an intellectual handicap may be seen in persons with seemingly above average intelligence who are unable to function as professionals maintaining a career. The thinking patterns of anorexic teens will need to be considered by therapists attempting to counsel them about nutrition.

Anorexic teens have also been described as wishing to stave off adulthood.[6] The question is whether the teens wish to avoid maturation or whether maturation eludes them? It has been noted that a driven, obsessional quality and a low tolerance for anxiety are common psychological characteristics of anorexic teens.[28,41] Exploration of their psychological state using the study of dreams and other methods has led to the conclusion that immature personality development in the teens leaves them without the adequate defenses or the complex cognitive abilities necessary for adulthood.[42,43]

Although most families with anorexic teens would describe themselves as normal and without problems until the manifestation of anorexia nervosa, these families often have a multitude of problems. The parents may have been dominating and intrusive.[10,25] They may have overlooked the *actual* (including the nutritional) needs and emotions of their children, even in times when the children may have been ill.[9] By adopting a "helpless" stance, the affected children may be thoroughly manipulative and involved in their parents' conflicts.[25] Both parents and children are locked into a system where problems go unresolved and responses are stereotyped. A main feature of the system is the child's developing illness and its utility in perpetuating the unresolved nature of the conflicts. Parents often do not establish a strong dyad that the family can depend on for support and use as a problem-solving model. Children grow up committed to maintaining the status quo rather than gaining independence. These latter two symptoms have been nearly universally noted by workers in the field, although the traits have not always been attributed to the basic family system.

Physiological State. In a certain number of cases, ranging from 10% to 40%, the anorexic teen is overweight when the disorder is initially manifest.[3,6,9,16] Heavy children are likely to experience puberty at an early age.[6,20] When this occurs in a young woman who is predisposed to anorexia nervosa by an anorexogenic family background,[16] it may be anxiety provoking to a severe degree. The anorexic teen is typically hypersensitive to either early or late developing breasts and hips.[3,6,9] She will not want to stand out from her peers in physical development, nor will she want the responsibility of managing the attention from young men that it will bring. In her mind the physical features of development may represent an accumulation of unwanted fat.

Young patients often recall a chance statement about their needing to lose weight by a relative or close friend or a weight-losing plan suggested by a health professional as the trigger for their initial weight-restricting behavior.[10] Disappointment related to personal ambitions, separations, loss of significant family members, and illness undermine the anorexic teen's self-esteem and have been shown to precede the weight-losing process.

The obvious difference between the anorexic teen and the average young woman who sets out "to lose a few pounds" is the degree of compulsivity with which the anorexic teen carries out her plans.[3,6,10] The anorexic teen is virtually obsessed with decreasing the amount of energy she retains in her body and increasing the amount she expends.

No diet has been demonstrated to be significantly more likely to be used by these young women, but a low intake of carbohydrate is most frequently mentioned in the literature.[3,6] The anorexic teen usually develops a personal philosophy regarding her diet, and she will limit her diet by eating food only from certain categories and in certain ways. The following are examples of such limited diets and limiting behaviors:

Eating foods with very low calorie content in relation to volume

Eating low-carbohydrate foods with almost no protein or fat

Eating high-protein foods with very little carbohydrate

Eating certain foods (regardless of caloric value) that are craved

Eating vegetables with a small amount of protein

Eating a few particular foods that are repeated to the exclusion of all others

Eating a particular pattern of the same foods at the same meal day after day

Eating food with the same utensils in a pattern

Eating food alone, never with family or friends

Eating foods mixed with particular condiments

Eating foods mixed in an unusual and, to most people, inedible fashion

Eating foods earned by doing an inordinate amount of exercise

The anorexic teen may manipulate the fluid or sodium content of her intake. In addition, she may force herself to vomit and misuse laxatives or diuretics to rid herself of food energy and weight. Vomiting may follow episodes of gorging.[3,6,8,10,25]

Exercise rituals are equally varied. Anorexic teens are so frequently involved in junior and senior high athletics that coaches should be educated about the disorder. Well-meaning coaches should be able to recognize which of their students may be exercising to their detriment by compulsively training beyond reasonable endurance while losing weight at a rapid rate. Such behavior should indicate the need to investigate the developmental progress of the teenager in a comprehensive fashion; it should not be regarded as a praiseworthy method for achieving success. A high percentage of young dancers may also be found to be anorexic when compared with an average population.[6,16] Possible elements of compulsive exercise are listed below[6,10,25]:

Excessive calisthenics before starting or ending the day

Excessive running, walking, swimming, bike riding, dancing, or any strenuous exercise

Overuse of an exercycle or other device

Limited rest and/or sleep

Use of caffeine or other stimulants

Amenorrhea. Although one would expect a woman in a state of starvation to become amenorrheic,[44] indications are that cessation of the menses occurs in some teens with anorexia before they have lost sufficient weight to cause an interruption of the cycle.[3,6,45] The speculation is that psychological factors are the probable cause since stressful states are known to interfere with the endocrine system regulating the menstrual cycle.[8,10,46] The psychological set of young women developing anorexia nervosa suggests that they may be dismayed by the onset of menses[3] and that at best they are ambivalent toward this manifestation of their approaching adult feminine status. It is possible that this orientation contributes to the precarious state of these young women's cycles. At any rate, the weight loss is generally sufficient to provide a physical basis for continued interruption of the menses.

Nutritional Status. The biochemical consequences of the early precipitous weight loss caused by a semistarvation diet are relatively undramatic when compared to the psychological changes.[44] During the initial phase of an anorexic teen's energy restriction, the body does not exhibit the effects of malnutrition to any measurable degree other than a decrease in weight.[25] Infections are not generally seen.[6,47,48] Deficiencies of specific nutrients have not been reported,[3] but they may exist subclinically depending on the food habits of the individual. If weight loss continues unchecked, the symptoms of severe starvation may become apparent. This indicates the possible onset of a crisis.

Intervention Strategies. A recognition of the developing symptoms of the person affected by anorexia nervosa is the most important early intervention strategy. Friends, school personnel, family, and health professionals are among those who observe the growing problems and can take steps to bring the individual into treatment. The unique combination of symptoms; the lack of expressed concern over severe weight loss; and the sudden inability to function in social, academic, or vocational situations identify the anorexic teen. Hyperactivity, denial of problems, and resistance to external interchange may mask the true nature of the problem, especially for the inexperienced observer.[3,6,10,25] Individual and family psychotherapy by experienced therapists will enable both the affected teen and her family to adopt more appropriate roles and will help the anorexic teen to complete the psychological developmental processes that have been arrested. Because of the complexity of the interactional and behavioral patterns and the severity of the effect on the patient, recovery from anorexia nervosa will require a great deal of time and effort even if treatment is initiated at an early stage following the manifestation of physical signs.

Other than general monitoring of height and weight, it may not be necessary to treat the patient physically at this stage. Refocusing her attention on the primary emotional and interactional problems rather than on the power struggle over food and exercise patterns will often enable the patient to abandon her compulsive striving for thinness.

The patient should have access to a professional who can answer her questions about nutrition and make sure that she has the information she needs to begin to regulate her eating patterns to meet her physical needs. Generally, the perspective of these young women is distorted to the degree that they have never learned normal regulation.[6,10] Outside intervention may be necessary to enable them to establish habits that teens are expected to learn by family modeling. Information should be given in the context of the anorexic teen's desire to change rather than imposed as a rigid system of dietary planning by a professional. The overall disorder should not be defined as solely a nutritional problem, although nutritional counseling is an important component of therapy.

A deterioration of the physical or mental state of the anorexic teen signals an impending crisis that will require more comprehensive management. A lack of progress toward positive family interaction patterns during the initial therapy or continuing avoidance of intervention will often lead to this deterioration.

There are a number of cases of anorexia nervosa in which the person is able to function at a level short of crisis throughout the teen years and thus avoid intervention.[6] Some of these women may carry their problems through adulthood and never receive therapy. Others may seek treatment to improve their ability to function successfully in life, even though the physical aspects of their disorder may not seriously impact their health.[6]

Crisis Stage

Psychological State. The anorexic teen in crisis is able to engender panic in family, friends, and professionals.[6,10] The family, which often has attempted to cope with her abnormal behavior in a circle of secrecy, may become desperate and seek medical aid.[6] They may have ignored her progressing emaciation until it has reached the point of crisis.[32] Often they present a cold and resistant front and are reluctant to establish a therapeutic relationship.[6,39] They usually have made authoritarian but ineffective attempts to "make her eat."[3,25]

The family generally sees the teen's bizarre eating behavior as the problem and fails to understand the ramifications of developmental or interactional patterns.[6,10,25,49] The family often seeks treatment that does not demand their involvement with the patient in therapy.

The anorexic teen, not having developed autonomy, has given herself over to ritualistic behaviors. Superficially, she appears to have tremendous control because of her refusal to deviate from her self-destructive stance. However, in reality the evidence points to an underlying inadequacy in relationships, conceptualization, and self-support.[6,10,12,25,42]

As she becomes truly cachectic, the psychological changes inherent in starvation are superimposed on the anorexic teen's disturbed psychological state. Many of the characteristics of the typical anorexic teen in crisis state have been seen in classical cases of starvation.[3,10,28] Keys and co-workers[44] found psychological changes were apparent when subjects had lost about 12% of body weight. The box on p. 114 lists some of the major characteristics of "semistarvation neurosis." Keys and co-workers[44] observed more severe symptoms of behavior change in subjects with less initial stability of personality. Theoretically, the psychological effects of starvation thus are great for anorexic teens since they are a psychologically vulnerable group.

Many patients resist what they see as intrusions by professionals.[6,50] They are secretive and protect the fact that they are carrying out their rituals. Their behavior may otherwise reflect the apathy typically seen in starving people. In obsessional preoccupation[10,32] they plan menus, read recipes, cook and serve food to others, cut or manipulate food before eating it, and record all that they eat.[6,8,25] They usually have a detailed knowledge of the energy value of foods. When forced, they may pretend to eat and then hide and dispose of the food.[8,10,25,28,32]

The anorexic teen has a fear of gaining weight ("weight phobia").[6] She may choose a low weight goal and then reset the goal when she has reached

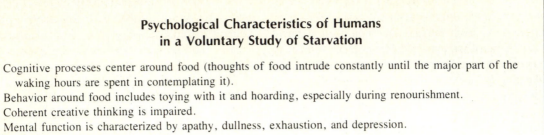

**Psychological Characteristics of Humans
in a Voluntary Study of Starvation**

Cognitive processes center around food (thoughts of food intrude constantly until the major part of the waking hours are spent in contemplating it).

Behavior around food includes toying with it and hoarding, especially during renourishment.

Coherent creative thinking is impaired.

Mental function is characterized by apathy, dullness, exhaustion, and depression.

Interest in sexual function is lacking.

Data modified from Keys, Ancel, et al.: *The biology of human starvation,* University of Minnesota Press, Minneapolis. Copyright © 1950 by the University of Minnesota Press.

that point. Finally, the therapist can discern that there is no limit that the teen considers low enough.[8]

Physiological State. In the crisis stage the psychodynamics of anorexia nervosa have led to a situation where the individual is unable to take care of herself. The physical state of starvation is superimposed on the other problems inherent in the disorder.[3] Although symptoms to some degree may be influenced by the particular food habits of the individual, they generally will fit into patterns that have been described for all anorexic teens. The physical signs of anorexia nervosa are listed below:

Fat-store depletion
Muscle wasting
Amenorrhea
Cheilosis
Desquamation
Dry skin
Hirsutism
Thin, dry, brittle hair
Alopecia
Degradation of fingernails
Acrocyanosis
Postural hypotension
Dehydration
Edema
Bradycardia
Bradypnea
Hypothermia
Constipation
Sleep disturbance

Although weakened and emaciated, the anorexic teen generally will continue excessive exercise routines.[28,51] She may complain that her stomach is "bloated."[10,28] Often "hunger gurgles" will be audible when she is quiet. Speech is breathy and is visibly difficult to produce.

The hair of the anorexic teen is dry and brittle and may fall out. At the same time, the body may become increasingly hirsute, with fine lanugo hair visible over the trunk, extremities, and perhaps the face. The skin is usually dry and scaly. Acrocyanosis (mottled blue or red coloration of the extremities) is seen. Cheilosis may develop. The condition of fingernails often deteriorates. Most strikingly, because of muscle wastage and lack of body fat, the skeleton becomes visible through the skin and the eyes appear sunken. The physical appearance of the anorexic teen thus resembles that of other starving persons such as those seen in natural and man-made disasters (for example, famine and war).*

*References 3, 6, 10, 25, 28, 32, 40, 49, 52.

Anorexic patients develop hypotension with blackouts or fainting spells as a result of severe weight loss. Bradycardia and certain cardiac irregularities demonstrable by electrocardiogram also accompany weight loss of this magnitude. The cardiac irregularities are reversible with improved nutrition and do not appear life threatening until an advanced state of starvation has been reached.[3,6,28,40,49]

Edema, especially in the lower extremities, is observed in anorexia, even though plasma proteins may remain normal. It recently has been thought that the development of edema is caused by a glomerular abnormality resulting from energy deprivation.[3,51] Fluid and electrolyte imbalances of a severe nature are life-threatening aspects of cachexia and must be corrected on an emergency basis.[25,49] The imbalances will be exacerbated when patients are vomiting, when they are abusing diuretics or laxatives, or when their dietary habits include extremes of fluid, salt, or other electrolyte intake.[3,6]

Biochemical changes are reflected in carotenemia, elevated serum cholesterol, leukopenia, and bone-marrow hypoplasia.[49,53] There may be hypocalcemia if vomiting occurs or if laxatives or diuretics are being misused.[3,6] The carotenemia is interesting in that it was not found in cachectic individuals who were not anorexic.[54] It is not known whether this is caused by a defect in the utilization of carotenoids or by the ingestion of large amounts of vegetables, which is customary in many anorexic teens.

Bradypnea is the major alteration in respiratory function.[25,40] Gastrointestinal tract changes include delayed gastric emptying and mild, nonobstructive jejunal dilation in certain anorexic teens.[6,49] These young women experience constipation as a result of diminished food intake.[40] They may, however, develop diarrhea if the malnutrition is sufficiently extensive to cause abnormalities of the gastrointestinal tract.[6,49]

The endocrinological abnormalities in anorexia are such that the body essentially reverts to a prepubertal hormonal state. As a result of hypothalamic change, the anorexic teen is amenorrheic, is unable to adapt to heat and cold, suffers sleep disturbances, and is unable to conserve body water. There is a lack of interest in sex.*

The measureable changes in pituitary and hypothalamic functions (Tables 5-1 and 5-2) are compatible with body responses geared to survival in the face of starvation. These abnormalities generally disappear with renourishment, although the psychological factors may lengthen the process.[49,56-59] Recovery in the nourished state can be interpreted to mean that the hypothalamic changes result from the starvation of anorexia nervosa and that anorexia nervosa is not caused by malfunctions of the hypothalamus. Conclusive data, however, are not available to support either hypothesis.[39,49]

During a crisis, professionals must monitor the physical state of the anorexic teen and take remedial action when there are signs that starvation is approaching a terminal state. The most outstanding of those signs are the following:

Imbalance in fluid and electrolytes (signifies inability of the body to maintain homeostasis)[10]

Severe cardiac abnormalities in the absence of electrolyte imbalances (signifies a wasted myocardium)[49]

Absence of ketone bodies in the urine (signifies a lack of fat stores for metabolic fuel)[25]

Concurrent infection (signifies increasing nutritional needs)[49]

Intervention Strategies. If the anorexic patient is unable to increase her energy intake after early intervention, a period of hospitalization may be necessary to avoid further deterioration of her mental and physical abilities caused by the severe starvation. One of the most pressing questions during the crisis of an anorexic patient is when hospitalization may be indicated.[10] Therapists must

*References 8, 36, 37, 40, 49, 55.

Table 5-1. Hypothalamic malfunction in anorexia nervosa

Symptom	Comment
Lack of thermoregulation Does not shiver or maintain basal body temperature in heat or cold Exhibits paradoxical response to heat or cold	Defect could be in temperature sensation or stimulus integration[8,36,49]
Abnormality in water conservation Unable to concentrate urine during water deprivation	Suggests defect in or near hypothalamus[8,36,49]
Delayed release of tropic hormones, luteinizing hormone (LH), follicle-stimulating hormone (FSH), thyroid-stimulating hormone (TSH), and prolactin	May be part of hypothalamic dysfunction since other cause is not evident[8,49]
Impaired carbohydrate metabolism	May be related to abnormalities in insulin degradation, growth-hormone and/or cortisol receptors, and glucagon levels[8]

Table 5-2. Pituitary end organ function in anorexia nervosa

Endocrinological Parameters	Proposed Mechanism
Elevated plasma growth hormone	Result of chronic hypoglycemia or hypoamino-acidemia[8,36,49,60,61]
Normal plasma prolactin[8,49]	Normal pituitary prolactin function[8]
Low basal 3,5,3'-triiodothyronine (T_3), normal thyroid-stimulating hormone (TSH), and normal free thyroxine (fT_4)[8]	Abnormality of the hypothalamus manifested by altered set point for thyrotrophin-releasing hormone (TRH) or TSH release and by delayed TSH release after exogenous TRH, with normal pituitary-thyroid axis[8,36,49]
Normal or elevated plasma cortisol with one-half subjects lacking diurnal variation[8]	Hypothalamic defect with intact pituitary-adrenal axis[8,36,49,60]
Low basal serum gonadotropins and prepubertal secretion pattern[8]	Lack of endogenous luteinizing hormone–releasing hormone (LRH) production*

*References 8, 36, 49, 57, 60, 62, 63.

monitor the condition of the anorexic patient to ensure that she obtains intensive physical care if the physical status warrants this. Observing her condition for physical signs is confusing. Although she is emaciated, she may continue to be hyperactive.[6] It has been demonstrated that even after losing a large percentage of body weight, human beings can move about and survive. Keys[44] found that after 3 months of semistarvation and an 18% loss of body weight, experimental subjects were able to perform an average of 36% of the total work on a treadmill they performed when normally nourished. After 6 months of semistarvation at

25% loss of body weight, they were still able to complete about 16% of the work they did before. Their mental state was quite compromised, however.[44] The deterioration of the body from starvation thus follows a continuum with few defined milestones until a terminal state has been reached.

For some clinicians, the decision to hospitalize an anorexic patient depends on her reaching a life-threatening physical state. However, if the goal is to renourish the individual so that she will be able to benefit from psychotherapy without ''semistarvation neurosis''[44] as many authoritative therapists recommend,[6,10,32] the anorexic patient must be hospitalized before a critical stage has been reached.

Most therapeutic programs for patients with anorexia nervosa can be categorized as psychotherapy,[10] milieu therapy (therapeutically structured environment),[40,64,65] behavior modification,[66-69] family therapy,[25,31] or eclectic therapy (various elements combined).[7,39,70] Drugs to alter mood, behavior, or appetite have been used in combination with other intervention strategies, but they generally are not used alone[3,36,49,70-72] and are thought by Crisp[6] to be dangerous. Programs will have a specific thrust based on the aspect of the problem that is seen as most important. Therapists who stress the importance of renourishment before intensive psychotherapy will see that as a key issue. Renourishing a self-starving anorexic teen, however, can never be completely divorced from the psychological strategies that will accomplish this.

Other therapists focus more on the psychodynamics of the patient's family situation, following the theory that improvement in interactions and personality structure will lead to improved nourishment. In this case the therapist helps the patient to give up her symptoms by beginning to deal with the underlying issues. Modern protocols are being developed that use a variety of elements at different stages of the disorder. Almost all of these protocols stress the necessity for consistent long-term care to completely rehabilitate the individual.[3,6,10,25,49] Such protocols are not often described in the literature because their eclectic nature does not lend itself well to controlled research.

The characteristics of anorexia nervosa are usually so distinct that there is no question about the diagnosis to those familiar with the disorder. This is true, in part, because the characteristics of the disorder are seen in not only the patient herself but also in her relationships with her family, peers, and total environment. However, it is important to rule out other abnormalities that occasionally have been confused with anorexia nervosa (for example,

inflammatory bowel disease, brain tumors, and primary endocrinological or metabolic abnormalities). A complete investigation should be made if the case appears atypical in any way.[25,49,73]

Most workers stress the need to begin informing and educating the patients and their families about the disorder on admission to the hospital.[3,6,25,32,40] Each program must come to terms with the presentation of food to the patient, a treatment component largely determined by the main theme of the program. If the program is based on behavior modification, food will be presented within a system of positive and negative reinforcers, usually contingent on weight gain. The reinforcers are usually tied to privileges that increase activity level. If the program has a parental theme, the inpatient personnel will present food firmly and helpfully.[69,70,72] Whatever the program, it may be difficult for professionals to maintain: anorexic teens usually will challenge even experienced staff[25,70,74] with behavior that ranges from protests to trickery and belligerence and that is punctuated by emotional outbursts.[3,10] It is important that all professionals dealing with anorexic patients function as a supportive team. They should have specific training in carrying out a therapeutic protocol by clinicians who have experience with eating disorders.[3,10,25,65]

Nutritional components of therapeutic regimens for anorexia nervosa in crisis are intertwined with the psychological aspects of the treatment. Certain principles can be observed that will apply regardless of the treatment modality. Renourishment obviously will begin with an increase in energy intake. For a person who has been taking in only 400 kcal/day, even 1000 kcal/day will be a step toward renourishment. To gain the patient's cooperation, it usually will be necessary to increase the energy level of the intake gradually. This is carried out by allowing approximately 1 week of observation before a specific treatment modality is initiated.[3,25,65] Descriptions of renourishment in cases of starvation emphasize a gradual increase.[52] Mention has been made of paralytic ileus and gastric dilation[3,49] as possible complications of renourishing too rapidly. However, such problems are seldom described in the literature concerning renourishment in anorexia nervosa. Many programs appear to have had no difficulty over the years in using a 3000 kcal dietary regimen.[6,39,66]

In some programs the patient will be allowed to choose anything available on the hospital menu.[66,72] Other programs impose rules, make additions to what is ordered, or serve an imposed menu.[3,6,25] In some cases consultation with a dietitian over menus is allowed, but in other programs the patient is prohibited from discussing food with the therapeutic team. The prohibition is held over from a former era when one professional was usually responsible for the care of the anorexic patient. On present-day therapeutic teams, however, the nutrition specialist can contribute to overall rehabilitation by counseling and educating the anorexic teen in addition to providing nutritional support in the physical sense.

If a diet is prescribed following the principles established for renourishing malnourished individuals,[75] it will have adequate protein to meet basic needs with additional energy made up of carbohydrate and fat. Stordy and co-workers[76] used a diet of 14% total energy from protein, 50% from carbohydrate, and 36% from fat. Indications are that about 7500 excess kcal are needed to add 1 kg (2.2 lb) of body weight when patients are reaching a weight close to normal for their age, height, and sex.[39,77] Initial gains are made with fewer calories per kilogram of gain. This difference is probably accounted for by the initial addition of water and protein, which requires less energy than the acquisition of fat. The thinnest patients and previously obese patients require less energy per kilogram of gain than patients whose weight is closer to normal or who were not previously obese.[77] Stordy and co-workers[76] have shown that this is probably the result of a better adaptation to excess energy on the part of those not previously obese.

If a patient refuses food, a nutritional supplement, which is prescribed and dispensed as a medicine, has been used.[10,32,70] If a life-threatening state is reached at any time, with the patient refusing oral feeding, nourishment by nasogastric tube or parenteral methods may be necessary. These methods will be presented as life-saving procedures and not as a punishment for refusing to eat. Nourishment by mouth is the preferred route and is possible in most cases.[3,49]

Edema generally appears with renourishment and can be a problem because of the anorexic patient's phobia of weight gain.[70,72,78] The edema is seen as proof to her that she will "expand" as she feared. Some anticipatory guidance can help her to accept such a development. Assurance that professionals will aid her in gaining weight, which is strengthening for her, but not in forming excess fat can help desensitize the issue.[3,70] Regular body measurements, if acceptable to the patient, may demonstrate that the professional is indeed interested in working with her to monitor changes in size and body composition and to help her in accepting a gain in weight. The patient should be told that initial weight following obligatory water and lean tissue gain may be more highly proportional in fat as indicated by research in starvation.[78] As with any other issue, this can be taken in stride if it is explained as part of the natural phenomena. It should be emphasized that the extent of the fat gain will be limited and eventually overcome by complete physical rehabilitation, including fitness improvement, when adequate amounts of strength have been regained.[72] The inclusion of a nutritionist or dietitian on the therapeutic team provides for attention to these physical aspects of care in a manner that does not subvert the psychotherapeutic goals of redirecting the focus of the patient's concern.

The goal for ending hospitalization often is a particular weight. This may be a weight that is adjudged to be above a dangerous level of undernourishment, that is 50% of the difference between admission and normal weight (for age, sex, and height),[25] or that is 100% of the normal weight.[6] Experienced therapists feel a change in attitude must accompany such a gain in weight to justify release from the hospital.

Therapeutic Goals. Whatever the style, intervention programs for anorexic teens will firmly manage the nourishing function for the patient's life and avoid power struggles over details. The programs provide the patient with a model for regulation of food intake, energy output, and other physical aspects of life. The psychotherapeutic component will be directed toward effecting a change in the underlying psychological characteristics of the anorexic patient and in the interactions within her family.[3,6,10,25]

Long-Term Recovery

Psychological State. The anorexic teen who has recovered from a starvation crisis by gaining a certain amount of weight to ameliorate her physical state will still have to deal with the developmental arrest that brought her to the crisis. This may require a period of several years.[6] She may still be hostile toward continuing therapy. She will often play out her dependence and independence needs in relationships with therapists, being at once demanding and dependent, independent and rejecting. She may periodically change therapists or completely resist therapy. There may be multiple crises, often triggered by the need to face new situations in life.[6,49] When she is living with her family, they will be involved in the total process. They will need to adopt altered patterns of interaction to facilitate the development of their daughter.

Although some anorexic teens avoid a full physical crisis, their developmental problems are no less crippling, and their need for support in developmental progress may equal that of the patient who has been hospitalized.[6] Similarly, those anorexic teens who were brought to therapy early enough to avoid a crisis will need support. There will continue to be problems concerning vocational choices and preparation; economic stability; relationships with peers; and especially the opposite sex, weight management, and body image.

Physiological State. In the long term the anorexic teen will often experience wide swings in weight from extreme thinness to obesity before she will be able to bring her life into control.[6] She may see herself as somewhat detached from her body and experiment with various food habits before putting food into a more normal perspective. She may keep herself sufficiently thin that she will not resume her menses.[3,6] She may feel bloated and have bouts of edema and carotenemia.

Intervention Strategies. In the recovery period the psychotherapeutic goals will be to facilitate normal development in the anorexic teen, to prepare her for a full adult role in society, and to enable her to function without depending on bizarre eating and exercise habits. She will need information and retraining about food and the physical aspects of life. Many of the techniques described later in the section on obesity in this chapter will be useful in this regard. Issues such as the state of nourishment necessary to maintain the menstrual cycle will often resurface from time to time as development proceeds. Returning to such issues will enable the anorexic teen to deal more capably with them as time goes on. One well-known program incorporates training related to food experiences in cafeterias, grocery stores, cooking, and entertaining and thus helps ready the patient for managing food in her environment. The objective is to help the anorexic teen put food in a reasonable perspective rather than to overfocus on food out of ignorance.[6] Such an approach can and should be incorporated into hospital treatment as discharge nears.

Most often the whole family will be involved in long-term therapy. However, if a family refuses or if the patient is an older, emancipated woman, she may be seen alone. There will usually be individual and family counseling sessions.[6,10] A team consisting of medical, psychological, and nutritional specialists may provide care, or the care may be left to a single therapist who will be responsible for all aspects of therapy.

Results of Intervention Strategies for Anorexia Nervosa

Because of the multifaceted problems seen in anorexia nervosa, the measurement of treatment outcome should encompass the physical, psychological, and socioeconomic states of the individuals. The following criteria should be used[79]:

Weight and dietary habits
  Weight and shape ideation
  Food intake
  Weight-for-height proportion
Menstruation
Sexual adjustment
Psychological adjustment
Social adjustment
Occupational status

To demonstrate the stability of the posttreatment condition, an estimated 2 years should elapse before the criteria are applied. A review of treatment outcome in 1980 shows that such criteria were not utilized consistently in studies published between 1954 and 1978.[79] Body weight was commonly used, but the use was inconsistent because normal body weight was not always defined. Most studies reported on eating habits, but few investigated concerns about shape and weight. One fourth of the studies did not report menstrual function. Most reported on psychiatric symptoms. Marital status was reported more frequently than the normalcy of overall sexual function. Social, interactional, and economic reporting was quite varied.[79]

As to the conditions found, in three fourths of the cases body weight was reported to be improved. Menstrual cycles were not regularly maintained, however, and psychiatric status as indicated by affective disorders and psychosocial adjustment was even less satisfactorily normal. The more favorable outcome was that patients were able to support themselves economically. It was not noted, however, whether they were able to maintain a level of affluence comparable to their family backgrounds and intellectual potential as seen in academic settings.[79]

Mortality was reported to be as high as 10% in former years but was 2% among those treated by Crisp.[6,80] This is probably a more accurate figure in relation to modern programs, which are based on a greater understanding of the disorder. Patients probably are recognized more readily at present and are hospitalized before a terminal state of starvation has been reached. The ultimate goal of enabling the anorexic teen to live a normal, productive life has not often been measured effectively and probably has not often been reached. It is estimated by Crisp that it requires a period of several years.[6] Thus long-term follow-up with attention to a wide range of issues will be necessary to obtain an accurate evaluation of treatment programs in the future.

BULIMIA

First called bulimarexia, bulimia is the most recently recognized eating disorder and includes gorging followed by vomiting.[26,81] Although these symptoms may be part of anorexia nervosa, they also comprise a separate syndrome. Therefore the following terminology can be used to make distinctions:

Bulimia—gorging and vomiting without starvation
Bulimarexia—gorging and vomiting accompanied by voluntary starvation
Gorging (binging)—eating abnormally large amounts of food

The person suffering from bulimia generally maintains close to normal weight (Fig. 5-1) while gorging and vomiting on a regular basis. The bulimic teen may have somewhat less severe distortions in body image and less restrictive weight goals than the anorexic teen. She is often older at age of onset. This syndrome should be differentiated from the recent habit of many normal teens who vomit occasionally as a means of controlling weight. A serious condition will become uncontrollable, and the psychological features of the disorder will impair the normal functioning of the teen. Bulimia sometimes develops after the patient has had a serious bout with anorexia nervosa or obesity. The bulimic teen is more likely to be fertile than the anorexic teen, and therefore certain young women will be bulimic during pregnancy.

Psychological State

As described in various clinical accounts (for example, unpublished papers, conference proceedings, and articles in the popular press), anxiety over separation is usually one of the important issues for the bulimic teen. Her self-esteem is extremely low and is tied to her feelings about her body. She demonstrates excessive need for control and approval. She thinks of herself as physically unattractive, although she is well groomed and has a normally attractive physique. She develops guilt over her habits and her secret feelings of inadequacy. Superficially, she may be very responsible and keep a heavy social schedule. In reality she is close to few friends and feels no one "really knows her." In contrast to the more rigid anorexic teen, the bulimic teen often demonstrates poor impulse control, abuses substances, and becomes enraged. By all accounts, the gorging, vomiting, and purging serve to release tension for the sufferers. However, the residual guilt is the basis for renewed tension that perpetuates an uncontrolled cycle.[26] Social isolation is also perpetuated because of the fear that the secret will be found out. If pregnant, the bulimic teen may be committed to protecting the fetus but retain ideas that inhibit normal nourishment of herself, her fetus, and the child after it is born.

Physiological State

The bulimic teen periodically eats large amounts of food and then voluntarily vomits. The binge,

however, is defined by the bulimic teen. Because of distortions in thinking about food, the binge may be as little as one doughnut or as great as a package of them. As the duration of the habit extends, it becomes easier for the bulimic teen to vomit. Eventually, the vomiting is a nearly automatic response. In addition, she may take laxatives or diuretics to purge herself of the energy she has ingested. Physical symptoms include the following:

Damage to the teeth

Irritation of the throat

Esophageal inflammation and possible tracheoesophageal fistula (All the above symptoms are caused by exposure of unprotected tissue to acidic vomitus.)

Swollen salivary glands (may be caused by acidic reflux or constant stimulation)

Rectal bleeding (caused by the overuse of laxatives)

Life-threatening-situations are rare. They are related to fistulas or ruptures in the upper gastrointestinal tract and fluid and electrolyte imbalances. Concerns during pregnancy are the adverse biochemical environment for the mother and fetus, the mother's abnormal weight-gain pattern (loss, lack of gain, inordinate gain), and the mother's unrealistic ideas about infant feeding.

Intervention Strategies

Specific strategies for intervention in bulimia are only beginning to be documented in scientific journals. The techniques most frequently mentioned are similar to those used in the long-term recovery period of the anorexic teen. The emphasis is on freeing the patient from guilt, facilitating gains in self-esteem, and helping her deal with anxiety. Challenging distorted goal setting based on perfection has been tied to this.[81] The woman's family or living partners ideally will be included in therapy. While she deals with the psychological problem, the bulimic teen will still have an eating disorder, and she will need reeducation to properly nourish herself. Physical and nutritional education can fill gaps in the knowledge these teens have about their body functions. Over time, myths about weight management can be dispelled and more normal eating habits developed. Because of distorted feelings about food, the bulimic teen may feel guilty each time she eats, despite the fact that food is necessary for life. The family often reinforces the guilt by a misguided overfocus on food, thinness, and the physical aspects of life. The bulimic teen may greatly restrict her food intake to match the ideal plan she conceives for herself. Binges thus may arise from the natural need for adequate food and the desire for additional gratification. With psychotherapists and medical specialists, the nutritionists on the professional team will help the bulimic teen see food in a more appropriate context and accept more realistic weight goals using the techniques described in the obesity section of this chapter. Helping the bulimic teen to understand the physiological processes of energy balance and nutrient functions is especially helpful. This education, however, must take place gradually, allowing time for alteration of the bulimic teen's own rigid system of beliefs. Family and individual psychotherapy will be necessary to deal with underlying causes of this obsessional behavior. Group therapy has been used.[81]

The bulimic teen who is pregnant can be helped to accept the idea that the baby she wants must be nourished. She can then be supported in learning to retain those foods that the fetus needs even if she cannot give up binging and vomiting totally. She should also be helped in learning to recognize natural hunger signals from her baby after it is born.

OBESITY

At the other end of the physical spectrum of eating disorders is the very heavy teenager. Unlike anorexic teens, people who are abnormally heavy do not fit into a homogeneous group and may be carrying excessive weight for a variety of reasons.[9,10,82,83] Factors leading to obesity can be broadly divided into those that are psychological and those that are physiological. In any individual a combination of these factors may be operative in the development and maintenance of obesity. Because of the cultural response to obesity, the adolescent whose obesity may be physiologically based will generally be subject to many of the same problems as those whose obesity is more psychologically based.[22,83-86]

Psychological Factors

Bruch[10] has described two basic forms of obesity that primarily result from psychological factors: *developmental* and *reactive*. *Developmental obesity* is an eating disorder comparable to anorexia nervosa in that it originates in the early life of the child. The families of developmentally obese teens fit Minuchin and co-workers' description[25] of the psychosomatic family. The family's attitudes and behavior thus stunt the child's psychological development and serve as primary causes of the obesity. The obesity itself further inhibits normal development, and this in turn leads to maintenance or increase of body weight.[10] The affected children are made to feel pressure, inappropriate responsibility, and specialness to an abnormal degree in family interactions.[10,20,87] They become rigid, isolated, and enmeshed.[10,20,87-89] They develop misperceptions about their basic physical needs and rely on coping skills based on the abuse of food.[9,10]

Although developmentally obese teens may not develop their full potential as self-competent, well-functioning adults, they are less likely to experience the complete developmental arrest that the anorexic teen does. There are other differences between the reactions of developmentally obese and anorexic teens, as well. For example, although obese teens tend to be perfectionists when establishing goals, they have negative attitudes concerning their ability to achieve those goals. Unlike the anorexic teen, the obese teen thus gives up easily rather than struggling to attain their goals.[87] This is obvious especially in their approach to weight management[2,10] and often in their academic performance.[88] Because their physical and psychological problems are not so extreme as the anorexic teens', the obese teens may never experience crises and may function at more or less stable levels throughout their lives.

The teen who is overweight is vulnerable to body-image disturbances.[14,21,22] The type of body-image disturbance appears to depend on the length of time the teen has been heavy, the amount of overweight that the teen carries, the teen's sex, and the circumstances surrounding the teen's unique development.[10,22,23,90] For example, teens who are heavy from childhood may react differently than those who have gained weight only during later adolescence.

Some teens think of themselves in an exaggerated sense as being "like a hippo."[10,84] Others misjudge their weight and the weight of those around them and think of extreme overweight as a more or less normal state.[10] For many, weight camouflages their developing sexuality and hides male and female characteristics. Weight may function in various ways as protection from a more complex life with which they cannot cope.[10,88,91] Like anorexic teens, many tie thoughts of success or failure to their weight status. They are unable to acknowledge any positive characteristics in themselves as they focus on what they see as negative aspects of their bodies.[22] They also appear inordinately sensitive to the societal value on thinness.[22] Rarely, there are teens who adjust very favorably to their obesity, both in the physical and psychological sense, without a disturbance of body image.

Reactive obesity refers to those situations where the origin of obesity is more short-term in nature. Obesity of this type is a reaction to stressful events in life.[10,92] The person affected will attempt to allay anxiety and depression by immediate gratification with food. Children who adapt to stress in this manner usually have family interactions similar to the developmentally obese but have avoided the more severe, long-term aspects of the disorder. Thus in times of stress they regress to the misuse of food in an effort to cope with crisis.[10]

Obesity Associated with Psychological Disorders. Obesity may be associated with severe psychiatric disorders in some teenagers. In others the overeating behavior may act as an emotionally stabilizing influence helping to maintain the person at a functioning level. Interference in such a situation, particularly without substitution of substantial support for the overeating behavior, can cause the disintegration of the person into an anxious or depressed state.[10,91-93]

Culturally Fostered and Behaviorally Based Obesity. The abundance of food and the lack of necessity to expend energy in our society make it very easy for children to gain unwanted weight.[21,83,85,88] In families where food-intake and exercise patterns are not appropriate for dealing with this situation, overweight can result without other specific psychological or physiological origins.[82]

Typical Patterns of Behavior in Overweight Teens. The usual overweight or obese teen is passive in interactions with others and with the environment.[10,88,89] This leads to social isolation and an increased dependence on the family for relationships,[10,83,88,89,94] even though the family interaction patterns may be unpleasant and the parents may exhibit intrusive and negative attitudes.

Adolescents often react to the stigma of obesity by adopting a stereotyped life-style with a narrow range of activities.[95] They feel the behavior of others toward them is affected by their overweight status. For example, if peers are unfriendly, the obese teens attribute it to their weight and disregard the circumstances. Their weight almost always figures prominently in their thoughts about themselves and in their decision-making processes. In addition to the obese teen's problems in social interactions, the eating functions of their lives also are generally distorted. For example, they may never feel comfortable eating in social situations. The isolation of obese teens leads them to opt out of many activities that would expend energy. They generally do not want to be seen wearing gym or swim suits or doing physical activities because they feel they are the object of attention and even ridicule.[20,22,88,93] Indeed, because most teens feel insecure about their own bodies,[14] they may actually direct teasing and cruel remarks at the obese teen. These remarks substantiate the obese teen's fears.[84] Because of this situation, the obese teenager usually spends an inordinate amount of time in passive pursuits such as reading and watching television. Both of these activities may be paired with eating. Commercial television, especially, fosters this behavior with frequent food-related cues.

Eating Patterns of Obese Teens. Although many studies of teens after they have become obese have shown that on the average they eat no more, and sometimes less, than their normal-weight peers,[20,21,96-98] they often have disturbed patterns of eating. Some of these patterns have been documented in scientific investigations, and others are readily observable in a clinic population. The more commonly occurring patterns are the following:

Consumption of an imbalance of high-energy and low-nutrient foods over low-energy and high-nutrient foods[21,22,99]

Interpretation of diverse feelings or situations as reasons to eat[10]

Susceptibility to eating cues unrelated to physiological needs[10,100,101]

Guilt related to eating under any circumstances

Lack of understanding of bodily needs for nourishment

Unwillingness to eat with others, including family members

Lack of structure in eating patterns[20]

Lack of sociability connected with eating patterns[20]

Night eating[10,100]

Binge eating[10,100]

Eating only in the latter part of the day after starvation in the early part[10]

Nausea described as connected with eating in the early part of the day[100]

Lack of any feeling of control over their food supply

Eating rapidly and indiscriminately[100]

Family Patterns. Parents in some families may be locked into a power struggle with the child, attempting in vain to control what he or she eats.[22,88] Overanxiety regarding slight overweight may actually contribute to growing obesity.[102] In other families overeating will be the main theme, with most interactions revolving around food. Family members may vie with each other to make sure they get their share. In some families the misuse of food is fostered by parents, grandparents, and others giving children food as a reward or in lieu of appreciation, love, and attention.[10,20] Families may have distorted views of body size and thus fail to recognize or be concerned with obesity in their children until it has reached an extreme degree. The value of heaviness in some cultures may place the child in a vulnerable position in the modern world where energy is easily taken in and physical activity easily avoided.

Physiological Factors

The genetic and biochemical factors that play a part in the disorder of obesity must be acknowledged, although not a great deal is known about the specific mechanism of such factors at present. It can be speculated that in certain individuals physiological factors are principally responsible for obesity. These factors have been frequently reviewed[82,96,102-109] and are summarized in Table 5-3.

One theory that cannot be overlooked is that individuals may be subject to a body-weight "set point." In other words, a certain body weight may be physiologically normal for them, and body

Table 5-3. Physiological factors observed in obesity

Factor	Proposed Mechanism	Recent Conclusions	Therapeutic Implications
Insulin insensitivity	Obese persons are less sensitive to the action of insulin, creating the state of hyperinsulinemia.[82]	Dietary factors and reversible changes in the metabolism of obese persons may be responsible for irregularities in body insulin levels.[82]	Moderation of simple carbohydrate and fat intake should be encouraged. Cyclical maintenance of obesity may be interrupted by factors such as exercise, which appear to alleviate insulin sensitivity independent of weight reduction.
Thyroid dysfunction	Faulty receptor sites impair the normal function of 3,5,3′-triiodothyronine (T_3) at the cellular level.[105]	Irregularities accompany and maintain obesity but are probably not a cause.[105]	In most cases thyroid medication is contraindicated.
Fat cell hypertrophy	As the body gains weight, the fat cells enlarge.[106]	The size of the fat cells can be reduced by increased energy output and decreased energy input.[110]	Reducing fat cells to normal size is a reasonable goal.
Fat cell hyperplasia	Number of fat cells increases when sufficient weight is gained.[106]	The heavier a body is and the longer it remains heavy, the greater the chance of an increased number of fat cells. The number of fat cells cannot be reduced with weight loss.[110]	Preventing an increase in the number of fat cells is a reasonable goal.
Thermogenesis	Obese persons produce less heat to dissipate energy.[111]	May be caused by specific mechanisms such as less brown fat or sodium-potassium–pump irregularity.[112,113]	Increase thermogenesis in any practical way (for example, exercise).
Brown fat variability	High cytochrome content of these adipocytes causes heat production[112]; smaller endowment leads to energy storage.	It is difficult to correlate particular amount with obese state in humans.	If operative, these mechanisms can only be overcome with extreme difficulty.
Sodium-potassium–pump irregularity	Lower number of sodium-potassium transporting units present in cells of obese persons.[113]	Irregularity may account for decreased energy usage in metabolism of obese persons.	Reduction of body weight, if possible, may lead to a state like starvation in persons with these irregularities.

Continued.

Table 5-3. Physiological factors observed in obesity—cont'd

Factor	Proposed Mechanism	Recent Conclusions	Therapeutic Implications
Genetic predisposition	Certain biochemical, morphological, and histological features are inherited.[107,114]	Differences may be aggravated by decreased energy output and increased energy intake.[107]	If obese persons have control of energy intake and output, psychological support for living with the status quo is a reasonable goal.
Physical set point	A feedback system alters intake and output of energy to maintain a particular body mass.[108]	As above.	As above.
Liproprotein lipase variability	Higher levels of lipoprotein lipase (LPL) in obese persons maintain obese state.[115]	Reduced persons have higher than expected levels of LPL, favoring return to the state of obesity.[115]	As above.

characteristics may be tuned to keep the body at that weight.[108] A postulated example involves the level of lipoprotein lipase, which favors adipocyte engorgement. Instead of falling to the expected lower level commensurate with reduced body weight, the level remains comparable to the higher body weight that the individual attained. Thus, like a thermostat, the process appears to lead to the maintenance of a certain weight.[115] The manner in which this is accomplished involves the physiology of fat cells.

Whether individuals are genetically predisposed to obesity or have gained weight through overeating, if they are in an obese state by the time they have reached adolescence, they are probably both hyperplastically and hypertrophically obese. The size, but not the number, of fat cells can be reduced. This limits not only the amount of reduction possible but also the possibility that the reduced state can be maintained.[106] Theoretically, levels of lipoprotein lipase influence this.

Further, a decrease in the amount of energy used in biochemical reactions may increase the amount of energy available in the system for storage as fat. The transmission of sodium and potassium between cells and the amount of energy used in heat production (thermogenesis) are being investigated as possible factors leading to these variations.[111,113] The amount of metabolically active fat (brown), as opposed to more quiescent fat, may be partly responsible for individual differences in heat production.[112]

Whether metabolic abnormalities such as insulin insensitivity or thyroid–receptor site irregularities occur as a cause or result of the obese state, they also tend to maintain high weight levels.[82,105]

In summary, it can be stated that there appear to be strong physiological factors that lead to and maintain obesity in teenagers. Based on present theory, the longer the teen has been obese and the greater the extent of obesity, the greater the effect of these factors. The adolescent whose obesity was originally caused by other factors (social, psychological, or familial) will be subject to problems of physiological obesity. This adds to the complexity of the obese state. At this point, study of the physiology of obesity has not yielded therapies that can be applied directly to improve these effects. The obese teenager will have to cope with physiological factors, some of which are probably not reversible. It can be hoped that future research will uncover specific therapies that can be directed toward specific physiological disorders.

Intervention Strategies

Evaluation. The individual combination of psychological and physiological circumstances by which an individual teenager has become obese must be identified so that intervention can be directed toward specific aspects of the problem. The degree of overweight must be considered. Chapter 3, especially Fig. 3-4, provides information about the evaluation of the size of heavy teens. Generally they will be overweight, obese, or morbidly obese. Some will suffer from hidden eating disorders such as bulimia or anorexia nervosa (recovery stage).

A thorough evaluation of all aspects of the teen's life will be necessary to develop a working understanding of an individual teen's weight problem.[88,94,116-118] Fig. 5-2 presents a guide for clinical assessment of eating disorders, including both psychological and physiological aspects. The information needed may best be gathered by a team of professionals.[94,95] If such a team is unavailable, the individual professional can call on other people who know the young person, such as school personnel, previous health-care providers, or counselors, for relevant information. Many of the aspects cannot be assessed immediately but will need to be explored over time. For example, many heavy teens will not feel sufficiently comfortable to undergo extensive body measurements initially. Since one of the main purposes of taking the measurements is to demonstrate change for the obese teen, the clinical usefulness of anthropometrics is decreased by forcing them on an unwilling teenager. If the diagnosis depends on the amount of fat versus muscle individuals are carrying, they generally are willing to have such measurements taken.

Another reason the evaluation cannot be completed immediately is that obese teens first coming to treatment often cannot describe precisely what they eat during the day because they have ignored this question over the years. It may take several months of focusing their attention before they actually will be aware of the food they consume. Others will be aware but unable or unwilling to report consumption accurately.

A physical examination of the obese teenager will disclose the stage of puberty and rule out any endocrinological abnormalities or complications of the obese state. Endocrinological disorders will rarely be found.[119] Most physiological abnormalities indicated by clinical laboratory measures associated with obesity will respond to weight reduction.[102,109] Laboratory and clinical tests other than those routinely done in general physical examination are not warranted.[20,119]

The most important aspect of an initial evaluation is whether the individual is committed to making changes, because only if the teen is a full participant in the process can any progress be made.[88,93,116] The teen's position on this must be assessed initially and with each visit. It is of no value for other people to have goals related to weight management if the teen is not ready to change the status quo.[88] The question needs to be, "Are you ready to make some changes?" rather than "Do you want to lose weight?" Many teens will truthfully answer "yes" to the second question but remain totally passive, the implication being that the process of losing weight is a passive one in which the professional administers treatment. A commitment to action provides the necessary realism to justify initiating treatment. From there on, further evaluation and treatment can continue simultaneously.

Reasons for Refraining from Instituting a Weight-Loss Program. A weight-loss program should not be instituted if there is a lack of commitment,[88] if it is likely to be another in a series of failures that is detrimental to the self-esteem of the individual,[88,116,120] or if the individual is obviously predisposed to obesity by overwhelming physiological factors.[83] If obese teens keep fit, maintain energy equilibrium, and are emotionally healthy, they will be candidates for weight loss only if they understand the physiological aspects of obesity and are determined to test the possibility of healthfully challenging those physiological factors. Those teens still growing in height should not be encouraged to lose.

Goals. The initial weight-related goal in a weight-management program is usually maintenance, that is, cessation of weight gain. In certain situations an even more basic change from *rapid gain* to *slow gain* is the appropriate goal. Immature teens who have not completed linear growth can bring weight and, more specifically, percentage of body fat into better proportion with height by holding their weight stable or by reducing gains to a low rate as height increases.[102] This eliminates nutritional risk to the adolescent from severe dietary restrictions at a time of rapid growth and development.[102,121] For teens who have stabilized their weight and are no longer gaining in height, the next step will be a slow, steady loss based on reeducation in the use of energy. A loss of 0.9 kg/week (2 lb/week) should not be exceeded.[117] If this appears insignificant to the teen, it can be pointed out that it would add up to more than a 45-kg (100-lb) loss over a 1-year period.

Short-term goals will need to be based not on changes in weight but on positive changes in food-related behaviors and attitudes with appropriate rewards built in. It especially is necessary to build a program around short-term, manageable goals[116] related to behavioral change since physiological factors may make actual weight loss a difficult, long-term achievement. The teen should be made aware that over the long term an energy deficit will eventually lead to weight loss, however slowly. Although this concept will be difficult for teens to accept, advancing psychological development on their part will lead to the ability to incorporate a longer range view of life.

Strategies Directed Toward Physiological Factors. Whatever the reason for an overweight teen's having accumulated additional weight, the method for altering the situation remains the same: decreasing the energy supply to the body and increasing the energy output until the appropriate state of deficit is established.[122] Insightful work by Björntorp,[123] Webb,[124] and others[125] warrants careful study. These researchers have pointed out that there is no way of knowing the exact use of energy by a particular body except by testing it over time. To lose weight a caloric deficit must be achieved at the cellular level. Because this is immeasurable under normal clinical circumstances, there is no set formula that assures weight loss. You cannot count calories of food energy being eaten and assume you know exactly what will be available within the biochemical system. Thus a deficit of 3500 calories calculated at the point of intake does not necessarily lead to a loss of 1 pound of body weight. This does not imply that the second law of thermodynamics is inoperative, but simply that energy from food may be used in a variety of ways once it is in the body. Certain mechanisms that may cause these variations are listed in Table 5-2. Thus both the physiological and psychological aspects of weight management are unique to the individual.

Eating Habits. Individual teens must be guided in learning the level of intake and output that produces weight gain, loss, and maintenance for them if the treatment is to be effective. An understanding of physiological factors must be incorporated. The teenager must be made aware that however bleak the physiological situation appears, the possibility of weight management has not been tested until the individual has control over energy intake and output. There is usually some potential for improvement in the diet that will help even those teens who are physiologically prone to obesity to become more fit and healthy, to stabilize their weight, and perhaps to lose small amounts of weight.

Strategies for dietary change need to address the following issues: (1) energy level and nutrient content of the food intake[116,118,122]; (2) circumstances surrounding eating related to timing, place, accompaning sociability, and emotions[116,117]; and (3) principles of nutrition, especially regarding weight management.[121,122,126]

Clinical experience shows that two basic facts about food intake are not consciously understood by many teens with weight problems. One is that the body needs food. Teens are used to eating food because they "like it," because "it tastes good," or because "it looks good." At the same time, they feel guilty about eating anything. Helping them to understand the need for a basic amount of food can help to liberate them from unnecessary guilt and can enable them to establish reasonable intake goals. The second fact, a refinement of the first, is that they must consider the nutrient content of the food they eat as well as the energy level. They are used to thinking of "calories" as bad and fail to realize that they can manipulate energy levels of intake while maintaining nutrient contents at necessary levels. Because teens are used to thinking of calories as mass, the current use by nutritionists of the term *energy intake* instead of *calorie intake* is especially important. This concept of calories as mass is especially prevalent in teens with eating disorders. That two such basic principles need to be taught to young people today shows how the role of food in our culture has been distorted.

Specific diets have rarely been successful in achieving long-term changes in eating behavior.[118,120,127,128] This is especially true for teens, who tend to rebel against authoritarian techniques and to hold a number of negative views about diets. *Food use retraining,* a series of habit changes planned jointly by the teen and the therapist and instituted in succession over time, will be more acceptable to most teens and is a more realistic way to approach a complex problem.[120]

Because eating habits have developed over a number of years, it is logical that the teen will need considerable time to make changes. Just as a teen cannot suddenly pick up a musical instrument and play it well but will need education, practice, and support to become proficient, most teens will not be able to adopt a new pattern as represented by a "diet" and perfect it immediately. Intensive treatment will usually need to be continued for a year or more to accomplish major dietary changes.[120] Breaking down the problem of misuse of food into small components makes change more probable.[120] For example, if a teen eats nothing throughout the day until after school and then overeats until bedtime, the logical step may be to add food earlier in the day. What habit will be the initial focus, how change will be accomplished, what foods will be eaten, and what motivations and rewards will be effective are developed and clarified in counseling sessions between the therapist and the teenager.

The therapist's objective is eventually to focus on each time and point in the day and environment where teenagers meet with food (for example, morning hours, school hours, after school, snack time, the dinner hour, night eating, parties, eating out, and family celebrations) and to help teens to retrain themselves in food's use. Most teens will have some reasonable habits that can be supported and used as a foundation for the emerging positive patterns.

Teenagers will need to be helped at every step to take responsibility for their own actions.[116] This process will educate teens about the steps necessary to bring eating habits under control. Coupled with psychological support, the process can lead to effective change. Even teens who are unsuccessful in retraining themselves during the adolescent period will have a model for the future, when they may be able to take greater control. Education regarding physiological factors of obesity will help teens to avoid the harmful quick-loss plans to which they are so vulnerable.[22,122]

An important component of this education involves informing the teen that rapid weight loss accomplished by either starvation or very low energy intake is ineffective. Since the loss is in lean body mass and fluids, it will inevitably be regained when normal eating is resumed.[103] The deprivation in such a regimen often leads to greater overeating. Thus the final result of a "crash" diet is often a net gain. It is not difficult to convince those who have had the experience a few times that such practices are ineffective, but it is important to support their impressions by teaching them the physiological reasons. Teens who will not be convinced that such methods are "unhealthy" will be deterred from using them by the knowledge that they will not lose fat. The propensity to use "diet aids" as described in Fig. 4-2 also needs to be countered by education designed to show their lack of effect, not by vague warnings about harm.

There are certain life-threatening situations where drastic measures will be necessary. As in cases of severe starvation, there are few clear signs that obesity has reached a critical stage. The physical condition should be monitored so that a rapid deterioration can be detected. The following are indications that hospitalization is warranted:

Sudden changes in cardiac and respiratory function

Inability to move, maintain balance, or travel

Rapid accumulation of weight because of the above

Inability to fit into furniture resulting in need to rest on floor

Ulcerations at pressure points and areas of friction

As with the anorexic teen, a period of separation from the family may break up a pernicious cycle leading to physical deterioration.

A comprehensive treatment using a modified fast as the dietary component is at present the most practical therapy.[129] Although it is still controversial whether lean body mass can be spared, such dietary methods appear less objectionable than other radical procedures.[103] The important elements of such a regimen are the behavioral and exercise components and the opportunities for constant monitoring of the biochemical state afforded by hospitalization. Educational and vocational components will often be necessary for the teenager, and individual and family counseling will be needed for those still living with a family.

Following weight loss, there will be a gradual renourishment of the individual until a normally balanced, moderate energy intake has been achieved.[129] Supported by counseling, this should accomplish the reeducation of the patient. The teen will also need to practice newly learned eating habits during increased periods of time outside the hospital setting. Plans should be made to assure that the environment to which the teenager returns will be improved over that in which morbid obesity developed. It may be necessary to help the family consider alternative placement if they feel they will be unable to make sufficient changes to meet the teenager's needs. This will be most appropriate at stages where emancipation is normal.

Energy Output. One of the most important concepts of weight management is that energy output must be increased.[1,110,116,126,130] Chapter 6 gives a full discussion of physical activity as an aspect of weight management. Again, individualized programs need to be developed with the participation of the obese teen to achieve a gradual increase in energy output.[1,126]

The fitness test in the box on p. 144 is designed to be a conservative tool that can safely be used with even the extremely obese. It can be used with or without professional help. Clinical experience has demonstrated that many overweight teens respond more favorably to fitness-improvement therapies than to those directed toward changing dietary patterns. Physically, it appears that increasing movement can be intrinsically rewarding, whereas denying oneself an accustomed food intake is more like punishment. Besides fitness testing and improvement, various strategies can be directed toward increasing energy output. These guidelines should be followed: (1) activities should be built into everyday life[114]; (2) the activities should be things the teen enjoys or finds useful[114]; (3) the teen should not be dependent on help from others or complex equipment; and (4) the activities should be unstressful in the sense that they do not cause embarrassing exposure.

Components of a Comprehensive Weight Management Program with Applicable Treatment Modalities

Food Management	Energy-Time Management	Psychosocial Adjustment
Food use retraining	Fitness testing and improvement programs	Supportive counseling
Nutrition education	Relaxation training	Family counseling
Behavior modification	Movement and dance therapy	Social skills training
Diet prescription	Expanded interest stimulation	Assertion training
		Psychotherapy
		Group support

Apart from designing all aspects of fitness improvement for the individual teen, a clinician will need to supply continuing support to enable the person to carry out such a program.

Strategies Directed Toward Psychological Factors. Weight management for teens should be a total rehabilitation program.[88,120] It demands a significant length of time[88,119,120] and must be individualized.[20,83]

Like the energy-output component, the psychological component of any weight-management problem cannot be overlooked.[88,92,120,130] In a short-term situation where the teen has a few pounds to lose, the problem is one of "motivation."[103] This can be provided in settings such as schools and many other community institutions. With extreme developmental obesity, changes usually will require extensive psychotherapeutic intervention, which includes the family when the teenagers are living at home.[10,20,92,119,120] For teens falling between the two extremes, a variable degree of supportive counseling will be needed to increase self-acceptance, to decrease stress, to facilitate development, and to enable adolescents to carry out weight-management strategies.* The teens need help in learning to experience the body's signals related to hunger and satiety and to adopt nondestructive coping mechanisms to re-

place the misuse of food. Techniques described in Chapter 10 will enable therapists of various disciplines to develop a relationship in which such goals can be accomplished.

Strategies such as camp settings,[131] supportive groups,[88,131] peer counseling, social skills and assertion training, body awareness experience,[132] and behavior modification[1,24,133,134] can be employed successfully with certain individuals. Groups and preplanned programs will help those adolescents with mild, relatively simple problems. However, none of these techniques provides a solution for all aspects of obesity. The techniques must be applied within the context of ongoing supportive counseling by professionals who assess the specific problems of an individual over time and choose the appropriate treatment modalities.[92] A team of professionals (see Chapter 10) will be best able to carry out a comprehensive program as described in the box above.[20,93]

Early reports declaring behavior modification techniques to be the answer to problems of weight control have not been upheld. Compliance appears to be extremely difficult for teens because of the need to reject control at this stage of psychological development. A recent review[135] holds out hope that behavioral specialists are becoming more aware of the need to consider a broader range of the circumstances surrounding human behavioral change. This could lead to the development of

---

*References 10, 20, 88, 92, 93, 102.

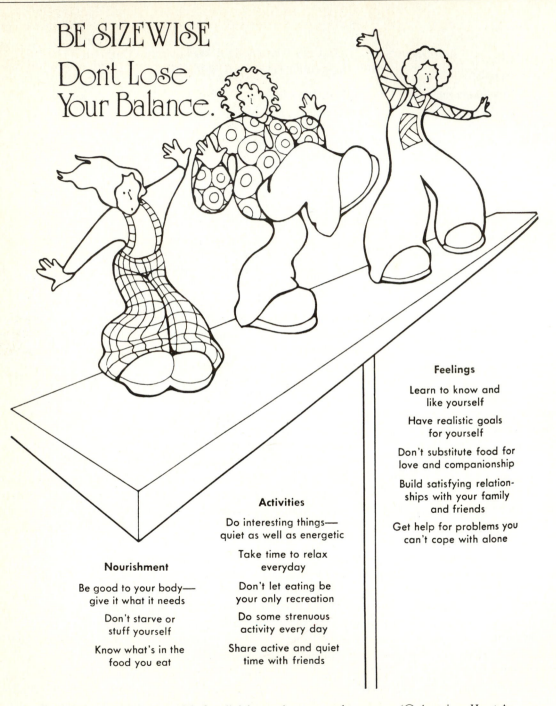

BE SIZEWISE
Don't Lose
Your Balance.

Feelings

Learn to know and
like yourself

Have realistic goals
for yourself

Don't substitute food for
love and companionship

Build satisfying relationships with your family
and friends

Get help for problems you
can't cope with alone

Activities

Do interesting things—
quiet as well as energetic

Take time to relax
everyday

Don't let eating be
your only recreation

Do some strenuous
activity every day

Share active and quiet
time with friends

Nourishment

Be good to your body—
give it what it needs

Don't starve or
stuff yourself

Know what's in the
food you eat

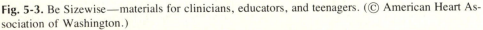

Fig. 5-3. Be Sizewise—materials for clinicians, educators, and teenagers. (© American Heart Association of Washington.)

more flexible techniques with less rigid time, content, form, and frequency constraints and greater individualization.[135] Clinicians would find improved behavioral techniques useful.

Parents need to be counseled to support their teenagers in learning to manage weight.[120] Education about the physiological factors surrounding overweight and rational approaches to management will help dispel detrimental myths parents hold. Helping them to develop a nonintrusive attitude toward their teens is of extreme importance. The counselor can demonstrate this by stressing the need for the teenager, not the counselor or the parent, to establish his or her own goals.

Education and Support in School and Community. Teachers, counselors, nurses, coaches, and other community leaders of adolescents have many opportunities to educate and support overweight teenagers.[126,130] Although they are rarely in the position to carry out therapy because of the complexity of the problem and the time demanded, there is much they can do. Curricula are being developed for the teaching of weight-management courses in schools. Such courses will be beneficial to the population as a whole and should not be limited to heavy teens. Appropriate goals are educational, not therapeutic. Concerning teens with weight problems, by encouraging them to increase healthful exercise and decrease unnecessary energy intake and by giving them positive support for development of realistic goals, adults can help the teens cope with their situation.

Those who have serious problems should be identified by screening for abnormal physical function, height/weight ratio, and psychosocial development. They should be referred to consulting dietitians, nutritionists, counselors, or physicians. Guidelines and educational plans for teenagers and those working with them are provided by the Be Sizewise* materials as illustrated by Fig. 5-3.

---

*Distributed by the American Heart Association of Washington, 4414 Woodland Park North, Seattle, Wash., 98103.

Outcome of Intervention Strategies

Reviews of the outcome of weight-management therapies for teens are uniformly gloomy.[22,120,136] In general such studies are designed as studies of *weight loss,* when informed workers in the field of adolescent health have stressed the importance of focusing on the other benefits of weight-management programs such as increased self-esteem.[20,88,93,102] A list of positive outcomes is included here to suggest realistic goals of comprehensive weight-management programs and educational projects for adolescents:

Increased self-esteem

Increased knowledge of nutritional principles of weight management

Increased knowledge of personal needs for nourishment

Improved control of food-related behaviors

Increased awareness of the role of exercise in weight management

Increased participation in energy-demanding activities

Increased awareness of the role of social and psychological factors in weight management

Increased participation in normal teen life

Improved ability to function in social situations

Improved ability to establish meaningful relationships

Greater ability to separate from enmeshing family

Improved body image

Ability to focus on aspects of themselves apart from weight

Ability to evaluate weight-loss plans

More realistic understanding of psychological and physiological aspects of their weight problem, including implications for their future goals

Greater readiness for bringing energy intake and output under control

Future research should be directed toward methods for accomplishing these more realistic expectations. These outcomes may not be labeled ''cost-effective'' or ''efficient,'' but they definitely contribute to the overall well-being of the patients as they prepare for adulthood.

SUMMARY

The spectrum of eating disorders affects adolescents physically, psychologically, and socially. Intervention strategies must be directed toward both the nutritional and developmental aspects of these disorders to be effective. Goals must be established in relation to all aspects. Helping patients put food into reasonable perspective in their lives will be a principal goal of nutritional therapy. A recognition of the amount of time required for effective intervention is of extreme importance in a basic understanding of eating disorders.

REFERENCES

1. Brownell, K.D., and Stunkard, A.J.: Behavioral treatment for obese children and adolescents. In Stunkard, A.J., editor: Obesity, Philadelphia, 1980, W.B. Saunders Co.
2. Lester, E.P.: Anorexia nervosa and obesity: recent developments, Can. J. Psychiatry 26:211, 1981.
3. Dally, P., and Gomez, J.: Anorexia nervosa, London, 1979, William Heinemann Medical Books, Ltd.
4. Crisp, A.H., Palmer, R.L., and Kalucy, R.S.: How common is anorexia nervosa: a prevalence study, Br. J. Psychiatry 218:549, 1976.
5. Duddle, M.: An increase of anorexia nervosa in a university population, Br. J. Psychiatry 123:711, 1973.
6. Crisp, A.H.: Anorexia nervosa: let me be, New York, 1980, Grune & Stratton, Inc.
7. Hasan, M.K., and Tibbetts, R.W.: Primary anorexia nervosa (weight phobia) in males, Postgrad. Med. J. 53:146, 1977.
8. Vigersky, R.A., and others: Anorexia nervosa: behavioral and hypothalamic aspects, Clin. Endocrinol. Metab. 5:517, 1976.
9. Bruch, H.: Developmental considerations of anorexia nervosa and obesity, Can. J. Psychiatry 26:212, 1981.
10. Bruch, H.: Eating disorders, New York, 1973, Basic Books, Inc., Publishers.
11. Fisher, S.: Body experience in fantasy and behavior, New York, 1970, Appleton-Century-Crofts.
12. Garfinkel, P.E., Moldofsky, H., and Garner, D.M.: The outcome of anorexia nervosa: significance of clinical features, body image and behavior modification. In Viger-

sky, R.A., editor: Anorexia nervosa, New York, 1977, Raven Press.
13. Garner, D.M.: Body image in anorexia nervosa, Can. J. Psychiatry 26:224, 1981.
14. Dwyer, J.P., and others: Adolescent attitudes toward weight and appearance, J. Nutr. Ed. 1(2):14, 1969.
15. Kaufmann, N.A., Poznanski, R., and Guggenheim, K.: Teen-agers dieting for weight control, Nutr. Metab. 16:30, 1974.
16. Garfinkel, P.E.: Some recent observations on the pathogenesis of anorexia nervosa, Can. J. Psychiatry 26:218, 1981.
17. Fransella, F., and Crisp, A.H.: Comparisons of weight concepts in groups of neurotic, normal and anorexic females, Br. J. Psychiatry 134:79, 1979.
18. Slade, P.D., and Russell, G.F.M.: Awareness of body dimensions in anorexia nervosa: cross-sectional and longitudinal studies, Psychol. Med. 3:188, 1973.
19. Casper, R.C., and others: Disturbances in body image estimation as related to other characteristics and outcome in anorexia nervosa, Br. J. Psychiatry 134:60, 1979.
20. Hammar, S.L., and others: An interdisciplinary study of adolescent obesity J. Pediatr. 80:373, 1972.
21. Huenemann, R.L., and others: Adolescent food practices associated with obesity, Fed. Proc. 25:4, 1966.
22. Dwyer, J.P., and Mayer, J.: The dismal condition: problems faced by obese adolescent girls in American society. In Bray, G.A., editor: Obesity in perspective, vol. 2, part 2, Washington, D.C., 1973, U.S. Government Printing Office.
23. Stunkard, A.J., and Mendelson, M.: Obesity and the body image. I. Characteristics of disturbances in the body image of some obese persons, Am. J. Psychiatry 123:1296, 1967.
24. Stuart, R.B.: Behavioral control of overeating: a status report. In Bray, G.A., editor: Obesity in perspective, vol. 2, 2 parts, Washington, D.C., 1973, U.S. Government Printing Office.
25. Minuchin, S., Rosman, B.L., and Baker, L.: Psychosomatic families: anorexia nervosa in context, Cambridge, Mass. 1978, Harvard University Press.
26. Pyle, R., Mitchell, J.E., and Eckert, E.D.: Bulimia: a report of 34 cases, J. Clin. Psychiatry 42(2):60, 1981.
27. Garfinkel, P.E.: Perception of hunger and satiety in anorexia nervosa, Psychol. Med. 4:309, 1974.
28. Casper, R.C., and Davis, J.M.: On the course of anorexia nervosa, Am. J. Psychiatry 134:9, 1977.
29. Anderson, A.E.: Atypical anorexia nervosa. In Vigersky, R.A., editor: Anorexia nervosa, New York, 1977, Raven Press.
30. Crisp, A.H., and others: The long-term prognosis in anorexia nervosa: some factors predictive of outcome. In

Vigersky, R.A., editor: Anorexia nervosa, New York, 1977, Raven Press.

31. Rosman, B.L., and others: A family approach to anorexia nervosa: study, treatment and outcome. In Vigersky, R.A., editor: Anorexia nervosa, New York, 1977, Raven Press.

32. Galdston, R.: Mind over matter: observations on fifty patients hospitalized with anorexia nervosa, J. Am. Acad. Child Psychiatry 13:24, 1974.

33. Garner, D.M., and others: Cultural expectations of thinness in women, Psychol. Rep. 47:483, 1980.

34. Mahler, M.S., Pine, F., and Bergman, A.: The psychological birth of the human infant, New York, 1975, Basic Books, Inc., Publishers.

35. Gesell, A., and Ilg, F.L.: Feeding behavior of infants, Philadelphia, 1937, J.B. Lippincott Co.

36. Vigersky, R.A., and Loriaux, D.L.: Anorexia nervosa as a model of hypothalamic dysfunction. In Vigersky, R.A., editor: Anorexia nervosa, New York, 1977, Raven Press.

37. Vigersky, R.A., and Anderson, A.E.: Conclusions. In Vigersky, R.A., editor: Anorexia nervosa, New York, 1977, Raven Press.

38. Bruch, H.: Psychological antecedents of anorexia nervosa. In Vigersky, R.A., editor: Anorexia nervosa, New York, 1977, Raven Press.

39. Russell, G.F.M.: General management of anorexia nervosa and difficulties in assessing efficacy of treatment. In Vigersky, R.A., editor: Anorexia nervosa, New York, 1977, Raven Press.

40. Silverman, J.A.: Anorexia nervosa: clinical and metabolic observations in a successful treatment plan. In Vigersky, R.A., editor: Anorexia nervosa, New York, 1977, Raven Press.

41. Smart, D.E., Beumont, P.J.V., and George, G.C.W.: Some personality characteristics of patients with anorexia nervosa, Br. J. Psychiatry 128:57, 1976.

42. Story, I.: Caricature and impersonating the other: observations from the psychotherapy of anorexia nervosa, Psychiatry 39:176, 1976.

43. Levitan, H.L.: Implications of certain dreams reported by patients in a bulimic phase of anorexia nervosa, Can. J. Psychiatry 26:228, 1981.

44. Keys, A., and others: The biology of human starvation, 2 vols., Minneapolis, 1950, University of Minnesota Press.

45. Frisch, R.E., and McArthur, J.W.: Menstrual cycles: fatness as a determinant of minimum weight for height necessary for their maintenance or onset, Science 185:949, 1974.

46. Rakoff, A.E.: Psychogenic factors in anovulatory women. I. Hormonal patterns in women with ovarian dysfunction of psychogenic origin, Fertil. Steril. 13:1, 1962.

47. Lucas, A.R.: On the meaning of laboratory values in anorexia nervosa, Mayo Clin. Proc. 52:748, 1977.

48. Bowers, T.K., and Eckert, E.: Leukopenia in anorexia nervosa: lack of increased risk of infection, Arch. Intern. Med. 138:1520, 1978.

49. Drossman, D.A., Ontjes, D.A., and Heizer, W.D.: Anorexia nervosa, Gastroenterology 77:1115, 1979.

50. Halmi, K.A., and others: Pretreatment evaluation in anorexia nervosa. In Vigersky, R.A., editor: Anorexia nervosa, New York, 1977, Raven Press.

51. Blinder, B.J., Freeman, D.M.A., and Stunkard, A.J.: Behavior therapy of anorexia nervosa: effectiveness of activity as a reinforcer of weight gain, Am. J. Psychiatry 126:77, 1970.

52. Burman, K.D., and others: Investigations concerning thyroxine deiodinative pathways in patients with anorexia nervosa. In Vigersky, R.A., editor: Anorexia nervosa, New York, 1977, Raven Press.

53. Hematology of anorexia nervosa, Nutr. Rev. 31:207, 1973.

54. Robboy, A.S., Sato, A.S., and Schwabe, A.D.: The hypercarotenemia in anorexia nervosa: a comparison of vitamin A and carotene levels in various forms of menstrual dysfunction and cachexia, Am. J. Clin. Nutr. 27:362, 1974.

55. Goldberg, S.C., and others: Pretreatment predictors of weight change in anorexia nervosa. In Vigersky, R.A., editor: Anorexia nervosa, New York, 1977, Raven Press.

56. Boyar, R.M., and Bradlow, H.L.: Studies of testosterone metabolism in anorexia nervosa. In Vigersky, R.A., editor: Anorexia nervosa, New York, 1977, Raven Press.

57. McArthur, J.W., and others: Endocrine studies during the refeeding of young women with nutritional amenorrhea and infertility, Mayo Clin. Proc. 51:607, 1976.

58. Moshang, T., and Utiger, R.D.: Low tiiodothyronine euthyroidism. In Vigersky, R.A., editor: Anorexia nervosa, New York, 1977, Raven Press.

59. Wakeling, A., DeSouza, B., and Beardwook, C.J.: Effects of administered estrogen on luteinizing-hormone release in subjects with anorexia nervosa in acute and recovery stages. In Vigersky, R.A., editor: Anorexia nervosa, New York, 1977, Raven Press.

60. Brown, G.M., and others: Endocrine profiles in anorexia nervosa. In Vigersky, R.A., editor: Anorexia nervosa, New York, 1977, Raven Press.

61. Casper, R.C., Davis, J.M., and Pandey, G.N.: The effect of the nutritional status and weight changes on hypothalamic function tests in anorexia nervosa. In Vigersky, R.A., editor: Anorexia nervosa, New York, 1977, Raven Press.

62. Boyar, R.M., and Katz, J.: Twenty-four hour gonadotropin secretory patterns in anorexia nervosa. In Vigersky, R.A., editor: Anorexia nervosa, New York, 1977, Raven Press.

63. Warren, M.P.: Weight loss and responsiveness to LH-RH. In Vigersky, R.A., editor: Anorexia nervosa, New York, 1977, Raven Press.

64. Abroms, G.M.: Defining milieu therapy, Arch. Gen. Psychiatry **21**:553, 1969.

65. Eckert, E.D., and others: Behavior therapy in anorexia nervosa, Br. J. Psychiatry **134**:55, 1979.

66. Argas, S., and Werne, J.: Behavior modification in anorexia nervosa: research foundations. In Vigersky, R.A., editor: Anorexia nervosa, New York, 1977, Raven Press.

67. Pertschuk, M.J.: Behavior therapy: extended followup. In Vigersky, R.A., editor: Anorexia nervosa, New York, 1977, Raven Press.

68. Stunkard, A.J.: New therapies for eating disorders, Arch. Gen. Psychiatry **26**:391, 1972.

69. Bruch, H.: Perils of behavior modification in treatment of anorexia nervosa, JAMA **230**:1419, 1974.

70. Maxmen, J.S., Silverfarb, P.M., and Ferrell, R.B.: Anorexia nervosa: practical initial management in a general hospital, JAMA **229**:801, 1974.

71. Needleman, H.L., and Waber, D.: the use of amitriptyline. In Vigersky, R.A., editor: Anorexia nervosa, New York, 1977, Raven Press.

72. Crisp, A.H.: A treatment regime for anorexia nervosa, Br. J. Psychiatry **112**:505, 1965.

73. White, J.N., Kelly, P., and Dorman, K.: Clinical picture of atypical anorexia nervosa associated with hypothalamic tumor, Am. J. Psychiatry **134**:323, 1977.

74. Morgan, H.G.: Fasting girls and our attitudes to them, Br. Med. J. **2**:1652, 1977.

75. Rutishauser, I.H.E., and McCance, R.A.: Calorie requirements for growth after severe under-nutrition, Arch. Dis. Child. **43**:252, 1968.

76. Stordy, B.J., and others: Weight gain, thermic effect of glucose and resting metabolic rate during recovery from anorexia nervosa, Am. J. Clin. Nutr. **30**:138, 1977.

77. Walker, J., and others: Caloric requirements for weight gain in anorexia nervosa, Am. J. Clin. Nutr. **32**:1396, 1979.

78. Brozek, J.: Starvation and nutritional rehabilitation, J. Am. Diet. Assoc. **28**:917, 1952.

79. Hsu, L.K.G.: Outcome of anorexia nervosa, Arch. Gen. Psychiatry **37**:1041, 1980.

80. Hsu, L.K.G., Crisp, A.H., and Harding, B.: Outcome of anorexia nervosa, Lancet **1**:61, 1979.

81. Fairburn, C.: A cognitive behavioral approach to the treatment of bulimia, Psychol. Med. **11**:707, 1981.

82. Bray, G.A., editor: Obesity in America, Washington, D.C., 1979, National Institutes of Health.

83. Hammar, S.L.: Obesity and the pediatrician, Am. J. Dis. Child. **125**:787, 1973.

84. Allon, N.: Self-perceptions of the stigma of overweight in relationship to weight-losing patterns, Am. J. Clin. Nutr. **32**:470, 1979.

85. Allon, N.: The stigma of overweight in everyday life. In Bray, G.A., editor: Obesity in perspective, vol. 2, 2 parts, Washington, D.C., 1973, U.S. Government Printing Office.

86. Hirsch, J.: The psychological consequences of obesity. In Bray, G.A., editor: Obesity in perspective, vol. 2, 2 parts, Washington, D.C., 1973, U.S. Government Printing Office.

87. Werkman, S.L., and Greenberg, E.S.: Personality and interest patterns in obese adolescent girls, Psychosom. Med. **29**:72, 1967.

88. Hammar, S.L.: The obese adolescent, J. Sch. Health **35**:246, 1965.

89. Monello, L.F., and Mayer, J.: Obese adolescent girls: an unrecognized ''minority group''? J. Clin. Nutr. **13**:35, 1963.

90. Stunkard, A.J., and Burt, V.: Obesity and the body image. II. Age at onset of disturbances in the body image, Am. J. Psychiatry **123**:1443, 1967.

91. Bruch, H.: The psychological handicaps of the obese. In Bray, G.A., editor: Obesity in perspective, vol. 2, 2 parts, Washington, D.C., 1973, U.S. Government Printing Office.

92. Steele, C.I.: Obese adolescent girls: some diagnostic and treatment considerations, Adolescence **9**:81, 1974.

93. Hammar, S.L., Campbell, C., and Woolley, J.: Treating adolescent obesity: long-range evaluation of previous therapy, Clin. Pediatr. **10**:46, 1971.

94. Stanley, E.J., and others: Overcoming obesity in adolescence, Clin. Pediatr. **9**:29, 1970.

95. Tobias, A.L., and Gordon, J.B.: Social consequences of obesity, J. Am. Diet. Assoc. **76**:338, 1980.

96. Mayer, J.: Overweight: causes, cost, and control, Englewood Cliffs, N.J., 1968, Prentice-Hall, Inc.

97. Johnson, M.L., Burke, B.S., and Mayer, J.: Relative importance of inactivity and overeating in the energy balance of obese high school girls, Am. J. Clin. Nutr. **4**:37, 1956.

98. Stefanik, P.A., Heald, F.P., and Mayer, J.: Caloric intake in relation to energy output of obese and non-obese adolescent boys, Am. J. Clin. Nutr. **7**:55, 1959.

99. Hinton, M.A., and others: Eating behavior and dietary intake of girls 12 to 14 years old, J. Am. Diet. Assoc. **43**:223, 1963.

100. Stunkard, A.J.: The pain of obesity, Palo Alto, Calif., 1976, Bull Publishing Co.

101. Rodin, J.: The externality theory today. In Stunkard, A.J., editor: Obesity, Philadelphia, 1980, W.B. Saunders Co.

102. Heald, F.P., and Kahn, M.A.: Teenage obesity, Pediatr. Clin. North Am. **20:**807, 1973.

103. Mahan, L.K.: A sensible approach to the obese patient, Nurs. Clin. North Am. **14:**229, 1979.

104. Stunkard, A.J., editor: Obesity, Philadelphia, 1980, W.B. Saunders Co.

105. Howard, A., editor: Recent advances in obesity research, I, Westport, Conn., 1974, Technomic Publishing Co., Inc.

106. Sjöström, L.: Fat cells and body weight. In Stunkard, A.J., editor: Obesity, Philadelphia, 1980, W.B. Saunders Co.

107. Foch, T.T., and McLearn, G.E.: Genetics, body weight and obesity. In Stunkard, A.J., editor: Obesity, Philadelphia, 1980, W.B. Saunders Co.

108. Keesey, R.E.: A set-point analysis of the regulation of body weight. In Stunkard, A.J., editor: Obesity, Philadelphia, 1980, W.B. Saunders Co.

109. Bray, G.A., editor: Obesity in perspective. vol. 2, 2 parts, Washington, D.C., 1973, U.S. Government Printing Office.

110. Björntorp, P., and others: Effect of an energy-reduced dietary regimen in relation to adipose tissue cellularity in obese women, Am. J. Clin. Nutr. **28:**445, 1975.

111. Sims, E.A.H.: Experimental obesity, dietary-induced thermogenesis and their clinical implication, Clin. Endocrinol. Metab. **5:**377, 1976.

112. Elliot, J.: Blame it all on brown fat now, JAMA **243:** 1983, 1980.

113. DeLuise, M., Blackburn, G.L., and Flier, J.S.: Reduced activity of the red-cell sodium-potassium pump in human obesity, N. Engl. J. Med. **303:**1017, 1980.

114. Huenemann, R.L., and others: Teenagers' activities and attitudes toward activity, J. Am. Diet. Assoc. **51:**433, 1967.

115. Schwartz, R.S., and Brunzell, J.D.: Increased adipose-tissue lipoprotein-lipase activity in moderately obese men after weight reduction, Lancet **1:**1230, 1978.

116. Young, C.M.: Dietary treatment of obesity. In Bray, G.A., editor: Obesity in perspective, vol. 2, 2 parts, Washington, D.C., 1973, U.S. Government Printing Office.

117. Halsted, C.H., and Stern, J.S.: ASCN workshop on obesity and its treatments, Sacramento, California, October 5, 1979, Am. J. Clin. Nutr. **33:**1326, 1980.

118. Munves, E.: Managing the diet. In Stunkard, A.J., editor: Obesity, Philadelphia, 1980, W.B. Saunders Co.

119. Daniel, W.A.: Adolescents in health and disease, St. Louis, 1977, The C.V. Mosby Co.

120. Coates, T.J., and Thoresen, C.E.: Treating obesity in children and adolescents: a review, Am. J. Public Health **68:**144, 1978.

121. Seltzer, C.C., and Mayer, J.: Body build and obesity: who are the obese? JAMA **189:**677, 1964.

122. Dwyer, J.P.: Sixteen popular diets: brief nutritional analyses. In Stunkard, A.J., editor: Obesity, Philadelphia, 1980, W.B. Saunders Co.

123. Björntorp, P.: Renaissance of a new frontier in obesity research, Acta Med. Scand. **196:**145, 1974.

124. Webb, P.: The measurement of energy exchange in man: an analysis, Am. J. Clin. Nutr. **33:**1299, 1980.

125. Webb, P., Annis, J.S., and Troutman, S.J.: Energy balance in man measured by direct and indirect calorimetry, Am. J. Clin. Nutr. **33:**1287, 1980.

126. Christakis, G., and others: Effect of a combined nutrition education and physical fitness program on the weight status of obese high school boys, Fed. Proc. **25:**15, 1966.

127. Van Itallie, T.B., Yang, M., and Hashim, S.A.: Diet and non-drug therapy. In Howard, A., editor: Recent advances in obesity research, I, Westport, Conn., 1974, Technomic Publishing Co., Inc.

128. Leon, G.R.: Current directions in the treatment of obesity, Psychol. Bull. **83:**557, 1967.

129. Lindner, P.G., and Blackburn, G.L.: Multidisciplinary approach to obesity utilizing fasting modified by protein-sparing therapy, Obesity and Bariatric Med. **5:**198, 1976.

130. Seltzer, C.C., and Mayer, J.: An effective weight control program in a public school system, Am. J. Public Health **60:**679, 1970.

131. Brandt, G., Maschhoff, T., and Chandler, N.S.: A residential camp experience as an approach to adolescent weight management, Adolescence **15:**807, 1980.

132. Harris, R., Nolte, D., and Nolte, C.: Effects of intervention on teenagers' physical and psychological identity, Psychol. Rep. **46:**505, 1980.

133. Mellin, L.: Shapedown: weight management programs for adolescents, San Francisco, 1983, Balboa Publishing Co.

134. Bellack, A.S.: Behavior therapy for weight reduction, Addict. Behav. **1:**73, 1975.

135. Wilson, G.T.: Behavior modification and the treatment of obesity. In Stunkard, A.J., editor: Obesity, Philadelphia, 1980, W.B. Saunders Co.

136. Collipp, D.J.: Obesity in childhood. In Stunkard, A.J., editor: Obesity, Philadelphia, 1980, W.B. Saunders Co.

Chapter 6

Physical Fitness, Athletics, and the Adolescent

L. KATHLEEN MAHAN

Adolescents are interested in how their bodies perform, and this interest in physical performance seems to be growing more popular, especially among teenage girls. Many of these teens are athletes or participate regularly in some kind of organized sport. These teens usually are fairly pleased with the appearance of their bodies and how they perform. Other adolescents, however, participate minimally in physical activity and are likely to be overweight. These teens are not experiencing positive feelings of physical fitness and are slipping into habits of inactivity. They will have less than optimal health in their adult lives because of their less than optimal fitness. These youth are concerned about their bodies, but their feelings usually are negative. They are likely to be unhappy with the shape and performance of their bodies and frustrated with not knowing how to improve them.

Because adolescents are developmentally in a phase of exploration and experimentation, they are easily attracted to products or programs that are novel and that promise quick changes in body shape and performance. Adolescents' rapid growth and consequent large nutritional requirements make them more physically vulnerable than others to the effects of these products, many of which result in poor dietary intake. It is important to edu-

cate teens in all aspects of physical fitness and its relationship to nutrition so that they can make wise choices and keep their perspective. Education that is geared toward teens' interest in body shape and performance will probably be well accepted and even enthusiastically sought.

PHYSICAL FITNESS

Physical fitness is hard to define, and the term is used loosely. Physical fitness involves both physiological and psychological factors. Only recently has there been any gain in scientific data about the physical component of fitness. Knowledge about the psychological factors is even more sparse. Is physical fitness the ability to get through the day, which may include watching a sport on TV, or is it being able to participate in that sport and do it well? Obviously physical fitness means something different to each person, but guidelines for measuring it objectively are being developed and improved rapidly.

In addition to the psychological and emotional state of an individual, other factors that influence fitness include the following: hormonal balance; amount of sleep; use of drugs, caffeine, alcohol, and tobacco; diet; exercise; and genetic factors such as heart size and strength, lung capacity, number of red blood cells, and composition of the muscle fibers.

Looking at physical fitness from a strictly physiological perspective, fitness can be described in terms of three components: body composition, muscular fitness, and cardiorespiratory fitness.

Body Composition

The body is made up of fat, muscle protein, interstitial fluids, bone minerals, blood plasma and cells, and small amounts of other tissues. In determining the level of physical fitness, it appears that there is a proportion of lean body mass to fat tissue that is ideal or at least better for health and performance. Several techniques of varying accuracy are used to determine the composition of the living body. Table 3-7 describes these techniques. Many usually are reserved for research purposes, but others, such as skinfold or fatfold measurements and body circumferences, have clinical usefulness as discussed in Chapter 3.

Standards for Fatness in Fitness. Most body fat exists in two compartments: *essential fat,* which is in the bone marrow, central nervous system, and other organs, and *storage fat,* which is in the adipose tissue, around the organs, and under the skin. It appears that the body needs a minimal amount of fat, and the essential fat is not subject to dietary changes. Even during prolonged periods of starvation, the leanest men had body fatness of 3% to 4% of body weight.[1] Storage fat, however, is subject to the influence of diet and exercise. In the male essential fat is about 3% of total body weight, but in the female essential fat is about 12% of total body weight. Because of this difference, Behnke[2] has proposed the concept of ''minimal body weight'' in the female. In the male minimal body weight and lean body weight are identical, but in the female minimal body weight incorporates both lean body mass and sex-specific ''essential fat'' in mammary and other tissues (Fig. 6-1).

In rare instances male athletes have been able to maintain body fat as low as the essential fat, and some female athletes or dancers maintain body fat levels at or below minimal weight in the interest of physical performance.[2] In most sports there appears to be no advantage in having excessive amounts of body fat, and most good male athletes have 5% to 8% body fat.[3] The exceptions are some wrestlers, weight lifters, and channel swimmers. (Swimmers with greater percentage body fat will be more buoyant and more protected against the cold water.) Athletes are concerned about the amount of fat in their bodies because fat does not produce energy for performance. Instead, it is weight that must be carried by energy-producing muscle tissue.

However, outside of athletic performance minimal body fat may not be optimal for health. For example, reproductive function seems to be affected by body fatness in the young female. The very lean young female, who frequently is an athlete, may have amenorrhea, dysmenorrhea, or anovulatory menstrual cycles.[4] Menses frequently will resume with a gain in body fatness. Menarche, the onset of menstruation, may also be delayed in very lean female athletes.[5] However, the factors of stress and hard training also can influence the menses and must be kept in mind.[6] Frisch[5] has theorized that the young female must achieve a body fatness of 17% before menses will begin and that the female who has ceased menstruating because of leaness must regain to 22% body fatness before menses will resume. This is discussed further in Chapter 1. Excessive leaness causes an alteration in the lean/fat ratio, and this could affect hormonal regulation of menstrual function.[6]

Regarding optimal fatness in men, recent findings from the Framingham study[7] indicated that adult males who were a small percentage overweight (based on standard weights in life insurance tables) had the lowest mortality rate. There was increased mortality only among those who weighed significantly more or less than average. This may mean that there is also a minimal level of fatness in the male below which health is not op-

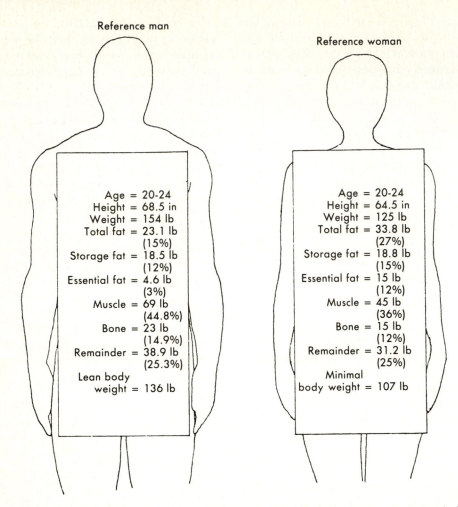

Reference man

Reference woman

Age = 20-24
Height = 68.5 in
Weight = 154 lb
Total fat = 23.1 lb
(15%)
Storage fat = 18.5 lb
(12%)
Essential fat = 4.6 lb
(3%)
Muscle = 69 lb
(44.8%)
Bone = 23 lb
(14.9%)
Remainder = 38.9 lb
(25.3%)
Lean body
weight = 136 lb

Age = 20-24
Height = 64.5 in
Weight = 125 lb
Total fat = 33.8 lb
(27%)
Storage fat = 18.8 lb
(15%)
Essential fat = 15 lb
(12%)
Muscle = 45 lb
(36%)
Bone = 15 lb
(12%)
Remainder = 31.2 lb
(25%)
Minimal
body weight = 107 lb

Fig. 6-1. Lean body weight in the male and minimal body weight in the female. (From Katch, F.I., and McArdle, W.D.: Nutrition, weight control and exercise, Boston, 1977, Houghton Mifflin Co. Copyright © 1977 by Houghton Mifflin Company. Used by permission.)

timal. Optimal fatness for health and longevity may be higher than optimal fatness for athletic performance.

At present we cannot state the optimal level of body fatness for an adolescent. However, in the clinical setting it can still be valuable to use skinfold or girth measurements as baseline information for monitoring changes in the amount of body fat in an adolescent over time.

Muscular Fitness

Muscular fitness, the second component of fitness, is measured in terms of strength, endurance, and flexibility. *Strength* is the ability of the muscular system to exert maximal force against an object or resistance all at once. Almost every sport requires muscular strength, but strength is also necessary to get through a busy day. *Endurance* is the ability to exert force, not necessarily maximal, over an extended period of time. Standing and holding an arm's load of books, for example, brings muscular endurance into play. *Flexibility* is the ability to use the muscles of the body throughout their range of motion. Good flexibility provides increased speed and agility and helps to prevent muscle or joint injuries.

Simple, effective methods for evaluating muscular fitness are available.[8-10]

Biochemical Aspects of Muscle Physiology. In studying muscular fitness it is now possible to look at the biochemistry of the muscle fiber itself. Skeletal muscle is composed of two types of muscle fibers: fast-twitch fibers and slow-twitch fibers. It appears that human beings are born with a predetermined number of the two types. The proportion of the different types of fibers varies with the individual and within a given muscle. Optimal performance in various types of sports seems to have some relationship to muscle-fiber type.

The *fast-twitch* fibers have a high capacity for anaerobic metabolism, especially in the production of adenosine 5'-triphosphate (ATP) from glycolysis, but they also fatigue rapidly because of their lower oxidative capacity.[1] Their contraction is rapid. Because of these characteristics, fast-twitch muscles are activated in short-term, high-intensity activities such as sprinting or weight lifting, which depend almost completely on anaerobic metabolism, and in stop-and-go sports such as tennis, basketball, and hockey. Anaerobic metabolism does not require oxygen.

The *slow-twitch* fibers contract more slowly than fast-twitch fibers. They contain higher lipid stores, many mitochondria (the sites of energy production), and a high concentration of those enzymes needed for aerobic (oxygen-requiring) metabolism.[11] These fibers have a much greater ability to generate ATP aerobically than do fast-twitch fibers. Slow-twitch fibers thus are important for endurance activities, such as long-distance running, that depend on aerobic metabolism for energy.[12,13]

Many sports require both types of fibers for best performance. Fast-twitch fibers are used at the initiation of exercise, before vasodilation, and when substrate delivery to slow-twitch fibers is minimal. As the exercise is prolonged, more slow-twitch fibers are recruited.

Effect of Training on Muscle Physiology and Metabolism. Training does not change an athlete's inherited proportion of muscle-fiber types. However, endurance training can increase the aerobic capacity of both types of fibers, especially of the slow-twitch fibers.[14] Sprint training can increase the size and efficiency of fast-twitch fibers, but the changes following sprint training are not nearly as great as those following endurance training.

Cardiorespiratory Fitness

Cardiorespiratory fitness, or aerobic capacity, is the third component of fitness. Cardiorespiratory fitness is the ability of the body to take oxygen from the atmosphere into the lungs and blood and transport it to the working muscle. At the muscle site, oxygen is used in the mitochrondria to oxidize carbohydrate and fat and to generate ATP, or energy. When cardiorespiratory fitness is low, muscles will not extract oxygen efficiently. The heart thus will need to pump more oxygen-carrying blood and will beat at a faster rate. As fitness improves, the heart and lungs become more efficient in handling oxygen, the heart needs to beat less frequently, and the pulse rate slows. With increased fitness there is greater ability to take in more oxygen: the athlete is able to work or play at a greater level of intensity without breathlessness and for a longer period of time without fatigue. Metabolically, there is an enhanced capacity for the aerobic production of ATP in the muscle, which will be discussed later in this chapter.

The effects of training before and during the rapid growth associated with puberty are not yet clear. There is evidence to suggest that training during puberty, as compared with training after, may be of greater importance in determining the ultimate dimensions of the oxygen transport system.[15-17] Other studies also have shown that, regardless of the type or intensity of the training, the previously untrained adult will not reach the high level of physical performance capacity observed in the individual who has trained since childhood.[18,19]

Because aerobic fitness is based on the ability to take up oxygen, this aspect of fitness is assessed by measuring the maximal amount of oxygen that is taken in during rest and during exercise. This maximal oxygen uptake during exercise is the Vo_2 max. Vo_2 max defines the point at which oxygen consumption and combustion can no longer keep up with the use of ATP by the contracting muscles.

At this point, oxidative, or aerobic, exercise can no longer continue. Oxygen uptake is measured as milliliters of oxygen taken in per kilogram of body weight per minute (ml/kg/min). It can range from 20 ml/kg/min in some sedentary or older people to 70 to 80 ml/kg/min in a top-notch athlete. However, it is more useful to compare teenagers against their own capacities over time than against a group norm. Because the measurement is based on the body weight, it is obvious that the lean person is going to have a better fitness score than the fatter person. The reason why women may have lower aerobic fitness scores than men is because of the

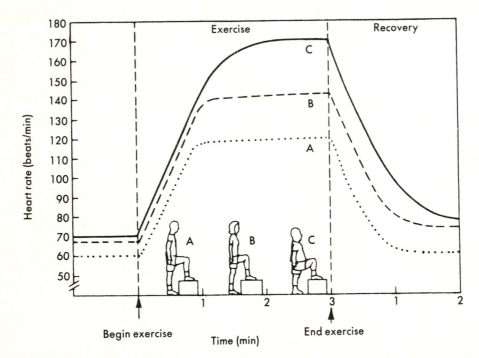

Fig. 6-2. Heart-rate response of three men of different levels of fitness to the same amount of exercise. *A* is in very good shape. He reaches a lower heart rate during the exercise and recovers and returns to his resting heart rate faster. *B* is in mediocre shape aerobically. *C* is sedentary and out-of-shape. His heart rate reaches 170 beats/min during the exercise, and it takes longer for him to recover and return to his resting heart rate. (From Katch, F.I., and McArdle, W.D.: Nutrition, weight control and exercise, Boston, 1977, Houghton Mifflin Co. Copyright © 1977 by Houghton Mifflin Company. Used by permission.)

greater percentage of body fat in the female. If the measurements are compared on lean weight alone rather than total body weight, aerobic fitness scores are comparable between men and women.

Aerobic capacity is measured most accurately in a laboratory by having the teen use an air-collection system while running on a treadmill. However, aerobic fitness can be measured less accurately in the clinical setting without elaborate equipment. It is still possible to give the teen a meaningful evaluation and a goal for improvement.

Because heart rate and oxygen uptake increase proportionately, maximal oxygen uptake and fitness level can be determined by taking the heart rate at rest and during a specified amount of exercise. The resting heart rate, the immediate postexercise heart rate, and the recovery heart rates (heart rates taken at certain times after the exercise is completed) are measured in beats per 10 seconds and multiplied by 6 to yield beats per minute. The *resting heart rate* for a teen is usually between 8 to 13 beats/10 sec.[20] The *immediate postexercise heart rate* is a measure of the body's ability to adapt to increased oxygen demands. The lower this heart rate, the greater the level of fitness. *Recovery heart rates* indicate the time it takes for the heart to return to its normal pace. The greater the level of fitness, the faster the heart rate returns to the resting heart rate, as illustrated in Fig. 6-2. The box on p. 144 presents a method for testing aerobic fitness and beginning a program of improvement suitable for even massively obese or unfit adolescents. A more specific method for aerobic testing that can be done in the clinician's office is given in Appendix J.

Physiology of Fitness

Fat Metabolism. With increased aerobic fitness there is an improvement in the action of the hormones, especially insulin, involved in the regulation of blood glucose and fat deposition and mobilization.[21-23] Instead of being stored as triglycer-

ide in the fat cells, excess blood glucose is better regulated and metabolized for energy production, thus reducing the amount deposited as fat. There is also an increase in the muscle fiber's ability to use fat as an energy source, as evidenced by increased lipoprotein lipase (LPL), which is responsible for the uptake of plasma triglyceride into muscle cells.[24]

Studies also show that the trained person is able to extract a greater percentage of energy from free fatty acids from fat stores in submaximal exertion. This is related to the action of the hormone epinephrine. Epinephrine stimulates the fat cell membrane and activates the enzyme hormone-sensitive lipase (HSL). HSL frees fatty acids from the fat cell to be utilized by the active muscle cells for energy. This process is inhibited by lactic acid produced during exercise when anaerobic metabolism (metabolism without oxygen) is functioning. Because this is the case more of the time in the untrained or unexercised person, the aerobically fit person can work or exercise longer aerobically. The aerobically fit person thus has less lactic acid buildup, less blocking of the action of epinephrine on the adipose cell, and a greater release of fatty acids for energy production.[25]

There is also a decrease in plasma insulin during physical training, which may be important in reducing fat deposition. This occurs after a single bout of exercise[23] even in those with hyperplastic obesity who have been unable to lose weight.[24] The reason for the effect is unknown, but it may be caused by hormonal balance changes or even muscle tissue changes such as an increased sensitivity of muscle tissue to insulin.[25]

It also has been found recently that exercise increases the level of high-density lipoprotein (HDL) cholesterol, which seems to protect against the development of atherosclerosis.[26,27] In addition, low-density lipoprotein (LDL) cholesterol, a risk factor for heart disease, decreases with exercise.[26] The HDL/LDL ratio can improve with exercise in both the obese and nonobese.[28]

Fitness: Testing and Planning Improvement Programs

1. a. Have client sit quietly and relax for 3 to 5 minutes.
   b. Take pulse for 10 seconds.*
   c. Record *resting heart rate (RHR)*: _____
2. a. Find intensity of exercise required to reach *training heart rate (THR)*† immediately after exercise. THR for teens is 20 to 22 beats/10 sec.‡
      Stop with the exercise that achieves 20 to 22 beats/10 sec. This is the exercise to use initially in the improvement program.

↑ Intensity increases	Run for 5 minutes
	Jog for 5 minutes
	Jog for 2 minutes—walk for 2 minutes—jog for 2 minutes
	Walk uphill or upstairs for 2 to 3 minutes
	Walk for 5 minutes at a more rapid pace
START	Walk for 5 minutes at a moderate pace

   b. Monitor pulse return toward RHR after each exercise level—it should be below 16 beats/10 sec by 5 minutes.

      _____   _____   _____   _____
      Immediate ⟶ 1 minute ⟶ 2 minutes ⟶ 5 minutes ⟶ . . .

3. *Improvement program:* To maintain THR for 15 minutes 4 to 5 days/wk:
   a. Work with client to design an individualized program that is comfortable for him or her.
   b. Plan 5-minute warm-up—move at level below the level that maintains THR.
   c. Exercise at intensity that maintains THR.
   d. 5-Minute cool down—back to warm-up speed—client should not sit or lie down immediately.
   e. Use a combination of exercise levels and types, if necessary.
   f. If the client is ill, he or she should begin after illness at lower intensity and return slowly to intensity achieved before illness
4. a. Retest every 3 to 4 weeks
   b. Increase intensity of exercise to maintain THR.
   c. Client can increase time spent doing the exercise by 5-minute increments, up to 30 minutes.
   d. When client has reached jogging level and maintained it for 6 to 8 weeks, increase THR to 22 to 25 beats/10 sec.
   e. Client can use any aerobic activities (for example, jogging, bicycling, skating, dancing) or combinations that the client prefers.

From Pipes, P.L.: Nutrition in infancy and childhood, St. Louis, 1981, The C.V. Mosby Co.; developed by Scott, B., and Rees, J., Adolescent Program, University of Washington, Seattle, Wash.

*10-second time segment is easiest to measure and use.

†*Maximum heart rate (MHR)* is approximately 200 beats/min for persons under 20 years of age (Cumming, G.R., Everatt, D., and Hastman, L.: Am. J. Cardiol. **41**:69, 1978). THR is 60% of MHR for persons with poor initial fitness, 75% of MHR for persons who are fit (that is, 60% of 200 = 120 beats/min = 20 beats/10 sec [20 to 22 beats/10 sec for normal variation]).

‡An adolescent of normal weight and in reasonable shape may want to start at 22 to 25 beats/10 sec.

NOTE: Contraindications for testing and initiating fitness program will be revealed by routine medical history and physical examination.

In addition, serum triglyceride levels were found to be lowered with aerobic exercise. However, the dietary approach to lowering serum triglycerides was found to be more effective than exercise.[29] Rigorous exercise, whether before or after a meal, also seemed to reduce postmeal lipemia.[30]

Thermogenesis. Originally termed luxuskonsumption, *thermogenesis* is defined as an increase in heat production and a dissipation of energy that results in the maintenance of stable body weight in the presence of excessive energy intake. Thermogenesis can be diet-induced, exercise-induced, cold-induced, or drug-induced, as seen with nicotine or caffeine. Thermogenesis is characterized by an increase in oxygen consumption.

The physiological basis for thermogenesis has not been explained, but thyroid hormone, norepinephrine, and the sympathetic nervous system seem to be involved. Thermogenesis is also related to the brown fat in the body. Brown fat, present in only small amounts in the body, is able to use excess energy to produce heat, thus preventing excess ingested calories from being stored as fat.[31]

Important to this discussion is exercise-induced thermogenesis. During the period after exercise, more oxygen is consumed than is required to support resting metabolism. This is known as recovery oxygen or the oxygen debt. After meeting the oxygen requirements for the initial restoration of creatine phosphate stores, the reoxygenation of myoglobin and hemoglobin, and the reconversion of lactate to glucose and glycogen, the body consumes and uses additional oxygen and energy. This excess intake cannot be explained, but the oxygen may be used by substrate cycles that lose heat and burn off energy in thermogenesis.[32] A bout of physical activity may raise the basal metabolic rate through thermogenesis by 25% for 15 hours after the exercise is over. There thus is a continued use of extra energy.[33] Therefore exercise is beneficial for weight control not only because of the energy expenditure during exercise but also because of energy expenditure after the exercise is over.

Appetite Control. Exercise has been thought to increase appetite, and the energy output from exercise thus has been downplayed in weight-reduction programs that focus on diets. In fact, *long* hours of physical labor or work do result in increased appetite and food intake to maintain weight. In normal-weight individuals as energy output increases, energy intake increases to maintain body weight. This is illustrated by animals in Fig. 6-3. However, there also is a low point of energy expenditure below which the energy intake does not decrease proportionately. Below this point, weight gain occurs.[34]

The effect of exercise on appetite control in humans is not as well studied, but it seems that a certain level of physical activity is necessary for maintenance of proper appetite regulation and appropriate body weight.[35]

In the short term, exercise decreases appetite. Most adolescents can attest to the fact that their appetite is depressed right after vigorous physical exercise. Epstein and co-workers[36] demonstrated this in school-age children. Food intake could be decreased in children by scheduling recess before rather than after lunch. Regular vigorous activity of moderate duration (1 to 2 hr/day) does not necessarily stimulate the appetite and cause increased energy intake.[1]

Weight and Fatness Control. Aerobic exercise has the benefit of increasing the percentage of body weight composed of lean body tissue.[2] The increase in lean body tissue from aerobic exercise is probably caused by muscular hypertrophy that may result from the increase in serum growth hormone during exercise.[37,38] Besides promoting growth of lean tissue, growth hormone has a fat-mobilizing function. The increase in growth hormone during exercise thus promotes deposition of protein in lean tissue and mobilization of fat. The end result is a loss of fat and an increase in the proportion of lean tissue.

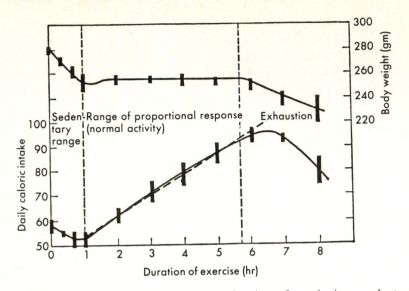

Fig. 6-3. Voluntary caloric intake and body weight as functions of exercise in normal rats. Regulation of food intake generally operates with precision only in the area of "normal activity." With low levels of exercise, an increase in exercise is not accompanied by an increase in food intake. At extremely low levels of activity, voluntary food intake is greater than at moderate levels. In the range of "normal activity," the regulation of food intake is functioning: food intake increases with activity and weight is maintained. At excessively high levels of activity, both food intake and weight decrease. (From the book, Overweight: causes, cost and control by Jean Mayer. © 1968 by Prentice-Hall, Inc. Published by Prentice-Hall, Inc., Englewood Cliffs, N.J. 07632.)

In addition to these changes, exercise causes an increase in energy expenditure from not only thermogenesis but also from energy used during the activity. The expenditure during activity is small compared with the caloric expenditure of basal metabolism, but if consistent it can account for a regular and significant expenditure of energy, a negative energy balance, and a reduction in weight. Exercise alone can reduce body weight, particularly body fat, even when there is no reduction in energy intake. Women lost up to ½ lb/wk when exercise was continued for 30 minutes daily.[39]

In contrast to exercise, diet or caloric restriction for weight control produces a 15% to 30% decrease in the basal metabolic rate (BMR) in both lean and obese persons. This adaptation begins to take place within 24 to 48 hours after caloric restriction is initiated, and it acts to prevent weight reduction. In one study the percentage of BMR change roughly paralleled the percentage of change in body weight. The average BMR drop was 12.3%, and the average weight drop was 13.3%.[40] During periods of energy restriction in animals, metabolic rate falls. BMR falls faster with each low-calorie episode and takes longer to return to baseline with refeeding.[41] It has also been shown in animals that when they are starved to lose weight and then fed again, they are more efficient metabolically in refeeding than they were as normal-weight animals.[42] In addition, during refeeding after energy restriction, there are increases in the ratio of body fat to lean tissue.[43] It is possible then that repeated attempts at weight reduction through diet may lead to a progressive slowing of

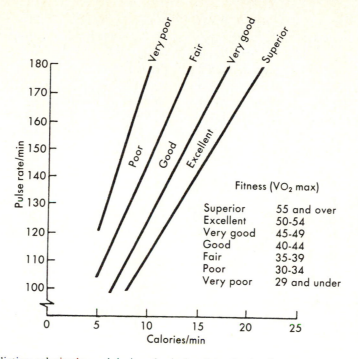

Fig. 6-4. Predicting calories burned during physical activity from pulse rate. (From Sharkey, B.J.: Physiology of fitness, Champaign, Ill., 1979, Human Kinetics Publishers, Inc. © 1979, Human Kinetics Publishers, Inc.)

weight loss and a more rapid regaining of lost weight as fat.[44] On the other hand, increased exercise for weight reduction increases resting metabolic expenditure and offsets the BMR decrease that accompanies energy restriction.

In addition, the protein tissue and water lost from dieting is greater than from exercise-induced weight loss. Exercise has a protein tissue–sparing effect. As much as 35% to 45% of the total weight lost may be lean tissue when weight is lost by caloric restriction alone.[45]

Energy Expenditure of an Activity. The energy expenditure of teens in a physical-activity program depends on their size and the intensity and duration of the activity. For physical activities that require movement of the entire body without support, such as walking, jogging, or stair climbing, the energy

expenditure is very dependent on the size of the individual. The obese teen will use more energy than the slender teen. These activities will promote the most weight reduction in the obese teen and should be encouraged. Many obese teens, even when in sports activities, do not move as much as their slim teammates and need to be encouraged to move more.

In addition to the adolescent's weight, the *intensity* of the activity affects the amount of energy used. Because the intensity is directly related to the amount of oxygen used, the greater the intensity, the more oxygen used and energy expended. The intensity of activity is measured in *metabolic equivalents* (MET), or multiples of the resting metabolic rate. One MET is equal to 3.5 ml oxygen/kg body weight/min. In general 1 L of oxygen used is equal to an energy expenditure of 5 kcal. Since the oxygen uptake is related to the heart rate, it is possible to determine the caloric expenditure of an individual performing a certain activity by measuring the heart rate during that activity. However, the level of fitness also needs to be considered. The caloric expenditure is less for those in low-fitness categories with high heart rates than for those in high-fitness categories with the same heart rate.[25] Fit subjects can use more energy and still have a lower heart rate as demonstrated by the graph in Fig. 6-4. By using this graph, it is possible to determine the energy expenditure per minute when the level of fitness and the pulse rate are known. This difference is another reason why the physically fit teen can control his weight better. The exercise performed by the fit teen uses more energy and thus promotes weight loss or weight maintenance.

A 70-kg (154-lb) male adolescent exercising at an intensity that raises the pulse to 100 beats/min consumes 1 L oxygen/min and thus expends 5 kcal/min. The same teen exercising harder so that his pulse is 170 beats/min consumes 3 L oxygen/min and thus expends 15 kcal/min (or 12.2 MET). Table 6-1 shows the pulse rates and energy expenditures for light, moderate, and heavy activity by a 70-kg (154-lb) adolescent. Appendix K gives the range of energy expenditures of various activities.

Table 6-1. Physical activity and energy expenditure for a 70-kg adolescent

Work Intensity	Pulse Rate	Kcal/min	Examples
Light	Below 120	Under 5	Golf, bowling, walking, volleyball, most forms of work
Moderate*	120-150	5-10	Jogging, tennis, bike riding, handball, basketball, hiking, strenuous work
Heavy	Above 150	Above 10	Running, fast swimming, fast rowing, wrestling, football, handball, squash, other brief and intense efforts

Modified from Sharkey, B.J.: Physiology of fitness, Champaign, Ill., 1979, Human Kinetics Publishers, Inc. © 1979, Human Kinetics Publishers, Inc.
*Preferred for weight-control benefits.

Designing a Fitness Program

Because training during adolescence may have a greater effect on cardiovascular capacity than training started later in life, the awareness of fitness and the beginning of an activity program for the teen is highly important for lifetime fitness. During adolescence, exercise should be systematic and vigorous because natural fitness levels, which are present in most normal-weight children, begin to fall off between 13 and 19 years of age in both boys and girls.[46]

Long-term adherence to exercise programs, especially among overweight persons, is usually poor. At its best, the rate of attrition is 25%.[47] Among teenagers the problem of adherence is even greater, and the reasons for dropping out of an exercise program are more complex. A changing body image, a lack of sustained interest in one activity, peer pressure, independence from parental advice, and a belief in personal infallibility influence the teen's attitude toward exercise. The overweight sedentary teen has even more reasons for disliking activity. These factors need to be considered in designing an exercise program and promoting adherence to it.

Because fitness programs require increased activity, it is useful to look at activity and energy expenditure as being of two types: routine and programmed. Routine activities are those done during the day that can be increased in frequency and duration. These would be activities such as walking, climbing stairs, standing, sitting, moving objects, and doing chores. Since these routine activities are done anyway, they are usually not perceived by the teen as being painful, time consuming, or requiring special skills or equipment. However, even these activities can be disliked and avoided by the heaviest teens. With a positive approach however, these activities can be increased in frequency and duration. Walking to the store, parking as far away from school as possible, using the stairs in buildings, and standing instead of sitting while waiting for the bus are examples of ways to increase energy expenditure by changing routine activities. Most teens do not think of such activities, and if brought to teens' attention they can mean a difference in energy balance.

Programmed activities are those that need to be planned or that require some attention to be included in a day's schedule. Bicycle riding, aerobic dancing, jogging, swimming, or any sport would be a programmed activity. This kind of activity requires a greater behavior change on the part of the adolescent, and the reasons for doing or, more importantly, not doing these activities can be complex. To be most beneficial for aerobic metabolism and weight control, the intensity, duration, and frequency of programmed activities should be specified or prescribed.

As discussed earlier in this chapter, *intensity* is important because it determines the energy or fuel source, the amount of oxygen consumed, and the amount of energy expended during the exercise. Intensity should be individualized depending on the present level of fitness. As the person becomes more fit, the intensity or strenuousness of the exercise should increase so that the appropriate heart rate is maintained.

The intensity of exercise is determined by using the *training heart rate* (THR). The THR is the heart rate that the exercising person must reach to achieve an increase in fitness, and it is based on a percentage of the maximal heart rate physically possible. The maximal heart rate is approximately 200 beats/min for persons under 20 years of age (193 to 204 beats/min).[48] The THR should be 50% of the maximal heart rate for those in poor physical shape (100 beats/min or about 17 beats/10 sec) and between 65% and 75% of the maximal heart rate for those in good physical shape (130 to 150 beats/min or 21 to 25 beats/10 sec). A THR of 60% to 75% of the maximal heart rate should be the goal for regular aerobic exercise to maintain fitness.

Exercising at about 50% to 55% of maximal intensity instead of at 60% to 75% results in greater fat catabolism and more weight-control benefits.[25] If the heart rate or intensity of the exercise is above 60% of maximal intensity, the body shifts to using more carbohydrate and less fat. Fat catabolism should be promoted for weight loss. In addition, the duration of the activity should be increased from 20 to 40 minutes per training session. To reduce body fat, the already fit person should exercise at 70% of the maximal heart rate.[25]

The heart rate should not be measured until after the activity has been maintained for 10 minutes. Before this time, the body is warming up, and the heart rate thus is not a good indicator of the activity intensity. If the heart rate is too high, the adolescent needs to slow down; if the heart rate is too low, the teen needs to speed up and increase the intensity of the exercise. There is no need to exercise at an intensity beyond the THR, but a heart rate below the THR means that an increase in fitness is not being achieved.

Duration of exercise can be prescribed in terms of time, distance covered (for example, in jogging or walking), or energy expended. The amount of energy expended can be used to determine the amount of activity necessary for a training effect because the energy expended depends on both the heart rate (intensity) during the activity and the length of time spent doing it. To achieve a training effect, an adolescent of low fitness should expend 100 to 200 kcal per training session. An adolescent of medium fitness, on the other hand, should expend 200 to 400 kcal per session, and an adolescent of high fitness should expend at least 400 kcal per session. Thus long-duration training (300+ kcal or 20+ minutes) is recommended to gain fitness and to derive the benefits of weight control and improved fat metabolism. In terms of time, exercise should be continued at a pace to maintain the THR for 20 minutes. It should be preceded by a 5- to 10-minute warm-up and followed by a 5- to 10-minute cool-down.

Frequency of exercise determines whether there will be a training effect and metabolic improvements. Two or three nonconsecutive sessions per week are enough to gain the training effect and maintain it. Exercise done less frequently than three times per week has training benefits only for those who are very unfit.

The program explained in the box on p. 144 should be designed to allow the teen to take an active part in its development. In fact, it may be approached from a behavioral-modification point of view with various steps that build on each other. The program should be compatible with the teen's state of fitness to prevent injury, discouragement, or eventual abandonment of the program.

NUTRITIONAL REQUIREMENTS FOR TRAINING

The nutritional requirements of the adolescent athlete are similar to those of the nonathletic adolescent with the exception of energy, carbohydrate, and a few vitamins and minerals. The basic nutritional requirements of adolescents are discussed in Chapter 3.

An important consideration, often forgotten by coaches and athletes in their zeal to perform, is the fact that the adolescent participating in sports may still be growing physically and psychologically.

This growth should not be jeopardized. Psychologically, this means that the teen should continue through the developmental stages. The adolescent's spirit of enthusiasm, self-exploration, and search for identity should be supported. Physically, it means that the body changes of adolescence should continue. There should be maintenance of stamina, energy, growth, and health. *Added* to this can be improvement of body composition, muscular fitness, and cardiovascular capacity for athletic performance.

Energy Requirements

For any teen, energy requirements depend on sex, state of maturation and growth, size, and type and amount of athletic training. Requirements change with changes in training and performance. A rough determination of daily energy expenditure is given in Appendix L. For some sports, such as archery, diving, golf, and weight lifting, there is relatively little increase in energy requirements if they are practiced for 1 hour or less per day. On the other hand, long-distance sports, such as long-distance running, swimming, and cross-country skiing, are high energy–requiring sports. Appendix K gives the energy expenditures of various sports and activities.

Energy requirements increase for different sports as the number of muscle contractions increases. The energy and oxygen required to initiate a contraction is greater than that required to maintain a contraction. Thus running and swimming, because of repeated contractions, require more energy than gymnastics, which relies to a greater extent on maintenance of contractions.

During periods of training that ranged from 70 minutes to a little over 3 hours, athletes were found to expend 25% to 36% of their total daily energy output.[49] In addition, as noted earlier in this chapter, the athlete exercising daily has an increased BMR after the exercise is over and may have a constantly elevated BMR during the period of intense training. Because the energy requirements of activity are added to those of growth, some adolescent athletes in heavy training may require either as much as 4000 to 5000 kcal/day or between 50 and 65 kcal/kg body weight/day.

Energy Production. Energy is produced by fission, a process that goes on inside the human body continuously. The end products of this fission are heat and chemical energy that power nerves and muscles. This chemical energy, *ATP,* is the fuel for all of the energy-requiring processes within the cell and the body. ATP is a molecule of energy because of its two phosphate bonds. These bonds are able to trap energy. When the bonds are broken, energy is released. When energy is needed instantaneously, stored ATP in the body is used. After ATP, the next most important energy source is *creatine phosphate (CP)*. It also has an energy-rich bond that, when broken, allows energy to be released. This energy can then be used to resynthesize ATP as it is needed. Because cells can store CP in greater quantities than ATP, it is called the "reservoir" of high-energy phosphate. However, the body's pool of ATP and CP is limited, and the energy released from these molecules will sustain "all-out" physical effort for only about 5 to 8 seconds.

For short but intense bursts of activity, such as sprinting for a bus, spiking a volleyball, or lifting a weight, this ATP and CP energy supply is crucial. To enhance the supply of ATP and CP in the muscles, athletes practice numerous bouts of short-duration exercise (lasting 5 to 10 seconds) using the specific muscles for which they want improved ATP and CP stores.

For activity lasting longer than a few seconds, there must be additional sources of energy from which to generate ATP. The next source is glycogen, which can be metabolized aerobically or anaerobically. During exercise of maximal effort that goes beyond 10 seconds, glycogen is being metabolized *anaerobically*. In this process of glycolysis, glycogen is broken down to glucose molecules. These glucose molecules are metabolized further to pyruvate, and two molecules of ATP are produced. Pyruvate then is metabolized to lactic acid, which can be changed back to pyruvate or can accumulate as lactic acid within the cell, as shown in Fig. 6-5. Glycolysis can be maintained for physical activity that requires an all-out effort for periods of up to 60 seconds. To increase the length of time for which anaerobic energy release can continue via this system, a training program should include repeated bouts of maximal effort lasting up to 1 minute alternated with 1- to 2-minute recovery periods. Each bout results in more lactic acid buildup. When the exercise is over or slows, the lactic acid is metabolized back to pyruvate and processed through the Krebs cycle using aerobic metabolism. The *trained* athlete can be recognized by an increased tolerance for lactic acid buildup and a highly developed system for dealing with this product of anaerobic metabolism. Table 6-2 gives the energy sources for various types of activity.

However, energy from glycolysis represents only 5% of the total amount of energy that can be produced when the glucose molecule is completely degraded to carbon dioxide and water. This complete degradation occurs in *aerobic metabolism*. As activity continues for longer than 4 minutes, the production of energy becomes mainly aerobic, and the energy for resynthesis of ATP comes from reactions that require the presence of oxygen. The pyruvate from carbohydrate metabolism and the breakdown products of fat and protein are metabolized via the Krebs cycle to carbon dioxide and water. Energy is released, and large amounts of ATP are produced (Fig. 6-5). Oxygen must be adequate for this process to proceed most efficiently. If oxygen is adequate, exercise can be continued in a "steady state" and fatigue is minimal. If the oxygen supply does not meet the demands, then aerobic metabolism is limited and some anaerobic metabolism takes place. The consequent buildup of lactic acid, if continued, eventually will cause fatigue. It is obvious then that the body's ability to sustain exercise for long periods of time depends

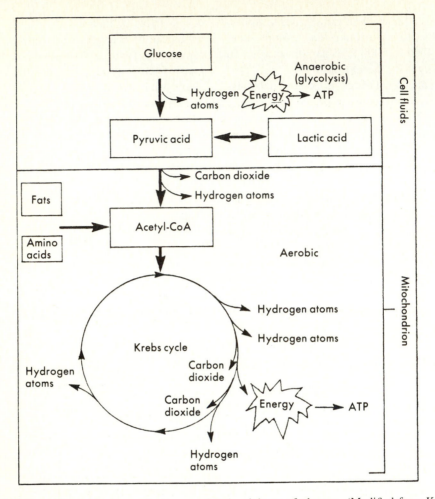

Fig. 6-5. Extraction of hydrogen during complete breakdown of glucose. (Modified from Katch, F.I., and McArdle, W.D.: Nutrition, weight control and exercise, Boston, 1977, Houghton Mifflin Co. Copyright © 1977 by Houghton Mifflin Company. Used by permission.)

Table 6-2. Predominant energy systems in activities of various durations

Time	Energy System	Activities
8 seconds or less	ATP-CP	High jump, shot put, tennis serve, golf swing, volleyball spike, 60- to 100-yd run, football, weight lifting
10 seconds to 90 seconds	ATP-CP and lactic acid	50- to 100-yd swim, 220- to 440-yd run, speed skating, gymnastic routine
2 to 4 minutes	Lactic acid and aerobic	Ice hockey, boxing, wrestling, press in basketball, 880-yd to 1-mile run, 200- to 400-yd swim
4 minutes and longer	Aerobic	Middle-distance and distance runs and swims, soccer, basketball, lacrosse, jogging

Modified from Katch, F.I., and McArdle, W.D.: Nutrition, weight control and exercise, Boston, 1977, Houghton Mifflin Co. Copyright © 1977 by Houghton Mifflin Company. Used by permission.

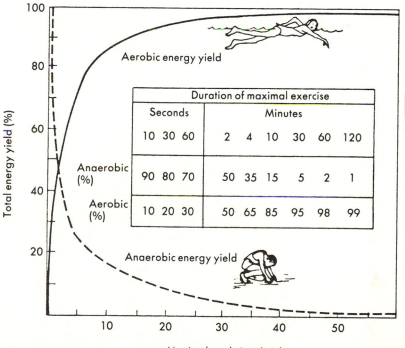

Fig. 6-6. Relative contribution of aerobic and anaerobic energy during maximal physical activity of various durations. Note that 2 minutes of maximal effort requires 50% of the energy from aerobic and anaerobic processes. (Modified from Astrand, P., and Rodahl, K.: Textbook of work physiology, New York, 1970, McGraw-Hill Book Co.)

on its capacity for aerobic metabolism. This in turn depends on the body's aerobic fitness as discussed earlier in this chapter. With training there is less lactic acid production during exercise because of increased capacity for aerobic metabolism. In the steady state, where the oxygen consumption meets the requirements of the working muscle, exercise could go on indefinitely if the athlete were motivated and if the loss of body fluids and depletion of body glucose and glycogen could be avoided. There are many levels of this steady state—it can range from a 6 min/mile pace for a marathon runner to a 20 min/mile walk for an obese adolescent.

The body makes a shift to greater aerobic metabolism with longer endurance exercise, as shown in Fig. 6-6.[18]

Energy Source: Carbohydrate or Fat? The energy source used during exercise depends on the intensity and duration of the exercise and the level of training of the athlete. During exercise of low intensity in which aerobic metabolism is predominant, energy is derived mainly from fatty acids that are oxidized to acetylcoenzyme A (acetyl-CoA). The acetyl-CoA is shunted into the Krebs cycle for further oxidation and release of energy. Since the body's store of lipid is far greater than its store of carbohydrate, as shown in Table 6-3, low-intensity exercise (less than 60% Vo_2 max), where the majority of energy expenditure is derived from the free fatty acids (FFA), can be maintained for long periods of time. As the exercise intensity or pulse

rate increases, carbohydrate becomes a larger fraction of the energy source. The longer the high-intensity exercise is sustained, the greater the percentage of anaerobic metabolism. The use of carbohydrate increases as a result. In an effort of high intensity (85% to 90% Vo_2 max), carbohydrate is the principal energy source, and the duration of the exercise is limited.[50] At lower intensities, fat metabolism spares glycogen. As the intensity increases, however, fat metabolism is replaced by glycogen or carbohydrate metabolism.

The first source of glucose for the working muscle is its own glycogen store. When this is depleted, glycogenolysis by the liver from its glycogen and then gluconeogenesis, primarily from the precursors pyruvic acid, lactic acid, oxaloacetate, and some amino acids, maintain the glucose supply. However, the liver cannot maintain blood glucose at high work intensities for prolonged periods of time, and hypoglycemia can occur. Ingestion of glucose during performance can help to prevent this hypoglycemia. At moderate work levels, ingested glucose can be used by working muscle, thus sparing muscle glycogen. At a marathon pace, however, ingested glucose has little sparing effect on glycogen. Even the trained athlete who has a higher than normal capacity for FFA mobilization and utilization is still using glucose for 10% to 20% of his or her energy needs after 3 hours of moderate-intensity exercise.

Exhaustion is correlated with depletion of glycogen stores and an inability of the body to maintain blood glucose. This depletion can occur during a long-distance event or during training when the athlete experiences a fatigue or "staleness." It develops over a period of several consecutive days of heavy training. During this time, the energy requirements and rate of glycogen burning exceed the athlete's intake of carbohydrate, and there is not enough time between workouts for complete resynthesis of glycogen. The muscle glycogen becomes lower with each day's workout until performance deteriorates and just the smallest amount

Table 6-3. Fuel reserves in an average man

Fuel	Tissue	Kilocalories	Grams
Triglyceride	Adipose tissue	100,000	15,000
Glycogen	Liver	200	70
	Muscle	400	120
Glucose	Body fluids	40	20
Protein	Muscle	25,000	6000

Modified from Newsholme, E.A.: Ann. N.Y. Acad. Sci. **301:** 81, 1977.

of exercise causes fatigue. The depletion can only be remedied by appropriate rest and carbohydrate ingestion. To avoid this situation, Foster, Costill, and Fink[51] recommend that, in addition to the usual diet, the athlete take in the extra energy required for training only as carbohydrate. This will ensure adequate carbohydrate intake and glycogen storage.

Muscle Maintenance Requirements

Protein. For centuries athletes have been advised to increase their protein intake to increase muscle mass and performance. This advice was based on the premise that increased protein enhances muscle growth and repair.[52,53] Because the training muscle is expanding its protein content as the muscle bulk and efficiency increase, adequate protein and energy intake is required. However, the need for protein is not greatly increased and certainly not to the extent that many coaches and promoters of protein supplements would have the athlete believe.

The studies on the protein needs of athletes are contradictory and are not well controlled.[54] No study conclusively shows a need for increased protein. Several reports have recommended the use of additional protein to develop the muscle mass. These reports recommend 2 to 2.5 gm/kg.[53,55] Others have recommended an increased protein intake to prevent sports anemia that may develop during the early months of a new training program.[55,56]

During a weight-gaining program, the athlete may require some additional protein (6 to 7 gm) to ensure the necessary amino acids for muscle synthesis, but this need would exist only during the period of muscle building. The total amount needed has been estimated to be 1000 mg nitrogen/day, which covers even the extremes in muscle development.[57]

To determine the amount of protein that the athlete needs, protein requirements are based on the following: obligatory nitrogen losses that occur daily, a factor for growth, a factor for individual variation, sweat nitrogen losses, and a factor to allow for incomplete protein. This determination is shown below for a 70-kg (154-lb) male adolescent:

28.7 gm	Replacement of obligatory nitrogen loss in urine, feces, skin, and other sites (assuming largest loss)
8.6 gm	30% Allowance for individual variation
4.8 gm	Allowance for growth (assuming most rapid growth)
7.5 gm	Replacement of nitrogen lost in sweat during 4 hours of vigorous exercise
6.3 gm	Allowance for increased muscle mass, as during some kinds of training
8.6 gm	Allowance for loss of efficiency of standard protein
64.5 gm	Total estimated protein requirement = 0.9 mg/kg*

The most liberal total estimate for a 70-kg (154-lb) male adolescent athlete who is still growing thus is 65 gm protein/day or 0.9 gm/kg/day. Sweat losses of nitrogen depend on the protein intake of the athlete. The greater the protein intake, the greater the sweat losses of nitrogen. Another factor to consider is that when skin nitrogen losses are high, as in high temperatures, there is a gradual decrease in urinary nitrogen loss.

This value of 65 gm of protein is at the upper extreme of the amount that an athlete would require. If it is compared to the RDA for protein, which is 56 gm/day, you can see that there is a difference of only 9 gm, the amount of protein in a little over 1 cup of milk. In addition, the figure for athletes includes several safety factors. Most athletes thus would not require that much protein.

---

*Data from Energy and protein requirements, Report of Joint Food and Agriculture Organization/World Health Organization Ad Hoc Expert Committee, World Health Organization, Technical Systems Series, no. 522, Geneva, 1973, World Health Organization; and Durnin, J.V.: Protein requirements and physical activity. In Pařízková, J., and Rogozkin, V.A., editors: Nutrition, physical fitness and health, Baltimore, 1978, University Park Press.

Even if the protein needs did approach the 60 to 70 gm/day level, the average athlete could easily obtain this amount from an ordinary diet, assuming that he or she was also meeting energy requirements. Since the average diet in the United States is 10% to 15% protein, an increased caloric intake to meet the energy requirements of activity will usually also provide enough protein. For example, the 70-kg (154-lb) male adolescent who eats an average of 3000 kcal/day would get 15% (450 kcal) of his intake from protein. This would provide 110 gm of protein, or 1.6 gm/kg. If the teen was in athletic training, his caloric requirement would increase perhaps to 4000 kcal/day, and the percentage of protein probably would still be the same. Thus 600 calories would be derived from protein. This would provide 150 gm of protein or 2.1 gm/kg, more than enough for muscle-mass development.

If the diet is too high in protein, it can lead to increased water loss, as water is excreted to rid the body of protein-breakdown products. Consequently, there is an increased need for water and a greater potential for dehydration.

Minerals. Athletes, especially those in endurance activities that stress aerobic capacity, appear to have less than optimal performance if they are anemic. Total body hemoglobin has been related to maximal oxygen uptake, and Haymes[52] has reported a linear relationship between maximal oxygen uptake and hemoglobin levels in both trained and untrained groups. Davies and co-workers[58] found that people with anemia had lower maximal oxygen uptakes as compared to control subjects.

There is still the question of whether iron supplementation in the healthy nonanemic athlete will improve endurance and performance. This has not been answered satisfactorily.[59,60] The data at this point do not seem to support the practice of giving routine iron supplements to athletes with normal levels of hemoglobin. However, it may also be wise to assess iron stores in the athlete by measuring serum ferritin and total iron-binding capacity

and to supplement if stores are low. The female athlete who experiences a heavy menstrual flow (greater than 60 ml of blood during a menstrual period) and thus a large iron loss should receive iron supplementation as a preventive measure.[61] The growing male athlete should pay special attention to the iron in his diet because of the iron requirements resulting from the growth of muscular tissue and blood. This is discussed further in Chapter 3.

What appears to be anemia (low blood hemoglobin) in athletes undergoing intense training is often a result of blood dilution. During periods of daily heavy training, sweating, and dehydration, plasma volume increases as a reaction to increased body sodium storage. Concentration of blood constituents, including hemoglobin, falls and results in an anemia. This anemia does not warrant increased iron intake or treatment. Sweat contains about 0.3 to 0.4 mg iron/L. In long-distance training in hot weather with a lot of sweating (8 to 12 L/day), this could mean a significant loss of iron.

Knowledge regarding the roles of other minerals in athletic performance is very sparse. The only definite recommendations that can be made at this time concern electrolytes, which will be discussed later in this chapter.

Vitamins. The literature on the use of vitamins in athletic performance has been reviewed thoroughly.[54,62] These reviews cite increased demands for the B vitamins because of their role in energy metabolism, which is increased in the exercising body. Buskirk and Haymes[63] suggest that if the number of mitochondria in the muscle cells increases with physical conditioning—and there is evidence that it does—then additional vitamin cofactors may be necessary to support the increased mitochondrial enzymatic reactions.

However, most athletes do in fact consume more of the B vitamins because of the increased caloric intake that is necessary to replace their large energy expenditure and to maintain their energy and weight balance. There is no doubt that deficiencies of the B vitamins decrease athletic performance,[54,62] but there is no solid evidence that supplementation with B vitamins in the replete individual will increase performance.[54]

The requirement for vitamin B_6 increases with increased protein intake, which has implications for athletes on high-protein diets. However, the same foods that would be plentiful on a high-protein diet, such as meat and other animal products, are also high in vitamin B_6.

Many athletes use huge amounts of vitamin C in attempts to prevent fatigue or to increase performance. One study showed that the heart rates of those on vitamin C supplementation were 8 to 10 beats/min lower than during the placebo trial. Generally interpreted, this is a sign of greater cardiovascular capacity and better heart function. Metabolically, the vitamin C supplementation was associated with increased turnover of catecholamines, reduced blood glucose concentration, and increased circulating FFA. The researchers concluded that vitamin C leads to a greater utilization of FFA as an energy source by the working muscle. This would have a glycogen-sparing and thus beneficial effect in long-lasting exercise. However, since the actual performance in this study was not significantly different, the value of vitamin C in athletic training is limited.[64]

Two other controlled placebo studies of the effects of vitamin C on performance provide evidence against its beneficial effect.[65,66] However, there is enough unknown about the mechanisms of vitamin C to warrant further research in this area.[54]

Vitamin E is probably the vitamin most widely used by athletes as a supplement for performance. It is theorized by its users that since vitamin E prevents unwanted oxidation of fatty acids, it is possible that supplementation with vitamin E will increase both the oxygen supply for other purposes, such as energy production in the citric acid cycle, and the fatty acid supply for energy. Hence vitamin E should be effective in endurance activities requiring an oxygen supply and fatty acids for energy. However, there is no objective evidence available to substantiate these proposed effects from vitamin E during exercise. On the other hand, there are several reports, including some very recent findings from well-controlled studies, that supplemental vitamin E exerts no effect on physical performance capacity.[67-69]

The reason why so many athletes still use vitamins may be that although drugs are illegal, vitamin and mineral supplements are not because they are considered food. Therefore an athlete searching for an ergogenic aid may well turn to vitamins because there is no risk of illegality in competition.

In summary, it does not seem that athletes require more vitamins, except in the case of B vitamins, than nonathletes. Even if they do, the athletes are usually consuming more vitamins than their nonathletic counterparts because they are eating more food to stay in energy balance. If the choices of these foods are reasonable and adequate, the athletes are getting more vitamins and thus meeting their possibly increased requirements.

Weight Gain

In some athletic events increased body mass is advantageous for stability, force development, protection, or thermal insulation. Typical athletes who may wish to gain weight are football players and others in contact sports, heavyweight wrestlers, weight lifters, and long-distance cold-water swimmers.

Thousands of young athletes every year spend their off-season time "bulking up" or gaining weight. In addition, an excessive diet may be augmented with drugs to increase appetite or with anabolic steroids to promote muscle buildup. Both drugs and steroids are inappropriate in the adolescent athlete. In a young athlete anabolic steroids can stunt growth through premature fusing of the growth zones of the long bones. The male teen can also develop acne, a deepened voice, excessive body hair, and enlarged breasts because some of the hormones are converted to estrogen. In older male adolescents the steroids can cause diminished testicular size, loss of potency, and a decrease in sperm production.[20]

Weight gain should not be viewed only as added pounds on the scale with no consideration for the composition of the weight gain. The goal should be to increase lean body mass, not body fatness, and young athletes must recognize that unless they augment their diet with a vigorous training program, they will gain body fatness in addition to muscle tissue.

Each pound of lean body tissue gain requires approximately an additional 2500 kcal over and above that expended.[70] By adding an additional 500 to 1000 kcal/day to the diet and performing vigorous exercise for 1 hr/day three times per week, the athlete can be expected to gain 0.45 to 0.9 kg/wk (1 to 2 lb/wk). This would be the maximal weight gain to be expected per week if the gain is to be only lean body tissue.[71] Periodic measurement of the skinfolds throughout the weight-gaining period will indicate to the nutritionist, coach, and athlete whether the weight gain is indeed lean body mass or body fat. Increasing weight and circumference measurements with identical or decreasing fatfold measurements would indicate growth in lean body mass.

In anticipating weight gain, the projected weight should be realistic. For example, a 16-year-old male adolescent measuring 177.8 cm (6 ft) and weighing 74.25 kg (165 lb) may be expected to gain an additional 4.5 to 6.75 kg (10 to 15 lb) of lean body tissue if he is well disciplined in increasing his intake and exercises hard.[71] Gains greater than this probably would be of body fat.

Young athletes trying to gain weight traditionally turn to high-calorie foods, such as beef, eggs, milk, dairy products, and desserts, that are also high in fat, particularly saturated fat and cholesterol. The result is a diet with atherogenic potential, especially when it is combined with weight gain. Athletes should be counseled in ways to increase their energy intake without increasing the saturated fat and cholesterol. This can be accomplished by doing the following: (1) beginning the program early so that there is time to gain the weight at a slower pace; (2) adding foods that are low in fat (for example, whole grain breads, cereals, and pasta, low-fat dairy products, fruits, and starchy vegetables such as winter squash, pumpkin, beets, carrots, peas, corn, and dried beans); and (3) using polyunsaturated fats (margarine and oils) as sources of fat.

Weight Reduction

For many more sports the competitive edge is a low body weight, and this often requires weight reduction. Again the concern is that muscle be maintained and that the weight loss be of fat and not water or lean tissue. The coach and athlete must be realistic in their expectations for an ideal body weight. It is important to remember that the adolescent may still be growing. Thus a weight that is too high at one time may be appropriate in several months after the teen has grown another 2 to 5 cm (about 1 to 2 in). Weight-reduction efforts should begin early so that a gradual weight reduction, no more than 0.9 kg/wk (2 lb/wk), will result in the eventual desired weight. A slow weight loss allows for reduction of body fat without the loss in muscle tissue and dehydration that comes with rapid weight reduction. Because 0.45 kg (1 lb) of fat contains approximately 3500 to 3750 kcal (7.7 to 9.5 kcal/gm fat),[35,72,73] to lose 0.45 kg fat/wk (1 lb fat/wk) the athlete would need to achieve an energy deficit of 500 to 535 kcal/day.

To obtain reduction in body fat alone, weight-loss efforts must be accompanied by aerobic exercise on a regular basis of at least three to four times per week. (The appropriate intensity for this exercise was discussed earlier in this chapter.) To achieve the 1000-kcal daily deficit necessary for a 0.9 kg/wk (2 lb/wk) weight reduction, the athlete should reduce energy intake by 500 to 700 kcal/day (but no less than 1800 to 2000 kcal/day for females and 2200 to 2400 kcal/day for males) and increase energy output by 300 to 500 kcal/day. Because of individual variation in energy metabolism, this is not an infallible method. However, it provides a *guideline* for the manipulation of energy intake and output to achieve weight reduction.

Fatfold measurements should be taken periodically to ascertain whether the weight loss is actually of body fat. Rapid weight reduction (greater than 1.35 kg/wk [3 lb/wk]) that it is not accompanied by skinfold reductions undoubtedly is caused by loss of lean tissue and loss of water. Reduction of skinfolds with weight reduction would indicate a loss of body fatness. The goal for body fatness should be reasonable based on the rate of growth and the sex of the adolescent. Minimal levels of body fatness are discussed earlier in this chapter. The method for calculation of body weight based on desired level of body fatness is shown in the box below.

In their zeal to lose weight, many young athletes, both male and female, may lose excessive weight or become extremely preoccupied with food and fatness. They usually feel under tremendous pressure to lose weight because of the unrealistic performance goals they set for themselves, their fear of not making the team (more so than of not winning), and the reinforcement they receive from the dominant persons in their lives. Coaches, teammates, and parents admire self-discipline, compulsiveness, and regularity in other aspects of sport training schedules. It stands to reason that the perfectionistic adolescent athlete who is constantly made aware of the threat of overfatness is highly vulnerable to becoming compulsive in this area as well. The result is often

---

Determination of Body Fatness and Optimal Weight

1. Weigh athlete (total body weight [TBW])
2. Using skinfold measurements or hydrostatic weighing, determine percentage of body weight that is fat (percentage body fat [PBF])
3. PBF × TBW = Weight of fat (F)
4. TBW − F = Weight of lean body mass (LBM)
5. LBM = (100% − PBF) (TBW)
6. Desired percentage for LBM = (100% − desired PBF)
7. $\dfrac{\text{LBM}}{\text{Desired percentage for LBM}}$ = Desired TBW for desired PBF

Example

65-kg female is 27% body fat. The goal for this athlete is to be 22% body fat. What should she weigh?
1. TBW = 65 kg
2. PBW = 27%
3. 27% × 65 kg = 17.55 kg of fat (F)
4. 65 kg − 17.55 kg = 47.45 kg of lean body mass (LBM)
5. 47.45 kg = (100% − 27%) (65 kg)
6. Desired percentage for LBM = (100% − 22%) = 78%
7. $\dfrac{47.45}{78\%}$ = 60.8 kg = TBW for 22% body fatness (PBF)

excessive dieting and extreme weight loss.[74] Young athletes with a rigid diet and rapid weight loss should be sought out by coaches and nutritionists working with athletes and counseled regarding the importance of gradual weight loss. More importantly, there should be an appreciation of the psychosocial development of teens and their consequent feelings of inadequacy regarding performance.

NUTRITIONAL REQUIREMENTS FOR PERFORMANCE

Although an athletic performance is more dependent on the athlete's training, it is apparent that the athlete's nutritional intake just before the event can also play a role in the performance. In the case of long-term events the nutritional intake during the event or game can have an effect. Let us look first at what the athlete can do in preparation for the event and then at the recommendations for optimal nutrition during the event.

Short-Term Events

Since the execution of short-term athletic performances primarily depends on the presence of adequate stores of ATP, CP, and readily available supplies of glucose, the carbohydrate intake just before an event is most important. Normal *muscle* glycogen stores usually are adequate for short-term performance, but inadequate *liver* glycogen can limit even short-term performance because of its hypoglycemic effect on the central nervous system. In preparation for short-term events the diet thus should be rich in carbohydrate for at least 1 day beforehand. Fruit juices, low-fat milk and dairy products, breads, cereals, low-fiber fruits, and starchy vegetables can be used in such a diet. To maintain as much carbohydrate as possible stored in the muscles, the training and exercise the day before should be kept to a minimum. This will allow the stores of ATP, CP, and glycogen to be at their maximum.

To achieve a feeling of lightness, the diet should be low in fiber and roughage so that the intestinal contents are minimal. The restriction of fiber and roughage in the diet should begin 24 to 36 hours before the event. Foods to avoid include the following: fruits and vegetables (especially raw ones with skins, stems, and seeds); whole grain breads and cereals (especially those containing additional bran, such as bran cereals and breads); dried peas and beans; nuts; and seeds.

Fats are another item to be considered in the diet. Because they take longer to digest, they may remain in the gastrointestinal tract and thus cause a feeling of heaviness. On the day of competition athletes should limit their intake of butter, margarine, mayonnaise, salad dressings, gravies, fatty meats, cheeses, cheese dishes, whole milk, ice cream, cream, bacon, sausage, fatty luncheon meats, pastries, pies, chocolate, and avocados.

Some athletes are disturbed by flatus during athletic events, especially if they are nervous. This can be avoided by eliminating gas-forming foods such as the following: cabbage, cauliflower, radishes, brussels sprouts, turnips, onions, rutabagas, green peppers, corn, dried peas and beans, apples, avocados, melons, and any other foods that may affect that individual.

The athlete performing in a short-term event does not need additional fluids or carbohydrate during the event. However, if the day includes several short-term events, such as several races or swim events, the time between the events should be used to replenish energy sources by consuming easily digested carbohydrates (for example, fruit juices, refined cereals and breads, and sugared drinks). Fluids should be taken freely throughout the day. Fluids will be discussed in the following section on the requirements during long-term events.

Long-Term Events

Carbohydrate and Glycogen. Performance in long-term, high-intensity athletic events of 1 hour or longer, such as long-distance running, cross-country skiing, bicycle racing, and some team sports like soccer and ice hockey, seems to be improved if the performing muscles contain higher than normal amounts of glycogen. Since muscles during exercise or work depend on a steady source of glucose for fuel and since carbohydrate is the most readily available fuel for use by the exercising muscle, it is a great advantage if the muscle has stored carbohydrate or glycogen to be used for energy. Even with prolonged exercise of 2 hours or more, when fats provide a sizable amount of the fuel for the muscle, there is still an obligate requirement for carbohydrate. In long-term, high-intensity events it appears that the depletion of glycogen from the slow-twitch muscle fibers accounts for exhaustion and fatigue.[75] For example, marathon runners often complain of exhaustion or "hit-ting the wall" at about the 20-mile mark. It is at this point for many runners that glycogen stores are depleted.

An exciting event in sports science was the discovery that the amount of glycogen stored in muscles could be increased with appropriate training and dietary manipulation.[76,77] A muscle biopsy of a person on a high-fat, high-protein diet showed less than 0.6 gm glycogen/100 gm wet muscle. The person could do a standard work load for only 60 minutes. After 3 days on a high-carbohydrate diet, muscle glycogen rose to 3.5 gm/100 gm wet muscle (Fig. 6-7), and the same standard work load could be maintained for 170 minutes. Preceding the 3 high-carbohydrate days with a period of exercise-induced depletion of glycogen reserves combined with a low-carbohydrate diet produced muscle tissue with glycogen at the level of 4 gm/

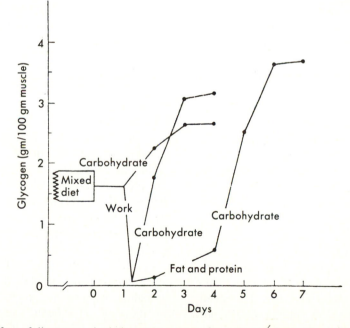

Fig. 6-7. Effect of dietary manipulations on amount of muscle glycogen. (From Williams, M.H.: Nutritional aspects of human physical performance, Springfield, Ill., 1976, Charles C Thomas, Publisher. Courtesy of Charles C Thomas, Publisher, Springfield, Ill.)

100 gm wet muscle, almost twice the normal amount, and the ability to work for 240 minutes.[78] It is still not clear why the muscle can accumulate above-normal levels of glycogen from diet manipulation, but this supercompensation is being used in the training of some athletes.

Using the original technique for maximal glycogen loading, the athlete begins a week before the athletic event with a low-carbohydrate, high-protein diet for 3 to 4 days combined with long, hard training to deplete the muscles of glycogen. This is followed by 3 to 4 days of a high-carbohydrate diet combined with light training to enhance the repletion of muscle glycogen and glycogen loading. The seventh day is the day of the event.

Most athletes are so miserable with light-headedness, weakness, and even nausea during the hard-workout, low-carbohydrate days that coaches often recommend a modified glycogen-loading regimen. Long exercise alone can adequately deplete muscle glycogen, and the low-carbohydrate phase is omitted. The difference in muscle glycogen between this modified regimen and the original is so small that it is not worth the discomfort to the athlete, especially during the week before an important event.[78]

The modified glycogen-loading technique (summarized in the box on p. 163) involves a long workout on the third day before the event. This long workout will deplete the glycogen stores. The workout must use the same muscles that will be used in the event, for only these muscles will supercompensate with glycogen. The workout is followed by a low-fat, high-carbohydrate diet in which, ideally, 80% of the calories is from carbohydrate. Since muscle and hepatic cells are most receptive to glycogen repletion right after depletion and since 60% of total storage occurs within the first 10 hours, the carbohydrate intake immediately after the endurance workout is most important. The workout should be in the morning to allow a full day for carbohydrate intake and glycogen loading. It takes 24 to 48 hours to bring glycogen levels back up to preexercise levels.

The high-carbohydrate diet should be rich in polysaccharides or starches to have the maximal glycogen-loading effect. Because they are released more slowly from the stomach, these carbohydrates produce a longer lasting insulin stimulation and thus more synthesis of glycogen from glucose.[79] Frequency of meals also may affect carbohydrate loading. Improved glycogen storage has been observed with two meals per day as compared to multiple smaller feedings with the same caloric value.[80]

The second day and the day before the event are easy, light-workout days. The athlete should eat a high-carbohydrate diet and drink at least 2 L of fluid per day. The water is necessary not only for the storing of glycogen but also for hydration. The athlete will have to drink beyond the point of thirst. Since 3 gm of water are stored with each gram of glycogen, a sign of good glycogen loading is a weight gain of a few pounds, possibly as much as 2.5 to 3.5 kg, caused by the 2 to 3 L of water stored with the maximal amount of glycogen.[81] In fact, athletes may complain of muscles that feel heavy or stiff, indicating that they are full of glycogen and water. Thus glycogen loading provides not only a source of carbohydrate during exercise but also a water reserve as glycogen is used and the water is released. It is also wise to avoid anything that would cause a diuresis during this period (for example, alcohol, caffeine, or diuretics).

The day before the race is again an easy-workout, high-carbohydrate day, but now the intake should be low in fiber to ensure that the intestinal tract is as residue-free as possible on the competition day. Emphasis on juices ensures a high-carbohydrate, low-fiber intake with good hydration.

The safety of glycogen loading is still questionable. Cardiac pain and electrocardiographical abnormalities have been reported in an older runner, and the long-range cardiac consequences of glycogen overloading of the heart muscle are not known.[82] In addition, the resulting weight increase from the water retention associated with glycogen loading may reduce the athlete's Vo_2 max.

Modified Glycogen-Loading Regimen

Third Day Before Race*

Exercise. Run 10 to 12 miles or work out at moderate intensity for 1½ to 2 hours to deplete glycogen stores.

Food Intake. After depletion exercise, eat predominantly low-fat, high-carbohydrate foods. Two or three *small* servings of protein-fat foods are acceptable, but the majority (70% to 80%) of caloric intake should be carbohydrate.

Minimize intake of salt and salty foods to avoid fluid imbalance and weight distortion.

Fluid Intake. Drink 8 or more glasses (8 ounces or more) of fluid, both water and juices. Drink beyond thirst. If traveling, especially by plane, carry a bottle of water.

Do not consume caffeine (coffee, tea, cola, cocoa, caffeine-containing medications), alcohol, or diuretic medications.

Weight. Weigh (nude) first thing in the morning. Weigh both before and after long run to assess fluid loss and drink to replenish.

Second Day Before Race

Exercise. Run an easy 3 to 4 miles or work out easily for 20 to 30 minutes.

Food Intake. Same principles as previous day.

Fluid Intake. Same principles as previous day.

Weight. Weigh (nude) first thing in the morning. If weight is down from previous morning, drink even more fluid.

Day Before Race

Exercise. Run an easy 3 to 4 miles or work out easily for 20 to 30 minutes or take a rest day.

Food Intake. Same principles as previous day. In addition, avoid foods high in fiber.

Fluid Intake. Same principles as previous days. Decrease intake of solid food and obtain proportionately more calories from juice and other sweet beverages.

Weight. Same principles as previous day. There will be a possible weight gain because of water retention associated with carbohydrate loading.

Day of Race

Food Intake. Eat no solid foods for 2½ hours before the start of the race. Food intake before this time should be light and consist of carbohydrate (for example, juice, white toast, and jam or honey). Quantity and frequency of food intake will depend on time of race start.

Fluid Intake. Until 1 hour before race start, drink 8 to 16 oz fluid/hr, preferably water and juice. Drink no caffeine or alcohol.

At 1 hour before race start, drink 1 to 2 cups of coffee or tea (4 to 5 mg caffeine per kilogram body weight). (Caffeine taken at this time has been shown to delay glycogen depletion and therefore increase endurance.) However, if significant adverse effects result from caffeine, omit this step.

From 1 hour to 15 minutes before race start, drink *no* fluids.

At 10 to 15 minutes before race start, drink 1 to 2 8-ounce glasses of *water*. Drink *no* sugar-containing beverages.

During race, drink frequently, preferably at every aid station. Considerations include heat, hills, and ability to tolerate fluids. Remember that thirst is not an adequate indicator of fluid need. Preferred beverages are water, replacement drinks, or very dilute juices.

After the Race

Eat and drink whatever sounds good. Carbohydrate is essential to replace glycogen, but now that the race is over it is not so critical to avoid fat, so enjoy favorite treats. Drink lots of fluid (at least 16 oz/hr) until weight returns to prerace level.

Developed by Edlefsen, J., formerly Nutrition Counselor, Sports Medicine Division, University of Washington, Seattle, Wash.
*It is possible that the glycogen-loading regimen could be used in preparation for endurance events other than running races.

The high-fat, high-protein diet during the first phase of glycogen loading could easily be high in saturated fat, total fat, and cholesterol and thus have atherogenic potential. Also, the ketosis resulting from this phase causes an increased water loss and the danger of dehydration during training. During this phase, carbohydrate is low and the energy needs are high because of the continued training. These energy needs are met by the breakdown of protein from muscle tissue, and this should not be done frequently. Therefore the full glycogen-loading regimen should be used judiciously if at all. The modified regimen in the box on p. 163 is preferred and is almost as effective. Even the modified technique should not be used any more frequently than every 3 to 4 weeks since it is impossible to obtain extremely high glycogen storage in muscles at more frequent intervals than this.[83]

The old tradition of taking a large spoonful of honey just before an event for "quick energy" is not a good idea in preparation for a long event. It appears that a large intake of sugar 30 minutes before an event results in impaired lipid mobilization, possibly because of the elevated plasma insulin following the carbohydrate intake. Elevated insulin causes an increased rate of carbohydrate utilization (in this case for energy requirements) and decreased lipid mobilization. Glycogen depletion thus occurs faster. Exercise time to exhaustion was reduced by 19% when exercise was performed at 80% Vo_2 max and the sugar was eaten 30 minutes before the start of the exercise.[51] Hypoglycemia can also result and is apparently of more significance in high-intensity exertion than in low-intensity exertion.[51] Athletes should be counseled to avoid ingestion of sugar within 1 hour before a race or event. Once exercise has started, sugar ingestion does not cause an increase in plasma insulin. In fact, during exercise, glucose ingestion helps to maintain the blood glucose and reduces the need for breakdown of liver glycogen.

During competition in cold conditions, there is an even greater demand for carbohydrate replacement because the body may be using energy both to keep itself warm and to perform. In these situations the replacement drinks can be more concentrated than usual, with 15 to 40 gm sugar/dl. The standard athletic drink thus would need to be consumed with less added water than recommended for hot-weather competition.[84] This is discussed in the following section on fluids and electrolytes.

Fluids and Electrolytes. For the athlete, during both training and long-term events, water is probably the most important of all the nutrients. Inseparable from water balance is the body's mineral or electrolyte balance. Physical exertion can cause tremendous water and electrolyte changes that require body adjustments. For example, during a marathon, a runner may lose as much as 2 L fluid/hr, most of it as sweat. Because water makes up 60% to 70% of the adolescent's body, this could represent as much as 3% of total body weight.

Water plays a number of important roles during physical exercise: (1) water transports nutrients and waste products to and from the cell via the bloodstream; (2) blood volume, which is dependent on fluid intake, is pivotal to the body's ability to dissipate body heat during exercise; and (3) water inside the cell provides the medium for the cell to conduct its activities, one of which is energy production.

During severe physical exercise when dehydration may occur, plasma water and blood volume fall. When the volume of blood is decreased, the body's ability to carry oxygen to the working muscles is lessened. The heart thus must beat more often to get as much blood and oxygen moving into the tissues as possible. This extra work for the heart means that the heart requires more energy. As a result, the exercise becomes even more intense and fatiguing. The body compensates by increasing capillary dilation and constriction. This allows the body to divert the limited blood volume from tissues that are not active to the muscles that are active and require oxygen.

The body uses water to cool itself by sweating. As sweat evaporates from the skin, it has a cooling effect. In a humid environment where the evaporation of body sweat is less, more sweat must be lost to get the same amount of evaporation and thus the cooling effect. Sweat that drips off the body does not have the same cooling effect as sweat that evaporates from the skin. In humid conditions or in the case of the person who sweats faster than the water is able to evaporate, the need for fluid replacement during exercise thus is very great. When body dehydration occurs, there is a reduction in the body's capacity to cool itself and body temperature rises.

Fluid and maintenance of blood volume also are important in helping the body move blood through surface capillaries so that heat can be dissipated directly from the skin. With dehydration and depletion of body blood volume, this process is compromised and body temperature will rise.

Because of these important functions of water, dehydration during physical exercise thus results in elevated body temperature and elevated heart rate. These effects are caused by the body's inability to supply the tissues with enough oxygen and to dissipate body heat fast enough. With a water loss of only 4% to 5% of body weight, the capacity for hard exercise will decline by 20% to 30%. When dehydration reaches 10% of body weight, there is severe risk of heat exhaustion and eventual circulatory collapse. If there is no fluid intake by 45 minutes after starting heavy exercise, body temperature begins to rise above the level it would normally attain with fluid intake and good hydration.

It is obviously important, then, to replace fluid during exercise to minimize dehydration and to maintain plasma volume, thus reducing the stress on the circulatory system and the danger of overheating. The best way to replace fluid losses during training or competition is to promote the fastest movement of fluid into the intestines where most of the fluid is absorbed. Cold drinks move into the intestinal tract faster. (Contrary to popular belief, many studies have shown that cold drinks do not cause stomach cramps.)[85] Fairly large volumes, rather than constant little sips, also seem to move in faster. On the other hand, it is not desirable to have excess water sitting in the stomach waiting to be absorbed, as this can be uncomfortable for the athlete. It is recommended that the athlete drink 150 to 250 ml every 10 to 15 minutes. This would be 1 cup about every 3 miles if the event was a road-running race. At this rate, absorption keeps up with intake.

Drinking a strong sugar drink is not a good way of replacing body water during competition because sugar retards movement of fluid into the intestines. For example, if an athlete drinks 1½ cups of water, only 30% to 40% of the volume is still in the stomach 15 minutes later. However, if he or she drinks 1½ cups of a soft drink, which would contain about 40 gm of sugar, about 95% of the volume is still in the stomach.[85] The maximal sugar content for an efficient replacement drink is 2 to 2.5 gm sugar/dl. Anything more concentrated than this will be absorbed at less than the maximal rate. Some of the athletic drinks are too concentrated for maximal absorption and should be diluted when used for rehydration during warm weather. ERG, Breaktime, and Body Punch are usually dilute enough to be used as is, but even these may sometimes need to be diluted further. Coca-Cola, to use another example, has 10.3 gm sugar/dl. Despite the testimonies of athletes, it thus theoretically should be far too concentrated for a fluid and carbohydrate replacement in warm weather. Orange juice, with about 10 gm sugar/dl, is also too sweet.

Recent experiments with oral ingestion of fluids have shown that it is possible to replace only 800 ml fluid/hr, which can be insufficient to meet the needs during long-term exertion where the fluid losses can exceed 2 L/hr.[86] However, it is important to replace as much fluid as possible during the event. The remaining replacement can be done afterward.

Within 15 minutes before a long athletic event

the athlete should drink 400 to 600 ml of water (1½ to 2½ cups). This will allow for maximal absorption of fluid. Because not enough time will have elapsed, this practice will also prevent the need to urinate before the event or, worse, during the first 15 minutes of the event. After exercise begins, the kidney slows down the making of urine to compensate for exercise and water loss. Between periods of exercising, water should be replaced. When there have been large fluid losses, the athlete cannot depend on thirst to determine fluid need and must drink past the point of thirst. Each pound of weight lost during competition indicates a fluid replacement need of 2 cups. (''A pint is a pound the world round.'')

Because body water homeostasis is so important, the body has mechanisms for assuring its maintenance. As glycogen is metabolized, an average of 0.45 mEq of potassium and 2.7 gm of water are released. In the presence of aerobic metabolism, 1 gm of glycogen yields an additional 0.6 gm of water. For every 1 gm of completely metabolized glycogen, 3.3 gm of water thus is produced and released from the cells. This water compensates for some of the water loss during athletic activity.

Electrolytes also are involved in body homeostasis. When the body sweats, it loses not only water but also electrolytes, principally sodium, chloride, magnesium, and potassium. The concentration of magnesium and potassium in the sweat is roughly the same as in the body fluids. The concentration of sodium and chloride in sweat, on the other hand, is roughly one third that of the plasma water. Thus sweat is quite dilute compared to other body fluids. During a long bout of heavy exercise with a large sweat loss (as much as 4 kg [9 lb]), the losses of sodium and chloride are the greatest, but even these losses reach only 6% to 8% of the body's total sodium chloride content. Each 500 ml of sweat contains about 1.5 gm of sodium. The potassium and magnesium losses are less, amounting to less than 1% of the body's total amount. Since the electrolyte losses on a percentage basis are much less than the water loss and since the concentration of the ions remaining in the body increases and accounts for immediate electrolyte adjustment, the need to replace water immediately during performance is much greater than the need to replace electrolytes.

The body also compensates for electrolyte losses. During the repeated bouts of heavy exercise and dehydration that might occur during the heavy-training and performance season for an athlete, the body adjusts to minimize electrolyte losses. Costill and co-workers[87] have shown that during repeated days of heavy sweating with fluid and electrolyte replacement as desired by the athlete, the kidney adequately reduces its excretion of water and electrolytes to prevent chronic dehydration and body electrolyte loss. During these repeated days of dehydration and uncontrolled replacement of electrolytes by food and drink, the body actually stores water and sodium in excess of the sweat loss. When the daily exercise bouts are terminated, the athletes quickly lose this excess water and sodium.[87] Even during repeated days of dehydration when athletes were given both low and normal potassium-containing diets, it was found that there was still very little change in either whole-body or muscle potassium.[88] The body was able to adjust and maintain proper body potassium levels on a wide range of potassium intakes.

As mentioned previously, in the body's attempt to maintain hydration during repeated days of sweating and dehydration, body sodium storage will increase. Thus the total body water, in this case extracellular, increases. As a result of this dilution of the plasma, the concentration of other blood constituents decreases. For example, the concentration of blood potassium may decrease and produce a false deficit of body potassium. In fact, little change in total body potassium occurs with repeated days of exercise and dehydration.

Usually sodium does not have to be replaced during competition. If it is present in the replacement drink, it should not be in high concentration. No more than 10 mEq sodium/L and 5 mEq potassium/L of solution are needed.[3] Because of the potassium released during glycogen metabolism, potassium does not need to be replaced during competition either. Both sodium and potassium usually can be adequately replaced with eating food and drinking as desired after the competition or training. However, in very hot weather when exercise is very vigorous, sodium replacement may need to be greater than the amounts that can be obtained from food. In this case it may be necessary to use salt tablets. However, tablets should be taken during the periods when the athlete is not exercising, not during the exercise. Salt tablets, if taken in excess, cause movement of fluid into the intestinal tract and possible nausea. They thus should always be dissolved in water first. Excessive sodium intake could lead to excessive water retention. Excessive sodium in the extracellular space may draw water from the intracellular space. This movement may balance the osmotic condition, but it also may compromise the performance because the cells will be partially dehydrated.[89]

Caffeine. When plasma FFA are elevated, there is a sparing of muscle glycogen and an enhanced capacity for endurance exercise.[90,91] Caffeine stimulates the mobilization of FFA. In trained individuals it was shown that consumption of 330 mg of caffeine (the amount in approximately 3 cups of coffee or 3 No Doz tablets) 60 minutes before beginning exercise resulted in an increase of 19.5% in total exercise time to exhaustion. Although oxygen uptake and heart rate were the same for both groups, those taking the caffeine considered the exercise to be easier despite not knowing whether they had taken caffeine. Fat oxidation, as indicated by respiratory data, was higher. Not only was more FFA being mobilized, but perhaps there was enhanced utilization of FFA by exercising skeletal muscle. It is possible that the athletes perceived the exercise to be easier after caffeine because caffeine reduces the threshold for neuronal excitation.[92]

If caffeine is to be used, and it is not recommended for children or the young teen, it should be taken 1 hour before competition. The amount would be 5 mg/kg. (1 No Doz tablet and 1 cup of coffee each contain 100 mg caffeine. Fig. 9-7 gives the caffeine content of various drinks and medications.) A 70-kg (154-lb) athlete would take 350 mg caffeine, or 3½ cups of coffee, to obtain the desired effects. If the athlete knows that caffeine has a detrimental effect because of nervousness or jitters, then the athlete should not take caffeine. Caffeine does function as a diuretic, so excessive urination may be another adverse effect.

Alcohol. In interpreting the extensive research related to alcohol and its effect on athletic performance, Williams[54] concludes that in events requiring fine neuromotor control, slight excesses in alcohol consumption may prove to be detrimental to performance. Small to moderate doses do not appear to have any significant effect on tasks involving maximal strength, local muscular endurance, or general cardiovascular endurance. Apparently, the various physiological changes produced by alcohol during a resting state are abrogated by the various neural and hormonal adjustments associated with the onset of exercise. One immediate effect is that since alcohol reduces feelings of insecurity, tension, and discomfort, it may elicit a greater self-confidence in the athlete. Although not actually performing better, the athlete may perceive that he or she is.[93] However, the idea that alcohol will improve performance is probably a misconception. Alcohol cannot be used as an energy source during exercise, does not influence Vo_2 max during exercise, and does not affect anaerobic energy expenditure through sources such as ATP or CP.[54]

Meals and Competition

No topic related to nutrition for athletes has more of a mystique than the pregame meal. This meal is overemphasized, for the high energy–demanding game is performed not only on the morning's intake but also on the intake of the 2 to 3 days preceding the event. However, for the athlete the pregame meal has a psychological aura. For this reason the meal is frequently unusual and may be ritualistic.

There is some scientific basis, however, for general recommendations for the athlete's pregame meal. The pregame meal should be eaten 3 to 4 hours before an event to allow for the food to move out of the stomach and be partially digested and absorbed. This also allows for plasma insulin to return to a "fasting" level and for mobilization of fatty acids during competition. The meal should be composed mainly of carbohydrate and protein. The amount of fat should be small because fat takes longer to digest and otherwise may still be in the stomach during the competition. The energy from the fat would not be available in time for the competition. For long-term aerobic events, the meal should be extra high in carbohydrate because carbohydrate is the most efficient fuel for exercise requirements. A reduced protein intake will mean a smaller load of protein-breakdown products to be excreted by the kidney and thus less water loss through urination. An appropriate pregame meal might be toast with cinnamon and sugar or jelly, a baked potato, spaghetti with tomato sauce, cereal with skim milk, or low-fat yogurt with fruit-sugar flavorings.

Fluid intake should be generous to ensure that the body is well hydrated before the event. For this reason the liquid pregame meal has been recommended by many coaches and used by many athletes. Although commercial liquid meals provide an easily digested, high-fluid, high-carbohydrate meal, there is no magic in choosing them for a pregame meal.

Nutritional intake following the event should be focused on rehydration, repletion of glycogen stores, restoration of electrolyte balance, and clearing of anaerobic metabolic products such as lactic acid. During this time, there is also repayment of the oxygen debt. The extra oxygen consumed in recovery from moderate exercise is associated with restoration of the ATP and CP high-energy phosphates that were depleted and not resynthesized during exercise. Later, in the "slow" component of recovery, lactic acid is reconverted to pyruvic acid and metabolized for energy through the Krebs cycle. It is also thought that some lactic acid is synthesized back to glycogen in the liver. Lactic acid is not a waste product, as it is frequently termed, but a potential source of chemical energy when adequate oxygen is present, as during recovery periods following competition.

Various studies have shown that 12 to 46 hours is needed for muscle glycogen repletion. This depends on the amount of carbohydrate in the diet.[77,94,95] Piehl[94] reported that 60% of the glycogen resynthesis occurs within the first 10 hours following the depletion. Thus the first day of high-carbohydrate intake in the loading regimen, or the afternoon and evening following athletic competition, is the most important for a high-carbohydrate intake. When possible, the postcompetition meal should be served in a relaxed and congenial atmosphere and should not be shortchanged. It is particularly important if there is further competition the following day.

Sodium can be replaced by salting food liberally and choosing foods high in sodium. Good sources of sodium include the following: canned soup, salted crackers, chips, snack foods, canned vegetables, vegetable juices, pickles, salted meats (such as cold cuts and frankfurters), and fast foods (such as hamburgers, french fries, and fish burgers). One-third teaspoon salt (sodium chloride) in a quart of water makes an acceptable sodium-replacement drink that is not too concentrated. Glucose added to the drink further aids the absorption of sodium from the intestine.

Potassium losses can be replenished by liberally eating foods high in potassium (for example, orange juice, bananas, potatoes, mushrooms, and most fruits and vegetables).

Rehydration is extremely important, especially

if sweat losses have been great and competition is anticipated again the next day. It has been claimed that it takes between 2 and 3 days for the body to be completely rehydrated after vigorous exercise.[96]

Injury

In the case of injury from athletic competition, attention should still be paid to the same factors: rehydration, replenishment of glycogen stores, and restoration of electrolyte balance. If surgery is considered and tissue healing will be necessary, adequate protein intake becomes important. In the event that the athlete will be unable to train at the previous level, attention should be paid to decreased energy intake so that appropriate body weight can be maintained. The intake reduction should be in the fat and refined carbohydrate component of the diet: pastries, ice cream, gravies, butter, candies, and soda pop. Injury recovery also may be a time of depression, boredom, and reduced activity, so the potential to gain weight is enhanced. Depression and boredom can lead to overeating, especially if the athlete is accustomed to a high energy intake, and this must be anticipated.

NUTRITIONAL ENVIRONMENT AND THE ADOLESCENT ATHLETE

Because the teenage athlete is so concerned with performance, ergogenic foods, or those thought to increase performance or enhance endurance, are talked about frequently. As depicted in Table 6-4, these foods range from bee pollen to wheat germ oil. They are a topic of conversation because they supposedly enhance metabolic processes associated with muscular contraction or energy production. Most of these foods and dietary practices are harmless to the athlete. The only danger these foods pose comes when they replace necessary foods that the athlete needs for body maintenance and repair and performance energy. Because of the athlete's excessive concern with performance,

hucksters of nutritional products take advantage of them. Most athletes, especially teenage athletes, will try anything at least once to see if it will affect performance. Athletes and coaches should be educated that there is no scientific evidence of advantage in these products. However, the product may have a psychological benefit for the athlete, in which case it is difficult to condemn it.

No matter how much the athlete knows about nutrition and the need for more energy and foods, if he or she does not have the time to eat or if nutritious, wholesome foods are not readily available, as may be the case in low-income homes, the athlete is not going to be well nourished. Even if the food is present, if a demanding training schedule does not allow time for appropriate meals and eating, the athlete will suffer. For example, the long-distance runner will frequently have two daily workouts, one in the morning before breakfast and one in the afternoon before dinner. The workout before breakfast may decrease the appetite for breakfast when it is available. Later in the morning, when the athlete is hungry, the athlete may be in school and not able to eat or have access only to vending machine foods, which are inappropriate except for their high energy content. In addition, the athlete may eat a small lunch in anticipation of the afternoon "hard" workout. The athlete may not want to "run on a full stomach." Allowing enough time after the workout so that the athlete feels hungry, dinner now must fulfill perhaps 50% of the athlete's requirements for protein, vitamins, minerals, and energy. A large, nutritious evening snack helps to meet these needs. If particular attention is not paid to the athlete's schedule and if wholesome high-calorie foods are not readily available, the tendency is for the teenage athlete to turn to easily obtained high-energy, low-nutrient foods that will at least satisfy the appetite. The optimal situation makes many nutritious snack foods easily available at home, on the practice field, and in the school.

The nutrition professional working with athletes

Table 6-4. Ergogenic foods

Food	Claims for Supposed Action or Effect	Conclusions on Effectiveness
Glucose, dextrose	Simple sugar that is source of quick energy and fuel for muscular contraction.	No evidence supports claims for increased performance; because of insulin-raising effect, may cause decreased use of fatty acids in long-distance events; may drain water into gastrointestinal tract and cause disturbance.
Honey	High source of fructose (40%), which supposedly is better than glucose for replenishing glycogen stores.	No evidence supports claims.
Gelatin	Credited with increasing muscle power and relieving fatigue because it contains glycine; glycine is a precursor of creatine. Some contend that gelatin thus helps form the high-energy phosphate phosphocreatine in muscles.	Literature shows no benefit to performance.
Lecithin	Phospolipid that supposedly possesses therapeutic properties of phosphorous, which plays significant part in functional efficiency of muscle and nerve tissue.	Good study shows ineffectiveness as an ergogenic aid.
Wheat germ oil Octacosanol	Supposedly increases oxygen uptake in the heart and skeletal muscle; glycogen metabolism is enhanced.	Much work by one author does not show conclusive results.
Phosphates Sodium phosphate Potassium phosphate	Because phosphates are involved in energetics of muscular activity, they are thought to be able to increase physical working capacity of humans.	No good evidence supports claim, but there may be placebo effect.
Alkaline salts Sodium citrate Sodium bicarbonate Tomato or orange juice	Supposedly increase blood pH and buffer the acidity buildup of lactic acid production during exercise.	Flatulence is a side effect. Biggest advantage, if any, would be in untrained athletes in anaerobic events where maximal work rate is of short duration (2 minutes or less).
Aspartates Potassium aspartate Magnesium aspartate	Have been used to counteract fatigue resulting from long marches, but action is unclear; may accelerate synthesis of ATP phosphocreatine and glycogen in muscle and thus enhance endurance capacity.	Studies do not substantiate claims for physical working capacity in trained men. More research is needed.
Bee pollen	Rich in carotene and contains all 22 amino acids, 27 minerals, and many enzymes; thought to enhance performance.	No scientific evidence showing an effect on performance other than possibly placebo effect. Ingestion can cause life-threatening allergic reaction in individuals sensitive to pollens.
B_{15}-pangamic acid	Chemical mixture isolated from apricot kernels and given the fraudulent name of vitamin B_{15}; supposedly increases respiratory ability by providing ''instant oxygen.''	Not really an identified chemical, although usually contains diisopropylamine dichloroacetate (DCA). DCA found to be weak mutagen. No tests on effectiveness, and use is possibly unsafe.

and coaches must make nutrition information available in a busy schedule. Many times the most effective place for the education is during or just before the practice session. The information provided must be relevant to performance to be appealing to the athlete.

SUMMARY

Physical fitness—composed of body composition, muscular fitness, and cardiorespiratory fitness—is important in the adolescent's physical and psychological development. Because of the nature of adolescent development, teens are particularly vulnerable to excessive claims for nutritional products and to compulsive eating behaviors that surround physical performance. This should be watched for closely in the teenage athlete.

Teens who are active as athletes have important nutritional requirements for extra carbohydrate, water, and electrolytes. These requirements must be met for optimal performance. The teenage athlete must receive guidance to eliminate some of the mystique surrounding certain foods, vitamins, and minerals. However, if these foods, vitamins, and minerals are assessed as being safe, they may be psychologically important in helping performance.

It is important that the athlete's environment be one that promotes positive eating and activity patterns. Besides enhancing physical performance, the environment should allow the teen to mature emotionally and psychologically.

REFERENCES

1. Katch, F.I., and McArdle, W.D.: Nutrition, weight control and exercise, Boston, 1977, Houghton Mifflin Co.
2. Behnke, A.R., and Wilmore, J.H.: Evaluation and regulation of body build and composition, Englewood Cliffs, N.J., 1974, Prentice-Hall, Inc.
3. Buskirk, E.R.: Diet and athletic performance, Postgrad. Med. **61**:229, 1977.
4. Dale, E., Gerlach, D.H., and Wilhite, A.L.: Menstrual dysfunction in distance runners, Obstet. Gynecol. **54**:47, 1979.
5. Frisch, R.E., and McArthur, J.W.: Menstrual cycles: fatness as a determinant of minimum weight for height necessary for their maintenance or onset, Science **185**:949, 1974.
6. Frisch, R.E., and others: Delayed menarche and amenorrhea of college athletes in relation to age of onset of training, JAMA **246**:1559, 1981.
7. Sorlie, P., Gordon T., and Kannel, W.B.: Body build and mortality: the Framingham study, JAMA **243**:1828, 1980.
8. Pipes, T.V., and Vodak, P.A.: The Pipes fitness test and prescription, Los Angeles, 1978, J.P. Tarcher, Inc.
9. Anderson, J.L., and Cohen, M.: The West Point fitness and diet book, New York, 1977, Avon Books.
10. Katch, F.I., McArdle, W.D., and Boylan, R.B.: Getting in shape, Boston, 1979, Houghton Mifflin Co.
11. Essen, B., and others: Metabolic characteristics of fiber types in human skeletal muscle, Acta Physiol. Scand. **95**:153, 1975.
12. Bergh, U., and others: Maximal oxygen uptake and muscle fiber types in trained and untrained humans, Med. Sci. Sports **10**:151, 1974.
13. Costill, D.L., Fink, W.J., and Pollock, M.L.: Muscle fiber composition and enzyme activities of elite distance runners, Med. Sci. Sports **8**:96, 1976.
14. Holloszy, J.O.: Adaptation of skeletal muscle to endurance exercise, Med. Sci. Sports **7**:155, 1975.
15. Astrand, P.O., and others: Girl swimmers, Acta Paediatr. Suppl. 147, 1963.
16. Baily, D.A.: The growing child and the need for physical activity. In Albinson, J.G., and Andrew, G.M., editors: Child in sport and physical activity, International Series on Sport Sciences, **3**:81, 1976.
17. Ekblom, B.: Effect of physical activity in adolescent boys, J. Appl. Physiol. **27**:350, 1969.
18. Astrand, P., and Rodahl, K.: Textbook of work physiology, New York, 1970, McGraw-Hill, Inc.
19. Bannister, R.G.: Limits of human performance, Basel, 1968, Documenta Geigy.
20. Gaillard, B., and others: Handbook for the young athlete, Palo Alto, Calif., 1978, Bull Publishing Co.
21. Holm, G., Björntorp, P., and Jagenburg, R.: Carbohydrate, lipid and amino acid metabolism following physical exercise in men, J. Appl. Physiol. **45**:128, 1978.
22. Björntorp, P., and others: The effect of physical training on insulin production in obesity, Metabolism **19**:631, 1970.
23. Björntorp, P., Sjostrom, L., and Sullivan, L.: The role of physical exercise in the management of obesity. In Munro, J.F., editor: The treatment of obesity, Lancaster, England, 1979, MPT Press, Ltd.
24. Borensztajn, J.: Effect of exercise on lipoprotein lipase activity in rat heart and skeletal muscle, Am. J. Physiol. **229**:394, 1975.

25. Sharkey, B.J.: Physiology of fitness: prescribing exercise for fitness, weight control and health, Champaign, Ill., 1979, Human Kinetics Publishers, Inc.

26. Huttunen, J.K., and others: Effect of moderate physical exercise on serum lipoproteins: a controlled clinical trial with special reference to serum high-density lipoproteins, Circulation **60**:1220, 1979.

27. Hartung, G.H., and others: Relation of diet to high-density lipoprotein cholesterol in middle-aged marathon runners, joggers and inactive men, N. Engl. J. Med. **302**:357, 1980.

28. Lopez, A., and others: Effect of exercise and physical fitness on serum lipids and lipoproteins, Atherosclerosis **30**:1, 1974.

29. Lampman, R.M., and others: Comparative effects of physical training and diet in normalizing serum lipids in men with Type IV hypolipoproteinemia, Circulation **55**:652, 1977.

30. Zauner, C.W., Burt, J.J., and Mapes, D.F.: The effect of strenuous and mild premeal exercise on postprandial lipemia, Res. Q. **39**:395, 1968.

31. Rothwell, N.J., and Stock, M.J.: A role for brown adipose tissue in diet-induced thermogenesis, Nature **281**:31, 1979.

32. Newsholme, E.A.: A possible metabolic basis for the control of body weight, N. Engl. J. Med. **302**:400, 1980.

33. Edwards, H.T., Thorndike, A., and Dill, D.B.: The energy requirements in strenuous muscular exercise, N. Engl. J. Med. **213**:532, 1935.

34. Mayer, J., and Thomas, D.: Regulation of food choice and obesity, Science **156**:328, 1967.

35. Mayer, J.: Overweight: causes, costs, and control, Englewood Cliffs, N.J., 1968, Prentice-Hall, Inc.

36. Epstein, L.H., Masek, B., and Marshall, W.: A nutritionally based school program for control of eating in obese children, Behav. Ther. **9**:766, 1978.

37. Sutton, J., and others: Hormonal changes during exercise, Lancet **2**:1304, 1968.

38. Eriksson, B.O., Persson, B., and Thorell, J.I.: The effects of repeated prolonged exercise on plasma growth hormone, insulin, glucose, free fatty acids, glycerol, lactate and β-hydroxybutyric acid in 13 year old boys and adults, Acta Paediatr. Scand. Suppl. **217**:142, 1971.

39. Gwinup, G.: Effect of exercise alone on the weight of obese women, Arch. Intern. Med. **135**:676, 1975.

40. Yang, M.U., and Van Itallie, T.B.: Composition of weight loss during short-term weight reduction, J. Clin. Invest. **58**:722, 1976.

41. Garrow, J.: Energy balance and obesity in man, New York, 1974, Elsevier Science Publishing Co., Inc.

42. Boyle, P.C., Storlien, H., and Keesey, R.E.: Increased efficiency of food utilization following weight loss, Physiol. Behav. **21**:261, 1978.

43. Szepesi, B.: A model of nutritionally induced overweight: weight "rebound" following caloric restriction. In Bray, G.A., editor: Recent advances in obesity research, vol. 2, London, 1978, Newman Books, Ltd.

44. Wooley, S.C., Wooley, O.W., and Dyrenforth, S.R.: Theoretical, practical and social issues in behavioral treatments of obesity, J. Appl. Behav. Anal. **12**:3, 1979.

45. Oscai, L.B.: The role of exercise in weight control. In Wilmore, J.H., editor: Exercise and sports sciences reviews, vol. 1, New York, 1973, Academic Press, Inc.

46. Cooper, K.H.: The aerobics way, New York, 1977, Bantam Books, Inc.

47. Pollock, M.L., Gettman, L., and Milesis, C.: Effects of frequency and duration of training on attrition and incidence of injury, Med. Sci. Sports **9**:31, 1977.

48. Cumming, G.R., Everatt, D., and Hastman, L.: Bruce treadmill test in children: normal values in a clinic population, Am. J. Cardiol. **41**:69, 1978.

49. Alexandrov, I.I., and Shishina, N.N.: Study of energy metabolism and nutritional status of young athletes. In Pařízková, J., and Rogozkin, V.A., editors: Nutrition, physical fitness and health, Baltimore, 1978, University Park Press.

50. Havel, R.J., Naimark, A., and Borchgrevink, C.F.: Turnover rate and oxidation of free fatty acids of blood plasma in man during exercise: studies during continuous infusion of palmitate-I-C^{14}, J. Clin. Invest. **42**:1054, 1963.

51. Foster, C., Costill, D.L., and Fink, W.J.: Effects of pre-exercise feeding on endurance performance, Med. Sci. Sports **11**(1):1, 1979.

52. Haymes, E.: The effect of physical activity level on selected hematological variables in adult women, Paper presented at the National AAHPER Convention, Houston, March 1972. Cited in Williams, M.H.: Nutritional aspects of human physical and athletic performance, Springfield, Ill., 1976, Charles C Thomas, Publisher, p. 164.

53. Travers, P., and Campbell, W.: The organism and speed and power. In Larson, L., editor: Fitness, health and work capacity, New York, 1974, Macmillan Publishing Co., Inc.

54. Williams, M.H.: Nutritional aspects of human physical and athletic performance, Springfield, Ill., 1976, Charles C Thomas, Publisher.

55. Yamaji, R.: Studies on protein metabolism in muscular exercise. I. Nitrogen metabolism in training of hard muscular exercise, J. Physiol. Soc. Japan **13**:476, 1951.

56. Yoshimura, H.: Anemia during physical training (sports anemia), Nutr. Rev. **28**:251, 1970.

57. Durnin, J.V.: Protein requirements and physical activity. In Pařízková, J., and Rogozkin, V.A., editors: Nutrition, physical fitness and health, Baltimore, 1978, University Park Press.

58. Davies, C., and others: Iron deficiency anemia: its effect on maximum aerobic power and responses to exercise in African males aged 17-40 years, Clin. Sci. **44:**555, 1973.

59. Schoene, R., and others: Effect of iron repletion on exercise-induced lactate production in minimally iron-deficient subjects (abstract), Clin. Res. **29:**452, 1981.

60. Finch, C.M.: Lactic acidosis as a result of iron deficiency, J. Clin. Invest. **64:**129, 1979.

61. Mayer, J., and Bullen, B.: Nutrition and athletic performance, Postgrad. Med. **26:**848, 1959.

62. Consolazio, C.F.: Nutrition and athletic performance. In Morgen, S., editor: Progress in human nutrition, vol. 1, Westport, Conn., 1971, AVI Publishing Co.

63. Buskirk, E., and Haymes, E.: Nutritional requirements for women in sport. In Harris, D.V., editor: Women and sport: a national research conference, University Park, Penn., 1972, The Pennsylvania State University Press.

64. Howald, H., and Segesser, B.: Ascorbic acid and athletic performance, Ann. N.Y. Acad. Sci. **258:**458, 1976.

65. Rasch, P., and others: Effects of vitamin C supplementation on cross country runners, Sportzärztliche Praxis **5:**10, 1962.

66. Grey, G., and others: Effects of ascorbic acid on endurance performance and athletic injury, JAMA **211:**105, 1970.

67. Lawrence, J.D., and others: Effects of tocopherol acetate on the swimming endurance of trained swimmers, Am. J. Clin. Nutr. **28:**205, 1975.

68. Sharman, I.: The effects of vitamin E and training on physiological function and athletic performance in adolescent swimmers, Br. J. Nutr. **26:**265, 1971.

69. Shephard, R., and others: Do athletes need vitamin E? Physician Sports Med. **2**(9):57, 1974.

70. Worthington-Roberts, B.: Nutritional considerations for children in sports. In Pipes, P.: Nutrition in infancy and childhood, ed. 2, St. Louis, 1981, The C.V. Mosby Co.

71. Smith, N.J.: Nutrition and the young athlete, Pediatr. Ann. **7**(10):49, 1978.

72. Heald, F.: Treatment of obesity in adolescence, Postgrad. Med. J. **51:**109, 1972.

73. Klafs, C., and Arnheim, D.: Modern principles of athletic training, ed. 5, St. Louis, 1981, The C.V. Mosby Co.

74. Smith, N.J.: Excessive weight loss and food aversion in athletes simulating anorexia nervosa, Pediatrics **66:**139, 1980.

75. Costill, D.L., and others: Glycogen depletion pattern in human muscle fibers during distance running, Acta Physiol. Scand. **89:**374, 1973.

76. Bergstrom, J., and Hultman, E.: A study of glycogen metabolism during exercise in man, Scand. J. Clin. Lab. Invest. **19:**218, 1967.

77. Hultman, E.: Physiological role of muscle glycogen in man with special reference to exercise, Circ. Res. **20** (suppl. 1): 99, 1967.

78. Bergstrom, J., and Hultman, E.: Muscle glycogen synthesis after exercise: an enhancing factor localized to the muscle cells in man, Nature **210:**309, 1966.

79. Costill, D.L., and others: The role of dietary carbohydrates in muscle glycogen resynthesis after strenuous running, Am. J. Clin. Nutr. **34:**1831, 1981.

80. Sherman, W.M., and others: Dietary influence on 24-hour muscle glycogen restoration following depletion (abstract), Med. Sci. Sports Exer. **12:**127, 1980.

81. Olsson, K.E., and Saltin, B.: Variation in total body water with muscle glycogen changes in man, Acta Physiol. Scand. **80:**11, 1970.

82. Mirkin, G.: Carbohydrate loading: a dangerous practice, JAMA **223:**1151, 1973.

83. Saltin, B.: Fluid, electrolyte and energy losses and their replacement in prolonged exercise. In Pařízková, J., and Rogozkin, V.A., editors: Nutrition, physical fitness and health, Baltimore, 1978, University Park Press.

84. Costill, D.L.: The drinking runner. In Higdon, H., editor: The complete diet guide for runners and other athletes, Mountain View, Calif., 1978, World Publications.

85. Costill, D.L., and Saltin, B.: Factors limiting gastric emptying during rest and exercise, J. Appl. Physiol. **37:** 679, 1974.

86. Bergstrom, J., and Hultman, E.: Nutrition for maximal sports performance, JAMA **221:**999, 1972.

87. Costill, D.L., and others: Water and electrolyte replacement during repeated days of work in the heat, Aviat. Space Environ. Med. **46:**795, 1975.

88. Costill, D.L., and others: Muscle water and electrolytes following varied levels of dehydration in man, J. Appl. Physiol. **40:**6, 1976.

89. Ryan, A.: Round table: balancing heat stress, fluids and electrolytes, Physician Sports Med. **3**(8):43, 1975.

90. Hickson, R.C., and others: Effects of increasing plasma free fatty acids on endurance (abstract), Fed. Proc. **36:**450, 1977.

91. Costill, D.L., and others: Effects of elevated plasma FFA and insulin on muscle glycogen usage during exercise, J. Appl. Physiol. **43:**695, 1977.

92. Costill, D.L., Dalsky, G.P., and Fink, W.J.: Effects of caffeine ingestion on metabolism and exercise performance, Med. Sci. Sports **10:**155, 1978.

93. Alcohol and athletes, Physician Sports Med. **7:**39, 1979.

94. Piehl, K.: Glycogen storage and depletion in human skeletal muscle fibers, Acta Physiol. Scand. Suppl. **402:**1, 1974.

95. Costill, D.: Muscular exhaustion during distance running, Physician Sports Med. **2**(10):36, 1974.

96. Greenleaf, J.E.: Involuntary hypohydration in man and animals: a review, National Aeronautics and Space Administration Publication SP-110, Washington, D.C., 1966, National Aeronautics and Space Administration.

Chapter 7

Nutrition and Chronic Medical Problems in Adolescence

MARGARET McINTYRE

GENERAL PRINCIPLES

The number of adolescents facing life with chronic illnesses or handicaps is increasing because of dramatic medical progress in the treatment of many serious diseases such as cystic fibrosis, leukemia, and chronic renal failure. It has been estimated that 7% to 10% of all children under 18 years of age have a chronic physical illness.[1] In addition to chronic illness, the onset of many diseases, such as ulcerative colitis, often occurs during adolescence. The problem of continued physical growth is a major concern in the adolescent. Ensuring optimal psychosocial development is also of utmost importance at this age. Skillful nutritional guidance and care based on knowledge of adolescent development, needs, and behaviors associated with chronic disease can be extremely beneficial to adolescents and their families.

The developmental tasks of adolescence—establishing independence, realizing one's identity, and preparing for adult self-reliance—are of special significance to adolescents with chronic diseases (see Fig. 7-2). The conflict between dependence and independence may be exaggerated by chronic illness. Dependence is often increased by the demands of treatment regimens such as pulmonary therapy in cystic fibrosis, insulin injection in diabetes, or dialysis in renal failure. Enforced reliance on parents for diet control can also foster dependency. Increasing responsibility for self-

care, such as management of the teen's own diet, will decrease dependence on others and allow the adolescent to continue development in this important area.

Essential to the task of developing identity and self-esteem is acceptance by peers. This is especially difficult for the teen who feels different because of illness. Eating ''different'' foods can be perceived as a stigma. The process of ego and self-esteem development seems to be affected by the duration and prognosis of the disease, with more severe problems seen in those with illness of long duration.[2] Kellerman and co-workers[3] have shown that poor prognosis heightens the adolescent's sense of anxiety and promotes low self-esteem that is not seen in adolescents with short-term illness.

Health problems, however, can also have a positive effect on adolescents' resolution of the developmental tasks of adolescence. With adequate support systems, many teenagers develop strengths and compensatory skills that enhance their coping ability.[4] They may develop a special tolerance for those who are different. They also may learn to assume a major role in planning and carrying out their health care. This role results in a degree of control that can be very useful in building self-esteem. A practical area for the adolescent to take responsibility is in the control and management of diet and eating patterns.

Self-image is closely related to perceptions of

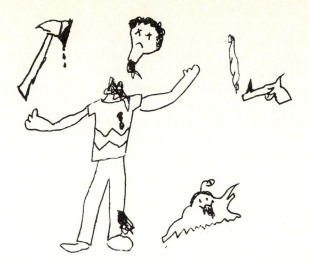

Fig. 7-1. Drawing by 12-year-old boy who has cystic fibrosis.

physical appearance. Figure drawings produced by adolescents may be useful in understanding how the teens see themselves. These drawings can also be an expression of patients' knowledge of their own bodies—a projection of their self-concepts and body images.[5] Many adolescents see themselves as ''damaged'' or otherwise devalued by their illness as illustrated by Fig. 7-1. Assault on body image may result in withdrawn behavior, self-pity, or aggressive acting-out behavior.

The use of an interdisciplinary team in the care and management of the child with chronic disease has special importance for the adolescent. The team can comprehensively address all aspects of the illness, including cognitive, emotional, and psychosocial. Team support can be invaluable both to the patients and to the team members because of shared information and feelings.

Inpatient Unit

Since adolescents have needs and problems different from those of young children and adults, a separate inpatient unit for the hospitalized adolescent is desirable.[6] The atmosphere in this unit can be conducive to adolescent psychosocial develop-ment. The staff benefits because patient manage-ment is facilitated and better overall care is pro-vided. Eating and mealtimes are important in the adolescent's hospital stay, and a separate adoles-cent unit provides opportunity for the dietitian to evaluate the adolescent's knowledge of nutrition and eating habits. Because teenagers value the op-portunity to select their own menus, they should be encouraged to do so whenever possible.

Group interaction helps adolescents move to-ward natural peer-group formation in the inpatient unit. In many settings a rap group is held regularly to ventilate feelings and share concerns.[7] Adoles-cents often focus on the issue of food as an expres-sion of their feelings of frustration, anger, and de-pression at being hospitalized and ill.

Approach to Nutritional Counseling

Poor compliance with diet instructions is not surprising in the adolescent who also is known for being noncompliant in the use of medications. This dietary noncompliance is often difficult for the nu-tritionist to assess. In the case of the diabetic who ''sneaks'' sweet snacks, for example, a rise in blood sugar may signify dietary noncompliance, but it also can be caused by nondietary factors.

Self-supervision by the teenager through diary keeping is one way of improving dietary compliance. Keeping a food record fosters independence and self-responsibility. Good, accurate nutrition education is also important so that the rationale behind the dietary measures is known and understood. When the nutritionist knows the family and has a feeling for how its members interact, compliance will also be facilitated. Home visits thus can be of great value. The nutritionist should try to establish alliances with chronically ill adolescents and should respect their independence and contributions.

An appreciation of the developmental stage of a patient will help the nutritionist in working with the teenager. Chapters 1 and 2 discuss these developmental stages. However, it is important to remember that it is common for a physiologically older adolescent with chronic illness to begin reacting and behaving as a younger adolescent. This regression may be temporary or long term.

Obesity sometimes accompanies chronic illness, especially when steroids are given as part of the treatment. Dietary restrictions in these cases can make a teenager feel deprived, depressed, and irritable. Encouraging the entire family to forgo fattening foods sometimes helps to alleviate the feeling of being different.

The goals of treatment for the chronically ill adolescent are the restoration of health (or the minimization of the effects of illness) and the promotion of normal physical and psychological development. Good nutrition management can be of great value in reaching these goals and is most effective when it is individualized, flexible, and sensitive to the teen's needs and feelings.

Drug-Nutrient Interactions

Drugs can increase nutritional requirements, inhibit nutrient synthesis, and produce malabsorption syndromes. They also can influence dietary intake by causing nausea, vomiting, diarrhea, and an altered sense of taste. Conversely, the teen's nutritional status can influence both the response to a drug and the effective dosage of a drug. Adolescents may be particularly vulnerable to some of these effects because of their increased nutritional needs during growth and their marginal or possibly inadequate diets. For example, the metabolism of folate is altered by some drugs. Because folate is destroyed in food processing (and thus is low in the snack and convenience foods that are widely eaten by teenagers), drugs may magnify already marginal folate nutriture.

Drug-induced nutritional deficiencies are more likely to be found in those needing many drugs or in those using drugs for long-term treatment of chronic disease. Teenagers with chronic disease need careful evaluation for nutritional deficits. Most drug effects are reversible with either proper nutrient supplementation or discontinuation of the drug therapy.

Appetite and Taste. Although amphetamines (such as methylphenidate [Ritalin] and dextroamphetamine [Dexedrine]) reduce appetite, they have not been effective in the treatment of obesity and are not recommended for teenagers as an appetite suppressant. The long-term use of such drugs for the control of hyperactivity may cause growth retardation. This retardation seems to be reversible with discontinuance of the medication during the summer months when ''catch-up'' growth can be seen.[8]

Many therapeutic agents for cancer cause loss of both appetite and sense of taste (see Table 7-2). In patients already debilitated by disease, the resulting decrease in intake can influence the prognosis of the disease and the response to treatment.

There are also drugs that increase appetite and thus food intake. These include steroids, insulin, psychotropic drugs, and certain antihistamines.[9,10]

Nutrient Absorption. Numerous drugs induce malabsorption by damaging the lining of the small intestine or by inactivating intestinal enzyme systems. A common aberration is the suppression of vitamin D metabolism, which leads to malabsorption of calcium. This effect occurs with the use of anticonvulsant drugs (for example, phenytoin [Dilantin], primidone [Mysoline], or phenobarbital) and is more severe with long-term treatment. If adolescents have been on such treatment for long periods of time, rickets and osteomalacia may result if there is not proper supplementation.[11] Antacids that contain aluminum (for example, Mylanta or Maalox) inhibit intestinal absorption of phosphorus and fluoride. In long-term use calcium excretion increases in the stool, causing skeletal demineralization. Antibiotics also impair absorption, affecting such nutrients as vitamin B_{12}, folic acid, fat, potassium, calcium, iron, carotene, and sodium.[11]

Mineral oil can make dietary carotene soluble. The carotene is then lost to the normal absorptive process and instead passes out in the feces.[11] Mineral oil also diminishes absorption of other fat-soluble vitamins and should not be used except on a short-term basis with adolescents.

Nutrient Metabolism. Isoniazid (INH), used as a prophylaxis in persons exposed to tuberculosis or in persons with a positive tuberculin test, inhibits the normal metabolism of vitamin B_6. Concomitant administration of pyridoxine (50 to 100 mg/day, depending on the dosage of the drug) is recommended for children over 11 years of age who are felt to be malnourished or vitamin deficient.[12]

Anticonvulsants may alter the metabolism of vitamin D, vitamin K, and folic acid. However, if folic acid supplementation is started after anticonvulsants have been given for some time, deterioration of seizure control may occur.[13] Dosages of up to 5 mg/day do not seem to have this effect.

Drugs can inhibit the synthesis of vitamins as well. Antibiotics can inhibit bacterial synthesis of vitamins in the gastrointestinal tract. For example, tetracycline can inhibit vitamin K synthesis. A drug history, including dose and frequency, should be included as part of a diet history, and appropriate treatment should be instituted. For further dis-

cussion of drug-nutrient interaction see references 14 and 15.

Substance Abuse and Nutrition. The increasing incidence of alcohol abuse among teenagers and the apparent spread of alcoholism across socioeconomic levels underlie the need for educating young people about the nutritional consequences and other hazards of alcohol ingestion. Alcohol abuse can cause anorexia (loss of appetite) and diminished food intake. It can also lead to tissue depletion of such nutrients as folate, thiamin, magnesium, and zinc. This depletion is caused either by the increased need for these nutrients to metabolize alcohol or by the diets of alcohol abusers, which are frequently deficient in these nutrients.

Narcotics, stimulants, and depressants may markedly disturb nutritional status, both because of the drugs' direct effects on body utilization and because the teenage abuser's life-style, including eating behavior, is often incompatible with obtaining an adequate diet. This is discussed further in Chapter 4. Nutritional support is an essential component of treatment in the rehabilitation of substance abusers.

IRON DEFICIENCY ANEMIA

As discussed in Chapter 3, iron needs are increased in adolescence because of accelerated growth and the onset of menses. Because of these increased demands, iron deficiency anemia can result.

Iron deficiency anemia is probably the most common nutritional disease seen among adolescents, and it is more prevalent in boys than in girls.[16] The *Ten State Nutrition Survey* showed that between 5% and 10% of teenagers had either hemoglobin or hematocrit levels that were below normal.[17] In addition, studies of children 1 to 18 years of age showed a higher incidence of anemia among the black population. In the *Health and Nutrition Examination Survey,* around 10% of the boys and 5% of the girls were found to be iron deficient. This study looked at hemoglobin, hematocrit, serum iron, and transferrin levels.[16] Other studies have found deficiencies in 10% to 27% of female adolescents and in 13% to 50% of males.[18] Brown and co-workers[19] found that there was a higher incidence of iron deficiency in girls over 15 years of age and in boys at 12 and 13 years of age.

Iron deficiency anemia is characterized as a microcytic hypochromic anemia because the red cells are small (microcytic) and pale (hypochromic). It is most commonly diagnosed by determining levels of hematocrit and serum hemoglobin. Standards are now available by developmental stage, sex, and race[20] as shown in Table 3-13. When possible, it is better to obtain more information about iron stores with additional tests because iron deficiency can occur without the person being anemic. In iron deficiency, serum iron is low and total iron-binding capacity (TIBC) is high. Transferrin saturation, which can be obtained by dividing serum iron by TIBC, is decreased with low iron stores. Values of 16% or less in girls and 20% or less in boys are considered inadequate.[21] Iron-poor bone marrow aspirate and a low serum ferritin also reflect reduced iron storage and can occur early in the course of iron deficiency before anemia develops.[22] In iron deficiency without anemia, plasma iron is less than 40 $\mu g/dl$, TIBC is more than 400 $\mu g/dl$, and serum ferritin is less than 12 ng/ml.

Iron deficiency not only causes anemia but is also a systemic disease. Clinical symptoms can include fatigue, weakness, and dysphagia (difficulty in swallowing).[23] Epithelial changes, such as glossitis, stomatitis, and koilonychia (spoon nail), can also occur, although these changes seem to be more unusual in adolescents than in the adult population.[24] Pica, especially pagophagia (eating ice), seems to be particularly related to anemia in children and adolescents. Iron deficiency can also lead to atrophy of gastric mucosa and decreased secretion of gastric acid. It can have tissue effects on the cardiovascular and musculoskeletal systems.[25]

Many clinicians feel that early iron deficiency short of anemia is related to a number of subjective psychomotor complaints. The relationship of behavior and iron deficiency has been widely studied[26,27] and is discussed further in Chapter 8.

When deficiency is found, a daily dose of 2 to 3 mg/kg of a simple ferrous salt, such as sulfate, gluconate, or fumarate, should be given. This should be given in divided doses three times a day between meals to avoid interference with chelating agents contained in foods. In practice, 300 mg given once daily is often prescribed for adolescents, who frequently fail to comply with iron-supplement recommendations. In fact, failure to take iron medications is the most frequent reason for failure to respond. Side effects of large doses of iron include nausea and constipation or diarrhea. An overt toxicity can occur with dosages of 200 to 250 mg/kg/day.[28] Delayed-release tablets are not as well absorbed in the small intestine, and large quantities of iron may adversely affect vitamin E absorption and produce imbalances in zinc and other minerals.[29]

Treatment with iron supplements is likely to produce only temporary improvement, and nutritional counseling is essential to produce long-term change and subsequent improvement in iron status. In Western countries the average diet contains 5 to 7 mg iron/1000 kcal.[30] However, because dairy foods, which are low in iron, form a significant amount of many teenagers' daily intake and because many foods popular with adolescents contain little iron, it is possible that adolescents' average daily intake is less than the norm. This problem is compounded in many adolescent girls because the need for iron increases at a time when the requirement for energy declines. In addition, many girls decide to follow weight-reduction diets at this time, further reducing the chances for an adequate iron intake.

Food sources of iron include liver, fortified cereal products, meat (especially red), fish, dried beans, green vegetables, and some dried fruits. Further discussion of the bioavailability and absorption of iron from food can be found in other texts.[31,32]

SICKLE CELL DISEASE

Sickle cell disease (SCD), or sickle cell anemia, occurs in approximately 1 in 1000 black persons. The course of the disease is variable, and the anemia may be intermittent or mild. Low body weight and a slight body build are characteristic of this disease. Ashcroft and others[33] found that children with SCD were smaller than control children. By young adulthood, however, there was no difference in height, suggesting that the increase in stature is greater than normal during adolescence. Considerable variation is seen in height, physical capability, and prognosis, but even with a mild course, teenagers tend to be emotionally affected by having a chronic disease that sets them apart from their peers.

The severity of SCD tends to increase with age, and good nutrition becomes a primary force in keeping the affected person in good health and in protecting him or her from infection. A balanced, high-quality diet with low to moderate iron intake should be advocated. Iron intake is limited because the liver already has increased iron stores as a result of the disease, and excess iron in the diet causes iron overload. Iron-rich foods, such as liver and iron-fortified cereal, should be excluded. The diet should be high in folate (400 to 600 μg/day) because the increased production of erythrocytes needed to replace those being destroyed by the disease increases the folic acid requirements. The nutritionist should be oriented to low-budget problems and should especially advocate low-cost sources of protein such as fish, eggs, and poultry. Since an abundance of liquids should be regularly consumed, the teenager with SCD should be reminded to keep a pitcher of water or fruit juice where it can be used regularly.

Zinc deficiency is often associated with poor appetite, short stature, and delayed puberty, all of which are seen in SCD.[34] Studies have shown decreased serum zinc in patients with SCD. In a study by Brewer, Brewer, and Prasad,[35] 25 mg zinc acetate/day reduced the number of sickle-cell crises from six to less than three a year. Zinc supplementation also has enhanced healing of leg ulcers that are seen in affected adults and adolescents.

Measurement of plasma zinc concentration is subject to wide variation and may not reflect body stores. It has been suggested that the activity of carbonic anhydrase (a zinc-dependent enzyme) may be a more stable indicator of zinc deficiency in children with SCD. Its determination should probably precede the selection of patients who may benefit from zinc therapy. Assessment of zinc status is discussed further in Chapter 3.

Prasad and co-workers[36] have observed increased plasma copper in patients with SCD. Zinc and copper compete with each other for similar binding sites on protein, and it is likely that increased plasma copper is a result of the zinc deficiency. Prasad and co-workers caution that zinc used for long periods of treatment of SCD may produce copper deficiency.

DIABETES MELLITUS

Juvenile diabetes (as opposed to adult-onset diabetes) is a widely used term that is being replaced by a new designation, *insulin-dependent diabetes mellitus* (IDDM).[37] IDDM is characterized by the development of ketosis in the absence of insulin replacement and is probably the most important chronic disorder of young people in the United States. Its onset is typically in childhood or puberty, and the incidence seems to be increasing. The clinical onset in adolescents is rapid, although the duration of symptoms before diagnosis may vary from a few days to many months.

Relatively little is known about the precise relationship of physiological pubertal changes to control of IDDM, but sexual maturation and the adolescent growth spurt usually increase requirements for insulin. The metabolic instability so characteristic of diabetes in adolescents can also be influenced by the erratic eating habits, the spontaneous bursts of physical activity, and the mental and emotional stress common in this age group.

Coronary disease is two or three times more common in the diabetic person than in the non-diabetic person.[38] For this reason, the goal of therapy for diabetic adolescents is to keep blood sugar levels within normal ranges and to avoid the appearance of vascular complications, which often occur as early as 5 years after the onset of disease. Kaufman and his co-workers[39] evaluated diabetic children in a summer camp and found that the subjects' cholesterol levels fell to a range seen in non-diabetic children when they ate a low-cholesterol (300 mg cholesterol/day), low–saturated fat diet with a polyunsaturated to saturated fat ratio of 1.0 (P/S 1.0).

Recently there has been emphasis on increasing the dietary fiber in the diabetic person's diet. A study of adolescents with IDDM showed that their blood glucose control improved on a high-fiber diet.[40]

Since microvascular complications of IDDM are decreased with normalization of blood glucose concentration,[41] it is important to be able to follow diabetic control as closely as possible. With the advent of the use of serum glycosylated hemoglobin (hemoglobin A_{Ic}) as an indicator of blood glucose control, it has been possible to evaluate control over the preceding 1 to 2 months,[42] rather than relying on blood sugar measurements alone, which reflect only the immediate glucose concentration and can fluctuate widely. The concentration of hemoglobin A_{Ic} has also been found to correlate inversely with the concentration of serum cholesterol and plasma triglyceride, suggesting that improved diabetic control may diminish the risk of premature heart disease.[43]

The diabetic diet is a normal, healthy diet that is adequate for the entire family. It should be satisfying, flexible enough to allow unlimited activity, and place no unnecessary emotional burden on the teenager or the family. Diet instructions for the adolescent, especially during the initial hospitalization, should not contain too much overwhelming detail. Following are the three important principles of diet planning for an adolescent with diabetes: (1) meals and snacks should be eaten at regular times; (2) foods high in sugar should not be eaten in large quantities; and (3) cholesterol and fat, especially saturated fat, should be limited. For a more detailed description of designing a diabetic diet for the young person see references 44 and 45.

Although the traditional diabetic exchange diet can be used with the adolescent, most clinicians favor a more liberal approach to diet with teens. In several studies[46,47] no difference in long-term control was found between children on an unmeasured or liberal ''no-concentrated-sweets'' diet and children on a strict exchange diet. The most restrictive aspect of the liberal diets is the necessity of eating at regular times, thus avoiding a pattern of feast and fast. For example, this diet abolishes sleeping late on weekends and skipping breakfast. Adolescents can be encouraged to take insulin and breakfast at the regular time and then go back to bed if they wish.

Usually both an afternoon and an evening snack are recommended for the teenager with IDDM. The snack should be high in protein and complex carbohydrate. Candy, sodas, sweet desserts, syrup, jelly, and other concentrated sweets should be avoided. Should artificial sweeteners be used? The only rational argument for their use has to do with the psychosocial aspects of the diabetic adolescent's life. Adolescents are often in settings where sweet beverages or foods are essential elements, and at such times artificial sweeteners may have a place.

Follow-up visits with the nutritionist should occur on a regular basis and should include opportunities to clear up misunderstanding, to clarify the diet, to listen to diet-related concerns, and to assist in the adjustment of the diet. This is often a long process for the teenager, and dietary instructions often must be repeated and explained many times.

Low self-esteem is a common problem among diabetic teenagers who find the dietary restrictions of IDDM a serious handicap. Denial is often used as a defense against the pain of feeling defective and different. Support or rap groups can be invaluable aids for diabetic teens in airing their feelings and in relating to peers in the same situation. The nutritionist can be an important member of the team working with such a group.

DENTAL CARIES AND GUM DISEASE

There is overwhelming evidence that dietary carbohydrates play a major etiological role in dental caries. Simple sugars (such as glucose, fructose, and sucrose) and polysaccharides, which are broken down into simple sugars by salivary amylase, are fermented by bacteria into organic acids that demineralize tooth enamel. Adolescents' propensity for snacking on refined carbohydrates is conducive to tooth decay. Since 80% of the average person's total incidence of dental lesions occur in the teenage years, this is the time to encourage habits of choosing alternatives to sugar-containing foods.[48] Paradoxically, these are also the years when access to and desire for carbohydrate-rich foods are very high. Many adolescents have been rewarded with sweets as they were growing up, and they continue to reward themselves in this way.

Studies in Vipeholm, Sweden, have shown that the *amount* of sugar does not seem as important in the formation of cavities as the timing of exposure. Sweets consumed with or at the end of a meal did not have the cariogenic effect of sweets consumed between meals.[49] Thus the task of the nutritionist would seem to be to alert young people to the detrimental effects of sugars consumed throughout

the day and to encourage them to choose snacks such as cheese and celery, nuts, vegetables and dip, whole grain crackers, and fruit. The availability of these kinds of foods in vending machines should be a priority health issue for the community.

Highly cariogenic foods have certain factors in common: (1) they are eaten frequently, often between meals; (2) they have the ability to lower the pH of tooth plaque; (3) they are adhesive or sticky and may be retained in the mouth for a long period of time; and (4) they contain sugar or other fermentable sugar. Foods containing 10% to 15% sugar (Table 7-1) are suspect and should not be eaten between meals.[50]

A common practice among adolescents is to snack before bedtime. This could potentially lead to the development of dental caries unless the teeth are cleaned before sleep. Reduction of the flow of saliva, which occurs during sleep, reduces the natural cleansing mechanism and permits greater fermentation of cariogenic material.[48] Therefore the importance of brushing and flossing teeth and

Table 7-1. Sugar content of some common snack foods

Snack Food	Sugar Content (%)
Dry cereals	1-68
Candies	
Chocolate bars	26.8
Hard candy	85
Chewing gum	36.9-84.7
Cookies	11-48.4*
Graham crackers	13.9
Ice cream	8.8-21
Cakes and pies	4.7-40
Snack puddings	10-15.4
Soft drinks	1.8-9.8

Modified from Caan, B.: Med. Clin. North Am. **63**:1087, 1979.
*Most cookies contain over 15% sucrose.

of good dental hygiene, particularly before sleep, should be repeatedly stressed throughout adolescence.

Other factors have recently been shown to alter the cariogenic potential of the diet. Fats and proteins, in particular, have been associated with cariostatic effects. Fats may aid in caries protection by altering the surface properties of the tooth enamel and by decreasing the solubility of sugars. Fats also may be toxic to oral bacteria. Proteins are thought to interfere with plaque formation and to inhibit the growth of bacteria by increasing the urea concentration in the saliva.[51] There is also evidence to indicate that cocoa products and dietary phosphates may produce cariostatic effects.[52,53] The mechanism of action of these foods is not yet well understood. However, their role as possible protective agents must be considered when making dietary recommendations.

Fluoridation of the water supply is common in the United States because of the anticariogenic effect of the fluoride on tooth enamel. However, when fluoride content is 0.7 ppm or less, fluoride supplements are recommended for children. After 12 years of age or after the eruption of the permanent molars, however, oral fluoride supplementation is of less value.

It is becoming apparent that the cause of dental caries is a complex process involving the interplay of several factors. The minerals of the tooth enamel should be viewed as being in constant equilibrium with the oral environment. It is necessary therefore not only to consider the presence of fermentable carbohydrate but also such factors as food solubility, mineral composition, and the buffering capacity of the oral environment.

Nutrients and Gum Disease

Gingivitis increases in prevalence during the teenage years, and periodontal disease often follows. Little is known about nutrition's role in periodontal disease, although deficiency in ascorbic acid has received a great deal of attention as being

an important cause of the disease. Vitamin A deficiency, which is widespread in underdeveloped countries with high incidences of periodontal disease,[54] has also been implicated. Inadequate intake of these nutrients in the teen years can have an adverse effect on the health of the gums in later life.

ACNE

Acne vulgaris is a chronic inflammatory disease of the sebaceous glands. It is very common and probably affects all teenagers to some extent. In most cases it appears to be a natural part of the developmental changes that occur during adolescence. In a small percentage of teens acne can become a physically and psychologically destructive disease. Dermatological complaints represent as much as 50% of all adolescent contacts for health care.[55] The age of peak incidence is 14 to 16 years of age in girls and 16 to 19 years of age in boys. The following are some of the factors believed to participate in the genesis of acne lesions: androgens, sebaceous gland size, sebum production, bacterial colonization and dyskeratosis of the follicular epithelium, stress, and menstrual cycle changes.[56]

The sebaceous glands of the skin are under hormonal control, and the rapid acceleration of hormone production is directly related to the skin changes of acne. In a longitudinal study by Lee,[57] levels of serum testosterone were higher in pubertal boys who developed acne than in controls who did not develop acne. In a study by Hurwitz,[58] testosterone levels in girls tended to be higher with each successive stage of acne. Stress may increase the severity of acne by increasing the androgen output of the adrenal glands.[58]

At the present time, medical treatment is aimed at counteracting these endocrinological and microbiological factors. Usually two or more topical agents, such as benzoyl peroxide and salicylic acid,[58] are prescribed. However, the greater the number of drugs prescribed, the less the compliance.[59] Systemic antibiotics are also used. These antibiotics seem both to reduce the amount of free fatty acids in the sebum by about 50% and to treat the bacterial component. Becker and co-workers[60] report a significant improvement with the administration of topical clindamycin hydrochloride or clindamycin phosphate in an 8-week trial. Oral isotretinoin (13-cis-retinoic acid), a metabolite of vitamin A, was shown to decrease lesions in a double-blind study by Peck.[61] However, the toxic side effects of isotretinoin limit its widespread use at this time; a topical form is used.

Estrogens in birth control pills are thought to counteract the acne-producing effects of androgens. The level of estrogen required, however, may be higher than that present in the pills,[62] and sometimes the acne worsens in girls using the pill.[59]

Very little information supports a relationship between diet and acne, although many persons still have misconceptions about the role of the teenage diet. Fads have incriminated specific foods such as candy, citrus fruits, chocolate, soft drinks, french fries, and sugar. In addition, some people erroneously believe that "greasy foods cause oily skin" and that acne is caused by "acid in the system." Cornbleet and Gigly[63] conducted a study that showed no significant differences in patients with acne who were fed high-sugar diets. Fulton and co-workers[64] studied the effect of chocolate on the composition and output of sebum and found no significant effect. Anderson[65] divided patients into groups according to the foods each patient believed aggravated his or her complexion. Each group was challenged with large quantities of the specific food. Nothing significant occurred during a 1-week follow-up period.

When teenagers feel that certain foods aggravate their complexion, these foods certainly should be avoided. However, broad dietary restrictions encompassing all sweets and soft drinks, all fried foods, or all seafoods and shellfish should not be suggested, as such advice often frustrates the patient and decreases overall compliance. Dietary facts and fictions should be discussed during the initial visit to the physician or nutritionist. It also seems reasonable to stress the importance of eating a well-balanced diet that provides optimal levels of nutrients.

Studies from Europe suggest that zinc is intimately involved in the metabolism of vitamin A and that zinc supplementation is valuable in severe acne.[66] In a study by Michäelsson,[67] oral zinc (135 mg/day) was administered alone and in combination with vitamin A (300,000 IU/day). A comparison group was administered vitamin A alone and in combination with a placebo. After 4 weeks, significant improvement in the acne was found in the groups on zinc. The addition of vitamin A caused no further improvement. There was no improvement with either vitamin A alone or the placebo.[67] Often the acne recurred when the treatment was discontinued. After 12 weeks, the mean acne score was reduced by 85%. Although the mechanism for the action of zinc is not known, it is possible that zinc may promote the increased production of retinol-binding protein, which in some indirect fashion improves the patient's acne. A daily intake of zinc below the recommended 15 mg/day is not uncommon in puberty, and males with severe acne had low serum zinc levels in this study.

Even with a combination of treatments, acne does not improve overnight. Cunliffe[62] suggests that continuation of a particular treatment for 3 months is required before effectiveness can be fully assessed. To avoid frustration and discouragement, this should be explained to the adolescent before a regimen is initiated.

PULMONARY DISEASE

Cystic Fibrosis

Cystic fibrosis (CF) is an inheritable chronic disease whose major feature is the dysfunction of all exocrine glands. It is usually diagnosed in early childhood. With great advances in the treatment of CF, this disease is no longer confined to early life and will be seen with increasing frequency in older patients. Mean survival age was 3 to 4 years in 1950, 10.6 years in 1966, and 21 years in 1980.[68] However, despite the increasingly optimistic prognosis, there is a persistent incidence of growth failure and malnutrition in CF.

Although the main feature of CF is usually pulmonary insufficiency, 80% to 90% of CF patients have gastrointestinal involvement. The organs of digestion are affected by an overproduction of thick mucus that obstructs the ducts to the pancreas, thus preventing pancreatic enzymes—trypsin, amylase, and lipase—from being excreted into the duodenum. Steatorrhea and malabsorption result. Fat-soluble vitamins, fats, and protein are poorly absorbed.

To help remedy the weight loss and the failure to gain weight that occur because of the malabsorption caused by the lack of pancreatic enzymes in the intestines, pancreatic enzymes (Pancrease, Viokase, or Cotazym-S) are taken orally. They are used with each feeding and should not be mixed with acid foods (such as citrus fruits and juices and tomato products) or carbonated beverages. Dietary protein should be high and fat usually should be moderate (70 to 100 gm/day). Dividing the total day's intake into six small meals can be helpful. However, the body of every patient with CF handles food or tolerates various foods differently, and nutritional treatment must be on an individual basis. Specific nutritional deficiencies are reviewed in an excellent article by Chase.[69] Chase states that when CF patients are assessed nutritionally, energy, essential fatty acids, protein, fat-soluble vitamins, water-soluble vitamins, and trace minerals are almost always inadequate. Nutritional evaluation of CF patients should be done at least yearly. It should include measurements of total protein, albumin, and zinc, a complete blood count, and anthropometric data (see Chapter 3).

Children with CF, particularly those with growth retardation, often have slightly low plasma zinc concentrations. Zinc deficiency should be considered when somatic and sexual growth failure occur in patients with CF. Treatment with oral zinc sulfate seemed to result in increased growth for a group of patients in Britain.[70]

Compliance with diet often drops in adolescence. This drop may be caused by adolescent rebellion. However, some patients report that the need for pancreatic replacement seems to diminish with age. Some also seem to be able to tolerate a normal diet, including as much as 70 to 100 gm fat/day, without discomfort. These effects have been seen by Lapey and co-workers,[71] who concluded that growth failure and the state of nutrition correlated more closely with the pulmonary state than with pancreatic insufficiency. Most adolescents can regulate their own diet, primarily on the basis of symptomatology, with help from the nutritionist when needed.

Asthma

Bronchial asthma is an episodic, reversible obstructive condition of the pulmonary airways that affects people of all ages. Although the severity often tapers off at adolescence, asthma can be a cause of school absence, interrupted social functioning, and avoidance of sports in the teen years. Articulation and hearing loss have also been found to be associated with bronchial asthma.[72] Asthma is often a manifestation of an allergic response, and most clinical attention has focused on the airborne allergens such as dust, mold, and pollen. Whether food antigens are also likely to provoke respiratory distress is still controversial.

Several investigators have looked at the association between milk sensitivity and asthma. Complete elimination of cow's milk and dairy products is reported to relieve the symptoms of asthma.[73] Chocolate, nuts, soy products, rice, corn, oranges, and oats have also been suspect in some individuals. At least one double-blind study has supported this,[74] but more studies are needed. The nutritionist should be open to the possibility that a food allergy might be involved.

The metabolism of theophylline, a drug commonly used in the treatment of asthma, can be affected by the composition of the diet. Feldman and co-workers[75] have shown that in children an increase in carbohydrate in the diet (78% carbohydrate, 0.5 gm protein/kg) prolongs the half-life of theophylline, whereas an increase in protein (3 gm protein/kg, 65% carbohydrate) shortens the half-life. Since this effect has also been demonstrated in adults, it is probably also present in adolescents.

Nutritional approaches to eliminate allergies will not supplant treatment for asthma. Medical treatment should be individualized and related to the acute attack, prevention, and continued care. Occasionally, corticosteroids are used as maintenance treatment, and the nutritionist should be aware of possible physiological side effects. Because of their effects on growth and bone formation, corticosteroids should be used for adolescents only when absolutely necessary. However, a recent report showed that although height growth was delayed in adolescents on steroids, the final adult height was normal.[76]

GASTROINTESTINAL DISEASE

Crohn's Disease

Crohn's disease, or granulomatous ileocolitis, was first recognized in 1932. It is a chronic disease mainly affecting young adults and is characterized by a necrotizing, ulcerating, inflammatory process. The age of peak frequency is between 15 and 35 years. The course is extremely variable, but complications tend to be frequent and severe as the patient becomes older.

Initial symptoms are usually weight loss, diarrhea, cramps, and abdominal pain. The disease has many features of a malabsorption syndrome. The disease can cause alteration of motility of the gastrointestinal tract and create areas of malabsorption and obstruction or fistulas. Adolescents with this disease are subject to growth retardation or delayed sexual maturation. When malabsorption or malnutrition is a prominent feature, serum albumin may be low, macrocytic anemia may be present, and alkaline phosphatase may be elevated because of protein loss, poor absorption of folate or vitamin B_{12}, and poor absorption of calcium and vitamin D.

One of the goals of treatment is preservation or restoration of adequate nutrition and growth. To facilitate this, a high-protein diet with vitamin B_{12} and iron supplementation is recommended. The major aim of nutritional therapy is to maintain metabolic homeostasis and to provide adequate energy, protein, and other substrates to restore normal growth or to permit catch-up growth to occur.[77] Therapies such as food supplements, nasogastric infusions (tube feedings), and gastrostomy infusions are used. In acute attacks of this disease, total parenteral nutrition has been advocated as primary therapy as shown in Fig. 7-2. It restores metabolic and nutritional homeostasis and allows the bowel to rest. When there is chronic intractability of symptoms, surgery is sometimes recommended. For the preoperative patient, parenteral nutrition decreases morbidity in those cases where there has been weight loss and debilitation for an extended period of time.[78]

Ulcerative Colitis

Although Crohn's disease can occur in any portion of the gastrointestinal tract, ulcerative colitis is limited to the colon and usually involves the surface and mucosal layers of the intestine. Like Crohn's disease, it has no known specific cause. Its course is usually variable and protracted. It is generally recognized as a disease of young adults, with 10% to 32% of cases occurring before 20 years of age. Many investigators feel that it is being seen with increasing frequency in adolescents.[79] Ulcerative colitis is a severe disease in the adolescent age group. Over 90% of the adolescents with ulcerative colitis have moderate to severe in-

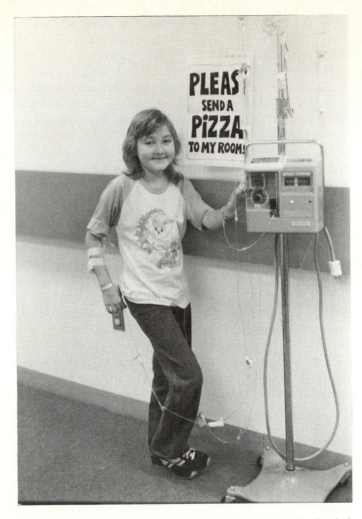

Fig. 7-2. Teenager receiving total parenteral nutrition who is asserting her independence.

volvement,[80] whereas less than 50% of adults with ulcerative colitis have this degree of activity.

Although short stature is more often seen in Crohn's disease, 20% to 30% of prepubertal patients with ulcerative colitis also have short stature.[77] Decreased energy intake is recognized as a major factor in growth retardation, and combined parenteral and oral feeding that provides 130% to 140% of estimated energy needs usually will promote growth. Some authors advocate an unlimited diet, but others suggest restriction of roughage and spices. A completely free intake for adolescents with ulcerative colitis is advocated by Davidson and co-workers.[79] This recommendation is based on the conviction that diet does not affect colonic symptoms and that freedom of choice is useful for overcoming anorexia and maintaining the best nitrogen balance. Folic acid deficiency is occasionally seen in patients whose diets have been restricted in fiber and leafy vegetables.[78]

Zinc deficiency may also be a factor accounting for growth failure of children with ulcerative colitis. This trace metal has an essential role in the metabolism of protein and nucleic acids. In patients with ulcerative colitis, zinc deficiency may have many causes, including chronic malnutrition and malabsorption, increased zinc excretion, and zinc loss through stools.[81] In a carefully controlled study, Nishi and others[82] found alterations in zinc metabolism in 28 of 30 patients aged 8 to 18 years with ulcerative colitis or Crohn's disease. Fourteen also had growth abnormalities. It would seem prudent to measure serum zinc levels in adolescents with ulcerative colitis or Crohn's disease and to consider zinc supplementation if levels are low.

There is no evidence that any specific diet prevents relapse in patients with ulcerative colitis. However, patients who have diarrhea despite optimal medical management should be tested for lactose intolerance, as lactose absorption can be abnormal in up to 20% of patients.[77]

For many adolescents with Crohn's disease or ulcerative colitis, the social complications of their physical immaturity are often more debilitating than the gastrointestinal manifestations.[83] For these patients it is extremely valuable to have the services of many professionals—psychologists, social workers, and nutritionists—in addition to physicians and nurses. Teenagers as a group may show poor compliance even under the best of circumstances, and the regimen must be kept as liberal and supportive as possible. It is important to help the patients develop self-awareness and perspective so that they can become allies in the treatment of their disease.

NEOPLASTIC DISEASE

Cancer is the leading nonaccidental cause of death in the 10- to 21-year-old age group in the United States. The types of common tumors differ from malignancies found in adults, with leukemias, malignant lymphomas, bone tumors, and neural lesions being the most frequently seen in adolescents.[84] In the past decade a significant improvement in survival has been observed in children and teens who are managed by aggressive use of multimodal therapies, including surgery, chemotherapy, and radiotherapy. Complex interactions occur between nutrition and cancer, many of them caused by cancer therapy, and there are signs that cachexia (severe protein and energy malnutrition) is a significant cause of mortality.[85]

Teenagers with cancer may be at particular risk for nutritional depletion because of added energy requirements for growth and continued development, because food preferences are strong, and because malabsorption is often severe and sudden in onset. In addition, the immature immune system is more susceptible to the effects of malnutrition in children than in adults.[86] The adolescent's immune system is probably somewhere between.

Nutritional problems can arise from the disease or the therapy and are best addressed as soon as possible after diagnosis. Thus it is advantageous for the nutritionist to be a part of the treatment team from the very early stages of disease. Nutritional assessment, including anthropometric data, levels of serum albumin and total protein, and a good dietary history, can be extremely useful and should be the first step in the nutritional management of the teenager newly diagnosed as having cancer. This can be followed with daily calorie counts and recommendations tailored to the needs of each individual. Oral alimentation is the preferred route of nutrition therapy. The principal goal is to avoid weight loss.

In working with teenagers and their families, the dietitian should emphasize both the quality and quantity of food. The best way to increase the consumption of food is to determine individual food preferences and provide as many highly preferred foods as possible. Satiety, an increased sense of fullness, is a common finding in cancer patients, so

Table 7-2. Anticancer agents used in adolescence

Drug	Category	Common Toxicity Affecting Nutritional Intake and Absorption	Other Effects
Doxorubicin (Adriamycin)	Antibiotic	Stomatitis, nausea, diarrhea	Alopecia, red urine, bone marrow suppression
Asparaginase (Elspar)		Nausea, vomiting, anorexia	Hepatic toxicity, pancreatitis
Cisplatin (Platinol)	Alkylating agent	Nausea, vomiting, anorexia	Kidney toxicity, possible hearing loss, bone marrow suppression
Fluorouracil (5-FU)	Antimetabolite	Nausea, ulcerations of mouth and gastrointestinal tract, diarrhea	Rash, bone marrow suppression
Cyclophosphamide (Cytoxan, Endoxan)	Alkylating agent	Stomatitis, nausea, vomiting	Alopecia, bone marrow suppression
Dactinomycin	Antibiotic	Stomatitis, vomiting, diarrhea, abdominal pain	Alopecia, bone marrow suppression
Methotrexate	Antimetabolite	Stomatitis, vomiting, diarrhea, anorexia, nausea, oral ulcerations, gingivitis	Alopecia, hepatic toxicity
Vincristine (Oncovin)	Vinca alkaloid	Nausea, vomiting, constipation, oral ulcerations	Alopecia, abdominal pain, jaw joint pain, joint pain

meals should be small and wholesome snacks readily available. In the hospital foods such as milk, juice, eggnog, cheese, peanut butter, pizza, and whole grain cookies should be accessible so that adolescents may eat whenever they are hungry. Often hunger is fleeting and passes quickly, especially during chemotherapy.

Nutritional supplements also have a place in increasing the nutritional intake of the teenage cancer patient. Preferences for the available supplements will differ. It has been recommended that the patient be presented with a tray containing a small sample of five or more liquid supplements and then encouraged to choose the one that is most palatable. A prescription then may be given for the use of this supplement. To arrive at the amount to prescribe, the dietitian estimates the average daily energy intake from food and calculates the total energy needs as shown in Appendix L. The difference is provided as supplements. When supple-

ments contain 1 kcal/ml, it is simple to determine the amount required. However, there are some new formulas that have 1.5 to 2 kcal/ml.

Anorexia, nausea, and vomiting are associated with nearly all chemotherapeutic agents as shown in Table 7-2. Radiation may further contribute to poor intake of food by causing ulceration of the oral mucosa. Malabsorption as a result of diarrhea is not uncommon. Food aversions and changes in taste, commonly seen in adult cancer patients, do not seem as prevalent in adolescents. In adults aversion to meats, sweets, chocolate, and hot coffee are commonly noted.

Learned food aversion is a special problem with patients receiving either radiation or chemotherapy. If a food is eaten shortly before the patient receives therapy, the nausea and vomiting resulting from therapy may be psychologically associated with the food eaten just before. From that time on, the patient may have an aversion to that food.[87]

It is easy to see that on multimodal or multidose treatment aversions to several foods could develop. The adolescent thus could be left with a very limited list of food choices.

The interrelationship of emotional variables should also be assessed. Changes in body weight and known symptoms of depression may be related. Fear of death, physical debilitation, body-image changes, social isolation, and pain may significantly interfere with eating behavior.

When weight loss is between 6% and 10% of usual body weight, when anorexia is present, when food intake is low, and when treatment is to be continued, total parenteral nutrition (TPN) is an alternative that is being increasingly used for nutritional support. It is well-tolerated by teens and is safe and effective, especially when managed by an expert nutritional team.[88] Excellent guides for its use are available.[89,90] Since TPN of less than 10 days duration is ineffective, patients should be treated for at least that length of time. Rickard and her co-workers[86] have shown that in a group of children 2 to 20 years of age TPN for less than 9 to 14 days did not replete weight or serum albumin concentrations. Use for 28 days, however, supported weight gain and increased serum albumin.

CARDIOVASCULAR DISORDERS

Cardiovascular diseases account for more than one half of the deaths in the United States each year. The major factors associated with risk of coronary heart disease are hypertension, hypercholesterolemia, and cigarette smoking. Obesity, sedentary living habits, and psychosocial tension are also factors, but they seemingly have less influence. Areas in which possible benefits may accrue from intervention are modifications of nutrition to affect hypercholesterolemia, hypertension, and obesity, encouragement of exercise, and programs to stop cigarette smoking. In addition to instituting dietary treatment of frank disease in the adolescent, it behooves the nutritionist to be alert to possibilities for preventive nutrition.

Hypertension

Essential hypertension in youth (as opposed to "secondary" hypertension, which is due to a known cause) does not have a precise clinical definition. There are no rules or guidelines on when to begin intervention, prevention, or treatment. However, essential hypertension clearly exists in youth and has its origins early in life. A family history of hypertension suggests a greater vulnerability to its development,[91] but usually there are no symptoms other than an elevation in blood pressure. As in all age groups, this measurement in adolescents has a high degree of variability and inaccuracy, making it difficult to diagnose hypertension with certainty. There is a diversity of opinion regarding the importance of an elevated measurement in teenagers. However, Londe and co-workers[92] found that there was no relationship between blood pressure and puberty in children 10 to 14 years of age and that the presence of hypertension in this age group should be regarded as a "suspicious finding."

Populations that freely salt their food show increasing blood pressures with age, and it is commonly assumed that blood pressure does rise with age. However, researchers found that in an Indian population in South America adolescents who consumed a low-salt diet failed to show a further rise in blood pressure as they grew older.[93] Chronic intake of salt in amounts well in excess of requirements may play a primary role in the pathogenesis of hypertension. Moreover, excessive salt intake might well aggravate the course of hypertension. Populations who eat small quantities of salt are relatively free from hypertension, so there is an epidemiological argument for limiting salt intake in children and adolescents. Counseling an adolescent to limit salt in the diet can have lifelong effects. Nutrition teaching can include the following: (1) explaining the difference between "sodium" and "salt"; (2) listing which foods have large amounts of sodium, which have added salt, and which are high in sodium through processing; and (3) pointing out the amount of salt in various fast foods. Learning to read nutrition labels can also be a skill taught to teenagers.

In teenagers, as in adults, elevated blood pressure is more common if a person is obese. Obesity is positively correlated with an increasing risk of developing hypertensive cardiovascular disease and hypertensive eye changes. The avoidance and prevention of obesity is the best course, but for the adolescent who is already overweight and hypertensive, supportive counseling that concentrates on changing dietary habits is indicated.

Most teenagers with chronic hypertension should be on long-term therapy. Since there is some concern about the long-term effects of the use of antihypertensive agents in the growing teenager, the possibility of controlling the blood pressure through dietary changes should be stressed. Getting the teen motivated is a challenge, particularly the asymptomatic teen. Compliance can be facilitated when there is a strong team consisting of physician, nurse, and dietitian or nutritionist.

Hyperlipidemia

Of the known risk factors for coronary heart disease, plasma lipid and lipoprotein levels are particularly relevant to teenagers because dietary modification, combined with drug treatment when necessary, has been shown to lower the levels of serum cholesterol in children and adolescents.[94] Various studies have shown that a plasma cholesterol level greater than 200 mg/dl and/or a plasma triglyceride level greater than 140 mg/dl places an individual at increased risk for developing early atherosclerosis.[95] High levels of high-density lipoproteins (HDL) may have a protective effect on the blood vessels, so these levels should also be measured, especially in teens from high-risk families (usually this means that a first-degree relative has had a coronary "incident" before the age of 50).

The critical time for cholesterol control seems to be during the second and third decades of life, and Breslow[96] suggests that primary prevention should occur ideally in the first and second decades.

The vast majority of individuals with hyperlipidemia do not have a recognizable pattern. In most individuals the diet contributes to the hyperlipidemia, but other environmental and genetic factors may also be involved. Hyperlipidemia may also occur in the presence of systemic disease. Prevention should be a total program of diet, physical activity, and maintenance of normal weight. Further discussion of treatment can be found in other texts.[97,98] The Dietary Goals outlined by the U.S. Department of Agriculture and the U.S. Department of Health and Human Services (see p. 73) and the Prudent Diet pattern advocated by the American Heart Association are both sensible lifetime plans. These guides both emphasize whole grain breads and cereals, fruits, and vegetables and the avoidance of fat, salt, and excess calories.

Motivating teens to reduce risk for future disease can be most effective within a framework of personal involvement and peer interaction. In one prototype program for teens,[99] screening for risk factors provides the "reality factor" that makes health education pertinent and appropriate. The study suggests that about half of all students screened will have one or more risk factors for heart disease, cancer, or stroke. The authors state that this type of program has a wide range of appeal and acceptance, from inner-city, depressed areas to upper-class, professional populations.

In an interesting study in a high school biology class in New Jersey,[100] very few tenth grade students (37%) knew that cholesterol is found only in foods of animal origin, and only 8% knew that saturated fat is not a type of cholesterol. Five to fifteen percent of teenagers have levels of serum cholesterol over 200 mg/dl.[95] This figure is lower in underdeveloped countries and higher in urban, industrialized countries. Habits that maintain a low-cholesterol diet clearly should be established during adolescence.

SUMMARY

Nutritional care of the adolescent who has a chronic medical problem is a challenge requiring patience, flexibility, and sensitivity to the adolescent's special needs. Consideration also should be given to the adolescent's stage of psychological development toward autonomy, responsibility, peer acceptance, and individuality. In addition, the nutritional care must provide for the adolescent's physical needs and maintain his or her growth and physical development to the extent possible. Adolescence is also a time when nutritional care can be directed toward preventing or delaying the onset of diseases such as hypertension and hyperlipidemia for which the teen may have a genetic predisposition.

REFERENCES

1. Seidle, A.H., and Altshuler, A.: Interventions for adolescents who are chronically ill, Child. Today **8:**16, 1979.
2. Hauser, S.T., and others: Ego development and self-esteem in diabetic adolescents, Diabetes Care **2:**465, 1979.
3. Kellerman, J., and others: Psychological effects of illness in adolescence, J. Pediatr. **97:**126, 1980.
4. Yaros, P.S., and Howe, J.: Responses to illness and disability. In Howe, J., editor: Nursing care of adolescents, Philadelphia, 1980, Lea & Febiger.
5. Becker, R.D.: Insight body-image problems, J. Curr. Adolesc. Med. **3:**36, 1981.
6. Silber, T.J., and Shearin, R.B.: Setting up adolescent inpatient units, J. Curr. Adolesc. Med. **2:**14, 1980.
7. Blum, R., and Chang, P.: A group for adolescents facing chronic and terminal illness, J. Curr. Adolesc. Med. **3:**7, 1981.
8. Safer, D.J., Allen, R., and Barr, E.: Depression of growth in hyperactive children on stimulant drugs, N. Engl. J. Med. **287:**217, 1972.
9. Roe, D.A.: Interactions between drugs and nutrients, Med. Clin. North Am. **63:**985, 1979.
10. Hartshorn, E.A.: Food and drug interactions, J. Am. Diet. Assoc. **70:**15, 1977.
11. Roe, D.A.: Drug-induced nutritional deficiencies, Westport, Conn., 1976, AVI Publishing Co.
12. Brin, M., and Roe, D.A.: Drug-diet interactions, J. Fla. Med. Assoc. **66:**424, 1979.
13. Norris, J.W., and Pratt, R.F.: Folic acid deficiency and epilepsy, Drugs **8:**366, 1974.
14. Roe, D.A.: Handbook: interactions of selected drugs and nutrients in patients, ed. 3, Chicago, 1982, The American Dietetic Association.
15. Krause, M.V., and Mahan, L.K.: Food, nutrition and diet therapy, ed. 7, Philadelphia, 1984, W.B. Saunders Co.
16. U.S. Department of Health, Education, and Welfare, Food and Nutrition Board, National Academy of Sciences–National Research Council: Iron nutriture in adolescence, Department of Health, Education, and Welfare Publication (HSA) 77-5100, Washington, D.C., 1976.
17. U.S. Department of Health, Education and Welfare: Ten state nutrition survey, 1968-70, Department of Health, Education, and Welfare Publication (HSM) 72-8134, Washington, D.C., 1972, Health Services and Mental Health Administration.
18. Gilman, P.A.: The anemias in adolescents. In Gallagher, J.R., and others, editors: Medical care of the adolescent, New York, 1975, Appleton-Century-Crofts.
19. Brown, K., and others: Prevalence of anemia among preadolescent and young adolescent urban black Americans, J. Pediatr. **81:**714, 1972.
20. Daniel, W.A.: Hematocrit: maturity relationship in adolescence, Pediatrics **52:**388, 1973.
21. Daniel, W.A., Gaines, E.G., and Bennett, D.L.: Iron intake and transferrin saturation in adolescents, J. Pediatr. **86:**288, 1975.
22. Jacobs, A., and Worwood, M.: Ferritin in serum: clinical and biochemical implications, N. Engl. J. Med. **292:**951, 1975.
23. Liebel, R.: Behavioral and biochemical correlates of iron deficiency, J. Am. Diet. Assoc. **71:**398, 1977.
24. Chu, J., O'Connor, D.M., and McElfresh, A.E.: Nutritional anemia. In Shen, J.T.U., editor: The clinical practice of adolescent medicine, New York, 1980, Appleton-Century-Crofts.
25. Oski, F.A.: The non-hematologic manifestations of iron deficiency, Am. J. Dis. Child. **133:**315, 1979.
26. Pollitt, E., and Leibel, R.L.: Iron deficiency and behavior, J. Pediatr. **88:**372, 1976.
27. Elwood, P.C., and others: Symptoms and circulating hemoglobin level, J. Chronic Dis. **29:**615, 1969.
28. Corman-Luban, N.L., Cananle, V.C., and Miller, D.R.: Anemia of adolescence. In Lopez, R.I., editor: Adolescent medicine: topics, vol. 1, Jamaica, N.Y., 1976, Spectrum Publications, Inc.

29. Llenda, M., and Ekvall, S.: Iron deficiency and toxicity. In Palmer, S., and Ekvall, S., editors: Pediatric nutrition in developmental disorders, Springfield, Ill., 1978, Charles C Thomas, Publisher.

30. Finch, C.A.: Iron nutrition, Ann. N.Y. Acad. Sci. **300:** 221, 1977.

31. Monsen, E.R., and Balintfy, J.L.: Calculating iron bioavailability: refinement and computerization, J. Am. Diet. Assoc. **80:**307, 1982.

32. Monsen, E.R.: Iron: a case study in nutrient availability. In Worthington-Roberts, B., editor: Contemporary developments in nutrition, St. Louis, 1981, The C.V. Mosby Co.

33. Ashcroft, M.T., and others: Growth, behavior, and educational achievement of Jamaican children with sickle cell trait, Br. Med. J. **1:**1371, 1976.

34. Daeschner, C.W., and others: Zinc and growth in patients with sickle cell disease, J. Pediatr. **98:**778, 1981.

35. Brewer, G.J., Brewer, L.F., and Prasad, A.S.: Suppression of irreversibly sickled erythrocytes by zinc therapy in sickle cell anemia, J. Lab. Clin. Med. **90:**549, 1977.

36. Prasad, A.S., and others: Trace elements in sickle cell disease, JAMA **235:**2396, 1976.

37. Rosenbloom, A.L., Kohrman, A., and Sperling, M.: Classification and diagnosis of diabetes mellitus in children and adolescents, J. Pediatr. **98:**320, 1981.

38. Kanel, W.B., and McGee, D.L.: Diabetes and cardiovascular disease: the Framingham study, JAMA **241:**2035, 1979.

39. Kaufman, R.L., and others: Plasma lipid levels in diabetic children: effect of diet restricted in cholesterol and saturated fats, Diabetes **24:**672, 1975.

40. Kinmonth, A-L., and others: Whole foods and increased dietary fiber improve blood glucose control in diabetic children, Arch. Dis. Child. **57:**187, 1982.

41. Cahill, G.F., Etzwiler, D.D., and Freinkel, N.: "Control" and diabetes, N. Engl. J. Med. **294:**1004, 1976.

42. Ditzel, J., and Kjaergaard, J.: Haemoglobin: A_{1c} concentrations after initial insulin treatment for newly discovered diabetes, Br. Med. J. **1:**741, 1978.

43. Calvert, G.D., and others: Effects of therapy on cholesterol concentration in diabetes mellitus, Lancet **1:**66, 1978.

44. Drash, A.L.: Nutritional considerations in the treatment of the child with diabetes mellitus. In Suskind, R.M., editor: Textbook of pediatric nutrition, New York, 1981, Raven Press.

45. Krause, M.V., and Mahan, L.K.: Food, nutrition and diet therapy, ed. 7, Philadelphia, 1984, W.B. Saunders Co.

46. Mozin, M.J., and others: Food habits of 215 diabetic children in Belgium, Acta Paediatr. Belg. **31:**56, 1978.

47. Birkbeck, J.A., Truswell, A.S., and Thomas, B.J.: Current practice in dietary management of diabetic children, Arch. Dis. Child. **51:**467, 1976.

48. Branham, R.L., and others: Nutrition and its importance in dental health, J. Fam. Pract. **6:**49, 1978.

49. Gustafsson, B.E., and others: The effect of different levels of carbohydrate intake on caries activity in 436 individuals observed for five years, Acta Odontol. Scand. **11:**232, 1954.

50. Newbrun, E.: Dietary carbohydrates: their role in cariogenicity, Med. Clin. North Am. **63:**1069, 1979.

51. Alfano, M.C.: Understanding the role of diet and nutrition on dental caries. In American Academy of Pedodontics: Changing perspectives in nutrition and caries research, New York, 1979, Medcom, Inc.

52. Kinkel, H.J., and Cremer, H.D.: The effect of cocoa ash and caries in the rate-comparison of ashed cocoa with a mineral mixture, J. Dent. Res. **39:**640, 1960.

53. Grenby, T.H.: Trials of three organic phosphorus-containing compounds as protective agents against dental caries in rats, J. Dent. Res. **52:**454, 1973.

54. Mallek, H.M.: Nutrition and the periodontal patient. In Randolph, P.M., and Dennison, C.I., editors: Diet, nutrition, and dentistry, St. Louis, 1981, The C.V. Mosby Co.

55. Brookman, R.R.: Adolescents on the surface, Med. Clin. North Am. **59:**1473, 1975.

56. Williams, M., and Cunliffe, W.J.: Explanation for premenstrual acne, Lancet **2:**1055, 1973.

57. Lee, P.A.: Acne and serum androgen during puberty, Arch. Dermatol. **112:**482, 1976.

58. Hurwitz, S.: Acne vulgaris: current concepts of pathogenesis and treatment, Am. J. Dis. Child. **133:**536, 1979.

59. Rasmussen, J.E.: A new look at old acne, Pediatr. Clin. North Am. **25:**285, 1978.

60. Becker, L., and others: Topical clindamycin therapy for acne vulgaris, Arch. Dermatol. **117:**482, 1981.

61. Peck, G.L.: Retinoids in dermatology, Arch. Dermatol. **116:**283, 1980.

62. Cunliffe, W.: Dermatology: acne vulgaris, Br. J. Hosp. Med. **20:**24, 1978.

63. Cornbleet, T., and Gigly, I.: Should we limit sugar in acne? Arch. Dermatol. **83:**968, 1961.

64. Fulton, J.E., and others: Effect of chocolate on acne vulgaris, JAMA **210:**207, 1969.

65. Anderson, P.C.: Food as the cause of acne, Am. Fam. Physician **3:**102, 1971.

66. Michäelsson, G.: Diet and acne, Nutr. Rev. **39:**104, 1981.

67. Michäelsson, G., and others: Effects of oral zinc and vitamin A in acne, Arch. Dermatol. **113:**31, 1977.

68. National Cystic Fibrosis Foundation: Patient registry, Rockville, Md., 1981.

69. Chase, H.P.: Cystic fibrosis and malnutrition, J. Pediatr. **95:**337, 1979.

70. Halsted, J.A., and Smith, J.C.: Plasma zinc in health and disease, Lancet **1:**322, 1970.

71. Lapey, A., and others: Steatorrhea and azotorrhea and their relation to growth and nutrition in adolescents and young adults with cystic fibrosis, J. Pediatr. **84:**328, 1974.

72. Baker, B.M., and Baker, C.D.: Difficulties generated by allergies, J. Sch. Health **50:**583, 1980.

73. Crook, W.G.: Food allergy: the great masquerader, Pediatr. Clin. North Am. **22:**227, 1975.

74. May, C.D.: Objective clinical and laboratory studies of immediate hypersensitivity reactions to foods in asthmatic children, J. Allergy Clin. Immunol. **58:**500, 1976.

75. Feldman, C.H., and others: Effect of dietary protein and carbohydrate on theophylline metabolism in children, Pediatrics **66:**956, 1980.

76. Martin, A.J., Landau, L.I., and Phelan, P.D.: The effect on growth of childhood asthma, Acta Paediatr. Scand. **70:**683, 1981.

77. Grand, R.J., and others: Reversal of growth arrest in Crohn's disease: a new approach, Pediatr. Res. **11:**444, 1977.

78. Rosenberg, I.H.: Nutritional support in inflammatory bowel disease, Gastroenterology **77:**392, 1979.

79. Davidson, M.N., Bloom, A.A., and Kugler, M.M.: Chronic ulcerative colitis of childhood: an evaluative review, J. Pediatr. **67:**471, 1965.

80. Patterson, M., Castiglioni, L., and Sampson, L.: Chronic ulcerative colitis beginning in children and teenagers, Am. J. Dig. Dis. **16:**298, 1971.

81. Wolman, S.L., Anderson, G.H., and Matliss, E.B.: Zinc in total parenteral nutrition: requirements and metabolic effects, Gastroenterology **76:**68, 1979.

82. Nishi, Y., and others: Zinc status and its relation to growth retardation in children with chronic inflammatory bowel disease, Am. J. Clin. Nutr. **33:**2613, 1980.

83. Daum, F., Boley, S.J., and Cohen, M.I.: Inflammatory bowel disease in the adolescent patient, Pediatr. Clin. North Am. **20:**933, 1973.

84. Steinherz, P.G., and Miller, D.R.: The adolescent with cancer. In Lopez, R.I., editor: Adolescent medicine: topics, vol. 1, Jamaica, N.Y., 1976, Spectrum Publications, Inc.

85. Van Eys, J.: Supportive care for the child with cancer, Pediatr. Clin. North Am. **23:**215, 1976.

86. Rickard, K.A., and others: Reversal of protein-surgery malnutrition in children during treatment of advanced neoplastic disease, Ann. Surg. **190:**771, 1979.

87. De Wys, W.D.: Nutritional care of the cancer patient, JAMA **244:**374, 1980.

88. Costa, G., and Donaldson, S.S.: Effects of cancer treatment on the nutrition of the host, N. Engl. J. Med. **300:**1471, 1979.

89. Dudrick, S.J.: A clinical review of nutritional support of the patient, Am. J. Clin. Nutr. **34:**1191, 1981.

90. Shils, M.E.: Principles of nutritional therapy, Med. Clin. North Am. **63:**1009, 1979.

91. Kilcoyne, M.M.: Adolescent hypertension: characteristics and response to treatment, Circulation **50:**1014, 1974.

92. Londe, S., and others: Blood pressure and puberty, J. Pediatr. **87:**896, 1975.

93. Lauer, R.M., and others: Blood pressure and its significance in childhood, Postgrad. Med. J. **54:**206, 1978.

94. Glueck, C.G.: Hypercholesterolemia and hyper-alpha lipoproteinemia in school children, Pediatrics **62:**478, 1978.

95. Stamler, J.: Population studies. In Levy, R.I., and others, editors: Nutrition, lipids, and coronary heart disease, New York, 1979, Raven Press.

96. Breslow, J.L.: Pediatric aspects of hyperlipidemia, Pediatrics **62:**510, 1978.

97. Breslow, J.L.: Diet, hyperlipidemias and atherosclerosis: pediatric aspects. In Suskind, R.M., editor: Textbook of pediatric nutrition, New York, 1981, Raven Press.

98. Krause, M.V., and Mahan, L.K.: Food, nutrition and diet therapy, ed. 7, Philadelphia, 1984, W.B. Saunders Co.

99. Williams, C.L., and Wynder, E.L.: Motivating adolescents to reduce risk for chronic disease, Postgrad. Med. J. **54:**212, 1978.

100. Podell, R.N., Keller, K., and Berger, G.: Cardiovascular nutrition knowledge and lipid levels among New Jersey high school students, J. Med. Soc. N.J. **72:**1027, 1975.

Chapter 8

Nutrition and Adolescent Behavior

L. KATHLEEN MAHAN

A variant of the idea that you are what you eat is the proposition that you behave the way you eat. The idea that behavioral problems, even crime and delinquency, might be caused by the nutrition of the problematic young person has captured considerable attention in the past decade. There are several reasons for this attention. First, it is common for many teens to have eating habits as described in Chapter 4, which raises suspicions that adolescents' diets are inadequate or at least not optimal. Second, the focus on our food supply as being overprocessed and lacking in nutrients backs up the "feeling" that many teens may not be getting all they require nutritionally. Third, looking at the diet for the cause of an adolescent's behavior gives the family an excuse for not considering family relationships or parenting issues as the cause of the adolescent's behavior. Fourth, because of the frustrating nature of adolescent behavioral problems, professionals and nonprofessionals are frequently caught looking for a simple solution, which a diet change seems to supply. To shed some light on this new, yet confusing approach to adolescent behavior, it is necessary to review both the *known* facts and the unproven theories about food and its effect on brain chemistry and behavior. Pioneering work in this area of nutrition has the potential for far-reaching changes in the approach to a person's food and environment.

COMPLEX NATURE OF BEHAVIORAL PROBLEMS IN ADOLESCENCE

Most adolescents go through this phase of their life with only minor behavioral problems. However, a small group of teens have a rocky course through adolescence and experience a great deal of physical and psychological stress that manifests itself in inappropriate behavior. Typical examples of problematic adolescent behavior are aggressiveness, learning disabilities, poor school performance, and hyperactivity. Lesser family annoyances include not getting along with the family, moodiness, and laziness. Problems of a more serious nature include depression, schizophrenia, and juvenile delinquency and crime. Adolescent behavioral problems are complex, solutions are not simple, and change is usually slow.

Behavioral problems in adolescents are caused by a combination of the internal changes of adolescence and various environmental factors, one of which is nutrition. The relationship between the nutrition environment and behavior is interactive. Nutritional intake and nutritional status can affect adolescents' behavior, and at the same time adolescents' behavior can affect what they eat and thus their nutritional status. For example, the behavior of adolescents who are not eating because of depression or who are not eating meals at home because of arguments with their family is likely to result in an inadequate diet and perhaps poor nutritional status. This, in turn, may affect the adolescents' behavior.

INFLUENCE OF PSYCHOSOCIAL DEVELOPMENT STATUS

Obvious factors, such as the family's eating patterns, economic status, cultural mode, and religious beliefs, influence which foods the adolescent will choose or be offered to eat.

Teens' psychological development, especially their body-image development as discussed in Chapter 2, also influences eating habits. Concern with body image, mainly its size and shape, can lead to excessive dieting and food aversion. This fear and guilt at eating leads to poor intake and possibly poor nutritional status. Teenage girls are especially susceptible to these pressures as discussed in Chapter 5. In a situation of constant dieting, perhaps combined with use of appetite-reducing drugs, there are prominent behavioral changes, and the teen can become apathetic, irritable, and excessively concerned with food.

Stress in the lives of adolescents affects not only whether they eat and how regularly they eat but also their nutritional requirements and how well they use what they consume. Stress, whether from infection, mild trauma, or psychological upsets, does have metabolic effects on the teen, and the result depends on the nutritional status of the teen and the frequency, intensity, and duration of the stress. School pressures, social worries, or family problems can cause a stress response in which norepinephrine and epinephrine are released. These cause an increase in urinary nitrogen excretion and a negative nitrogen balance. Scrimshaw and co-workers[1] studied adolescent males in a university examination situation and found that about one third of the group showed a statistically significant increase in nitrogen excretion. They also found that after the examinations there was a period of positive nitrogen balance to make up for the protein loss.[1] Additional studies have also shown that there are other nutritional responses to stress related to vitamin and mineral status.[2] Adolescents under constant psychic stress who already may have a low protein intake could possibly be in negative nitrogen balance much of the time. Since it is possible that during this same time the teens' nutritional intake is also poor, their nutritional status is in double jeopardy.

INFLUENCE OF NUTRITION ON NEUROLOGICAL FUNCTION AND BEHAVIOR

Knowledge of the influence of food and nutritional status on neurological function and behavior is expanding rapidly, but the gain in knowledge is not rapid enough to prove or disprove all of the many theories that are proposed to explain the relationships between eating and behavior. Let us first consider what is known in this area and then discuss the theories.

Neurotransmitters

The brain has 100 billion neurons or brain cells that are linked by a quadrillion connections or synapses. These synapses reorganize like growing ivy as a result of learning. The chemicals that pass across these synapses are called neurotransmitters. These *neurotransmitters* are the chemicals of the brain and the nervous system. They allow for the transmission of an electrical impulse across the synapse from one neuron (nerve cell) to another or from a neuron to a muscle or secretory cell outside of the nervous system. Successful functioning of the nervous system depends on the ability of the axon of one nerve cell to release sufficient quantities of neurotransmitter into the synapse to be picked up by the receiving or adjacent neuron. This is illustrated in Fig. 8-1.

Neurotransmitters are made from various amino acids and other substances. Until recently it was

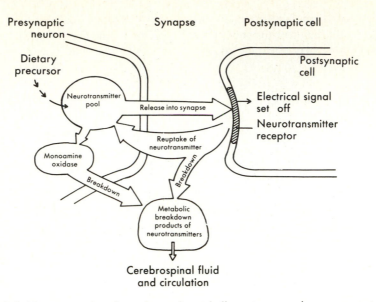

Fig. 8-1. Neurotransmitter formation and metabolism at synapse in nervous system.

assumed that the level of these neurotransmitters in the brain was not influenced by the brain level of the precursors from which they are made and certainly was not influenced by the level of the precursors in the bloodstream. However, it was an exciting discovery to find that the brain levels of neurotransmitters are affected quite rapidly by the level of their precursors in the brain and that the brain levels of the precursors are influenced by the diet.[3,4] Whether an increase in brain neurotransmitters also means a change in the amount of the neurotransmitter secreted into the synapse and whether or not this affects behavior is still debatable.[5] Also unknown is the duration of the effect of diet on the brain precursor or neurotransmitter level. Plasma levels of amino acids fluctuate during a 24-hour period depending on food intake, but the relationship is not completely understood.

Of the 10 to 15 compounds thought to function as neurotransmitters, the 5 primary ones are the amines—serotonin, dopamine, norepinephrine, epinephrine, and acetylcholine—that are synthe-

sized from the amino acids tryptophan and tyrosine and the molecule choline. Other possible neurotransmitters are γ-aminobutyric acid (GABA), whose precursor is glutamic acid, and the amino acids glycine and glutamic acid themselves. Not all of the neurotransmitters are subject to dietary influence. Thus far only acetylcholine, serotonin, dopamine, and norepinephrine appear to be subject to dietary control. Most of the information known about neurotransmitters comes from work in animals, and study of the relationships in humans is in the beginning stages. Table 8-1 summarizes what is known about neurotransmitter and dietary relationships.

The relationship of dietary choline content to brain choline levels and acetylcholine formation is straightforward: choline in a meal increases brain choline levels and thus increases brain acetylcholine levels.[6] When lecithin has been used as the source of choline, it is in highly purified form, not the form of most commercially available lecithin that health food stores are promoting.[10]

Table 8-1. Neurotransmitters, their precursors, and their possible relationship to diet

Neurotransmitter	Metabolic Precursor	Experimental Evidence and Relationships	Remarks
Acetylcholine	Choline or lecithin, which contains choline[6]	Has been used to treat manic-depressive illness, Friedreich's ataxia, Huntington's chorea, tardive dyskinesia, and Alzheimer's disease.[7] Thought to be related to memory.[8,9]	Choline in meal leads to elevated brain acetylcholine. Effects do not appear to be long-lasting. Commercially available lecithin does not contain phosphatidyl-choline in high enough amounts to affect brain choline levels.[10] Lecithin is found in eggs, meat, fish, and legumes.
Serotonin	Tryptophan	Appears effective in improving sleep and depressed mood.[3,12,13] Tryptophan-free diet reduces brain serotonin levels and reduces aggressive behavior in rats.[14] Tryptophan seems to promote sleep,[15,16] especially when given with carbohydrate.[17,18]	Protein in almost all foods contai_ 0.5% to 1.5% tryptophan. High-carbohydrate meal leads to elevated brain tryptophan.
Catecholamines Dopamine Norepinephrine Epinephrine	Tyrosine and possibly phenylalanine	Tyrosine has been used in treatment of depression, Parkinson's disease, and some kinds of hypertension.[7,20,21]	High-protein meal results in increased brain tyrosine.
γ-Aminobutyric acid (GABA)	Glutamic acid	—	A part of monosodium glutamate that in large amounts causes "Chinese restaurant" syndrome in some people.
Glycine and glutamic acid	Possible neurotransmitters themselves	—	—

The synthesis of the neurotransmitters serotonin, norepinephrine, and dopamine is also affected by the diet, but the relationship is not a direct one as it seems to be with choline and acetylcholine.

The precursors tryptophan, tyrosine, and other large neutral amino acids, such as phenylalanine, are passed into the brain by a common transport system. These precursors all compete with one another for entry as illustrated in Fig. 8-2. The protein in almost all foods contains relatively small amounts of tryptophan (0.5% to 1.5%) but much larger proportions of the other amino acids. A high-protein meal, although increasing blood tryptophan levels, retards the uptake of tryptophan into the brain by disproportionately increasing the plasma concentrations of the other amino acids that compete with tryptophan.[10] The greater the protein content of a particular meal, the more difficult it is for the tryptophan to enter the brain after the meal. On the other hand, a high-carbohydrate meal, which causes the release of insulin, results in elevated brain tryptophan and serotonin concentrations. The blood tryptophan's entry into the brain is facilitated because the release of insulin leads to a reduction in the blood levels of the other large neutral amino acids that compete with tryptophan for brain uptake. Tryptophan thus can pass into the brain without competition. The single meal that most effectively elevates the tryptophan and thus brain serotonin levels is one that completely lacks protein.[4] However, chronic consumption of a tryptophan-poor diet, one containing only corn protein for example, reduced the amount of amino acid in the whole body, including the brain.[11]

The precursor of norepinephrine and dopamine is tyrosine. Like tryptophan, tyrosine is a large neutral amino acid that must compete with other similar amino acids for transport into the brain. However, unlike tryptophan, whose brain level is not increased by the ingestion of protein, a high-protein meal leads to an increase in brain tyrosine, dopamine, and norepinephrine.[19]

It must be remembered that the precursors of the

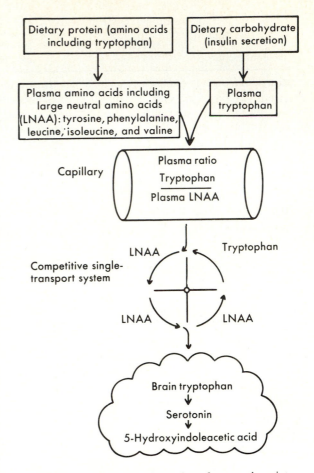

Fig. 8-2. Absorption and uptake of tryptophan into brain.

neurotransmitters interact with each other. For example, treatments designed to increase serotonin synthesis, such as tryptophan administration or a high-carbohydrate meal, may also decrease tyrosine uptake into the brain and thus brain synthesis of norepinephrine.

In addition, the hormonal changes of adolescence conceivably could further influence the metabolism and brain level of neurotransmitter precursors. These changes thus could possibly influence behavior.

Neuropeptides

Besides neurotransmitters, there are also neuropeptides, or amino acid chains, that are thought to have a role in the central nervous system. These include the peptide hormones (for example, gastrin and cholecystokinin) that are historically associated with the gastrointestinal tract and that are now believed also to be present in some areas of the brain. Other known neuropeptides are the endorphins and enkephalins that modulate pain perception, mood, and food intake.

In addition, there are some peptides that are found in the bloodstream in very small amounts and that are not made by the body.[22] These peptides, present in the hydrolysates of wheat gluten and α-casein, have been shown to have morphine-like activity. They have been called "exorphins."[22] Many factors, including permeability of the intestinal wall, deficiencies in intestinal enzymes, and permeability of the brain to exorphins, obviously are involved in whether exorphins play a role in brain function and subsequent behavior.

Opiates are known to induce a relaxed state, drowsiness, and sleep under the appropriate circumstances. The common experience of sleepiness after a heavy meal could be caused in part by the action of opiate-like exorphins produced by the body during the initial stages of food digestion. The behavior of babies after feeding is particularly striking in that they often fall asleep almost immediately. The high exorphin content of pepsin digests of casein may represent a mechanism for inducing sleep in the human, particularly the infant, after a meal. The neurotransmitter role for a food peptide is intriguing, and much more work needs to be done in this area.

Chronic Undernutrition

Although the physical and mental effects of severe malnutrition in young animals and children are documented and reviewed elsewhere,[23-26] very little research has focused on the problem of less severe chronic undernutrition and how it affects the older child and possibly the teenager's behavior.

Barnes[27] and Levitsky[24] have used the term *functional isolation* to describe the relationship between undernutrition and environmental stimulation that produces long-term behavioral changes of disinterest and lack of contact with the environment in infants and children. The consequence of this apathetic behavior is the functional deprivation of the individual of experiences that are necessary for cognitive development. It seems that the nutritional deficit causes alterations in the development of the central nervous system and that the lack of energy, when combined with a poor home environment, stunts the child's emotional growth. The child withdraws and adapts to the physiological stress of the nutritional deficit by developing behaviors that remove and insulate him or her from the environment and that then inhibit later development of appropriate patterns of social interaction. The individual will avoid new experiences and environmental stimuli that might be frightening or aversive and that would result in an elevated level of emotional response. These behaviors could decrease performance on tests of learning, even though the child's capacity to learn, or intelligence, has not been impaired by early malnutrition.[27] Studies of teenagers who were malnourished in early childhood showed impairment on intelligence tests when compared with children form a comparable environment without malnutrition.[28]

Lack of Environmental Stimulation

In studying the effect of malnutrition on neurological growth, development, and function, it is difficult to determine how much of the damage or poor performance is due to a lack of nutrients and how much is due to the nonstimulating, nonsupportive, and often harsh environment that may accompany malnutrition. Environmental stimulation seems necessary for optimal brain growth and intellectual capacity.[24,25,27,29] For example, an 8-

year study of Mexican school children showed that intellectual performance when a child entered school was related to his or her nutritional history as determined by body measurements. After 4 to 5 years of school attendance, however, differences in IQ were related more to socioeconomic conditions and the regularity of school attendance than to malnutrition.[30] Environmental enrichment can overcome the effects of malnutrition.[31,32]

Also to be considered is how the child's nutritional status may affect the manner in which caregivers respond to the child and alter the child's early experience in developmentally significant ways.[33] It would seem that this foundation of parent-child interaction could have a significant effect on later parent-teen interaction and on the teen's relationships with others in authority.

Vitamin Deficiencies

Severe deficiencies of the water-soluble vitamins result in neurological and behavioral changes, even when they are not combined with general malnutrition. As tests used to assess vitamin nutriture become more specific and sensitive, it is becoming clear that even less severe inadequacies of some of these vitamins could possibly cause subtle changes in the behavior of an individual.[34-36]

For example, vitamin B_6 has been studied for its possible role in behavior, particularly depression. Vitamin B_6 is necessary for the conversion of the amino acid tryptophan to the vitamin niacin and the conversion of tryptophan to the neurotransmitter serotonin. The conversion of other amino acids to neurotransmitters also requires pyridoxal phosphate, a form of vitamin B_6. Since serotonin deficiency has been suggested as being involved in depression, a deficiency of vitamin B_6 may contribute to the production of this depression.[37]

Evidence suggests that estrogen and other steroids compete with pyridoxal phosphate for binding sites, thus causing redistribution of vitamin B_6 among the apoenzymes and increasing the require-

ment for vitamin B_6. Vitamin B_6 deficiency has been reported in women using oral contraceptives, and current evidence indicates that as many as 50% of women using oral contraceptives will experience mild to moderate depression, irritability, tiredness, and emotional debility.[38] The teenage girl taking oral contraceptives might be in double jeopardy because of the effect from the pill and the possibility that her dietary intake of vitamin B_6 could be low if she also is dieting excessively and not eating properly. Chapter 9 contains further discussion of the use of oral contraceptives and their effects on metabolism.

Table 8-2 summarizes *possible* behavioral and neurological effects of various vitamin deficiencies. Unfortunately, many of these effects, such as irritability and anxiety, are vague and nonspecific and could be caused by a number of different influences. They are also common among teenagers. Any suspicion that they might be caused by nutritional inadequacies should be confirmed with biochemical and functional tests of the individual. There is always the possibility of a vitamin deficiency, especially as our perception of the early effects of vitamin deficiency sharpens. Adverse behavioral changes can precede specific clinical findings in a number of vitamin deficiencies.

Mineral Deficiencies

Iron. Many of the minerals required by the body function as enzyme cofactors, so it is plausible that their excess or deficiency could affect an adolescent's behavior. The mineral that has been studied the most with regard to its effect on behavior is iron.

Clinical observations of iron deficiency anemia in children, adolescents, and adults include the following behavioral changes: irritability; fatigue; weakness; anxiety; restlessness; decreased attentiveness, purposeful activity, and persistence; and impaired cognitive abilities. These symptoms are often dramatically remedied within several days of beginning iron therapy, long before there is any significant impact of iron repletion on the hemoglobin mass. From these observations has come the idea that iron deficiency may modify behavior outside of its role in oxygen transport as hemoglobin. It is theorized that it is the repletion of critical components of other iron compartments that is responsible for this rapid salutary effect of iron therapy.[39,40]

Since hemoglobin deficiency per se does not seem to be the agent for the behavior changes, researchers have considered other enzymes and pathways that require iron for normal function as possibly being abnormal and a cause for the behavioral changes. Iron is involved with enzymes critical in oxidative metabolism, DNA synthesis, and neurotransmitter synthesis and catabolism. For example, the metalloflavoprotein monoamine oxidase (MAO) catalyzes the oxidative deamination of various amines and appears to play a role in regulating the synaptic and extraneuronal levels of neurotransmitters. The activity of this enzyme is reduced in iron-deficient rats and is rapidly restored to normal function by iron repletion.[41]

Until recently it was believed that these iron-dependent enzymes were not affected until very late in the development of iron deficiency anemia. However, with more sophisticated technology it is now apparent that certain iron-related enzyme derangements may precede the development of anemia.[42] For example, iron-deficient children have been shown to excrete excessive amounts of the neurotransmitter norepinephrine in their urine, an abnormality that does not occur in other types of anemia and that is reversible within 1 week after institution of parenteral iron therapy. The implication of this finding is that the behavioral disturbances noted in iron-deficient children may be caused by deranged catecholamine levels in the central nervous system.[43]

Voorhees and co-workers[43] speculate that the progressive deterioration in school performance noted by Webb and Oski[44] in iron-deficient adolescent boys but not in girls is related to the fact that

girls have been found to have significantly higher mean platelet and plasma MAO activity than boys. Perhaps boys are more vulnerable to the consequences of iron deficiency than girls because of their lower physiological levels of MAO combined with decreased MAO activity resulting from the iron deficiency.[43]

From their work with iron-deficient (by transferrin saturation), nonanemic preschool children, Leibel, Pollitt, and Greenfield[45] suggest that the locus of the iron-related disturbance in mental performance in these children is at the level of information reception and not at the level of internal processing or information retrieval. There was no significant difference between the iron-deficient group and the controls with regard to IQ, but the iron-deficient children took more time to learn and made more errors in those aspects of the memory test dependent on attention. After restoration of transferrin saturation to control levels after 4 to 6 months of iron therapy, there were no differences in performance.[45]

From their work with rats, Massaro and Widmayer[46] speculate that perhaps iron deficiency produces a set of behaviors or a learning strategy that is competitive or inconsistent with environmental learning. The net effect then is a disturbance in the way in which information is learned or in what is learned in a particular situation. The effect this has on long-term learning ability is unknown.[46]

Since 15% to 20% of the population of the United States under the age of 20 years is iron deficient, iron deficiency should be considered as a possible factor in behavioral changes in teens.[47] The *Ten State Nutrition Survey* showed that the diets of teenagers are very likely to be low in iron.[47] In addition, because teens are in a phase of rapid growth, the iron requirements are very high, particularly for teenage boys. This is illustrated in Table 3-12.

Zinc. The importance of zinc as related to behavior has not been studied as extensively as iron, although several researchers have noted marked

Table 8-2. Somatic, neurological, and behavioral effects of some vitamin deficiencies

Vitamin	Effects of Deficiency			Situations Where Intake May Be Inadequate
	Somatic	Neurological	Behavioral	
Thiamin (B$_1$)	Poor appetite Loss of tone of gastro-intestinal tract Constipation Cachexia Edema Cardiac failure Beriberi	Wernicke's encephalopathy Peripheral neuropathy Polyneuritis	Mental depression Apathy Anxiety Irritability Korsakoff's psychosis	Alcohol abuse Poor diet, particularly one low in whole grain and fortified carbohydrate and high in refined carbohydrate and sugar
Riboflavin (B$_2$)	Cheilosis (cracks at corners of lips) Scaly shedding around nose and ears Nasolabial seborrhea Sore tongue and mouth Burning and itching of eyes Light sensitivity Ocular lesions Angular stomatitis	EEG abnormalities	No specific behavioral effects reported	Poor diet, particularly if other B vitamins are inadequate
Niacin, nicotinic acid, niacinamide (B$_3$)	Anorexia Glossitis Diarrhea Dermatitis Pellagra	Neurological degeneration Tremor Loss of position sense Spasticity Exaggerated tendon reflexes Progressive paralysis of lips, tongue, mouth, pharynx, and larynx Abnormally increased skin sensitivity Abnormal sensations such as burning or prickling	Symptoms associated with pellagra: Apathy Depression Anxiety Hyperirritability Mania Memory deficits Delerium Organic dementia Emotional lability	Poor diet, particularly if very low in protein
Pyridoxine, pyridoxal, pyridoxamine (B$_6$)	Weakness Abdominal pain Cutaneous lesions Lymphocytopenia	Lack of muscle co-ordination Convulsions EEG changes	Depression Nervous irritability Hyperacusia	Use of oral contraceptives or other estrogen-containing medication Poor diet Use of isoniazid or cycloserine (used to treat tuberculosis) Pregnancy

Nutrient	Physical signs	Neurological effects	Behavioral effects	Causes
Pantothenic acid	Gastrointestinal disturbance; Burning feet; Muscle cramps	Neuritis; Lack of motor coordination; Staggering gait; Numbness; Paresthesia	Restlessness; Irritability; Depression; Fatigue	Very poor diet, especially one low in all B vitamins
Biotin	Dermatitis; Anorexia; Anemia; ECG changes; Muscle pain	Abnormally increased skin sensitivity	Depression; Extreme lassitude; Somnolence	Consumption of many (about 24) raw egg whites daily for a long time
Cyanocobalamin (B₁₂)	Macrocytic anemia	Combined systems disease (diminished vibratory and position sense, abnormal EEG, and motor weakness)	No specific behavioral effects reported. Symptoms may occur as with other deficiency states: Irritability; Depression; Confusion; Memory loss; Hallucinations; Delusions; Paranoia	Strict vegetarian diet; Pernicious anemia; Chronic consumption of large doses of vitamin C
Folic acid, folacin, pteroylmono-glutamic acid	Megaloblastic anemia	No CNS symptoms reported after second year of life. Symptoms in infants: Mental retardation; Lack of muscle coordination; Continuing writhing movements	Forgetfulness; Insomnia; Apathy; Irritability; Depression; Psychosis; Delirium; Dementia	Severe, chronic gastrointestinal disorders; Use of anticonvulsants (phenytoin); Use of oral contraceptives; Use of cancer treatment drugs; Poor diet, especially one lacking fresh fruits and vegetables
Vitamin C (ascorbic acid)	Weakened cartilage and capillary walls; Cutaneous hemorrhage; Sore, bleeding gums; Anemia; Poor wound healing; Poor bone and tooth development; Scurvy	No CNS symptoms reported	Lassitude; Personality changes such as those occurring in physically ill persons: Hypochondriasis; Depression; Hysteria	Poor diet, especially one lacking fresh fruits and vegetables; Hyperthyroidism; Pregnancy; Neoplastic disease; Wound healing; Tuberculosis; Stress

Modified from Lipton, M.A., Mailman, R.B., and Nemeroff, C.B.: Vitamins, megavitamin therapy and the nervous system. In Wurtman, R.J., and Wurtman, J.J., editors: Nutrition and the brain, vol. 3, New York, 1979, Raven Press.

lethargy, slowing of activity, apathy, and decreased sexual activity in zinc-deficient men and women.[48-50] Poorer learning, more aggression, and less exploration is seen in animals experiencing zinc deficiency during various times in their life span.[51] Recently it has been postulated that there is a neurotransmitter role for zinc. This obviously requires much more research.[52]

Influence of Hunger on Behavior

The effects of rather severe chronic undernutrition on the behavior of animals and children have been discussed. An additional question arises: what is the effect of hunger, whether acute or chronic, on behavior? Among adolescents, the practice of not eating breakfast is a common occurrence. Some "dieting" teens skip both breakfast and lunch. Many teens fast throughout the day and then eat the majority or perhaps all of their calories within a period of 4 to 6 hours at the end of the day. What is the effect of hunger throughout the day, whether self-imposed or not, on the teens' behavior?

In a resting state the brain burns 10 times more oxygen and glucose than any other part of the body. Although the brain makes up only 2% to 4% of the body weight in adolescence, it generates 20% of the body's total energy requirements. In states of concentration, tension, or anxiety, the energy expenditure is even greater.

The brain has a higher metabolic rate than other organs, and within the brain different parts of the brain have different metabolic rates. The adult human basal metabolic rate is 0.4 ml oxygen/100 gm tissue/min. Energy expenditure can be measured in milliliters of oxygen per minute because of the constant ratio between energy production as ATP and oxygen consumption. This is further discussed in Chapter 6. By looking at Table 8-3 one can see that the higher brain centers require more energy per minute than do the lower brain centers.[53] The higher the brain area, the higher the metabolic rate. Higher areas consume four to five

Table 8-3. Metabolic rates of brain centers

Brain Center	Rate (ml oxygen/100 gm tissue/min)
Spinal cord	1
Medulla	2
Limbic system	3
Motor cortex	4
Posterior cortex	5-6
Frontal cortex	7-9

times more oxygen and glucose than do the lower areas.[54] The medulla, the lowest part of the brain, which is responsible for vegetative functions, matures prenatally and consumes 2 ml oxygen/100 gm/min. On the other hand, the frontal cortex, which organizes, integrates, analyzes, and evaluates, matures during the period of 18 to 20 years of age and consumes 7 to 9 ml oxygen/100 gm/min. The other areas of the brain fall between these two extremes in their rates of oxygen and glucose consumption. Performance is a function of the ratio of energy supplied to (S) and energy demanded by (D) the brain (S/D). *Energy Supply* is determined by the amount of oxygen, nutrients, blood, and depressants in and the metabolic efficiency of the system. *Energy demand,* on the other hand, is determined by the rate of metabolism of the brain area involved, stimulation, dissonance, stimulants, and temperature.

Munro[55] proposes that as the energy supply to the brain decreases or as the brain's demand for energy increases beyond the supply, brain function regresses down the hierarchy given in Table 8-3. Thus the frontal cortex, which requires the most energy, experiences functional deterioration first. Frontal functions of organization, regulation, analysis, and evaluation deteriorate. Without these functions, people are apathetic, see only their own points of view, consider only the present, and act as if they have been programmed by rewards or punishment.[56]

As the S/D ratio decreases, the following sequence of changes in nerve function occurs: (1) increased reactivity (interest or motivation), (2) hyperreactivity, (3) loss of synaptic transmission with increased arousal, (4) massive release of neurotransmitters and the spread of polarization with maximal arousal, (5) retraction and clumping of vesicles and mitochondrial damage with decreasing responsivity, and (6) at an S/D ratio of 0.5, irreversible structural damage.

Nerves do not consume ATP in reacting but rather in reestablishing the negative potential after discharge and in absorbing the neurotransmitters. In a situation of brain energy deficit (BED), nerves remain in a stable excited state and muscles remain contracted. Munro[55] proposes that it requires more energy not to react and to inhibit impulsive responses to distractions than to act. In brain energy deficits there is less ability to inhibit reaction, so the result is hyperactivity, overreaction, and labile emotions.[55,57]

Munro[55] states that the greatest differences in achievement between disadvantaged and middle-class children in the United States begin to develop in the fourth grade.[58] It is at this age (11 to 14 years) that the frontal cortex matures and the child enters Piaget's stage of formal operations (see Table 2-1). Munro[55] concludes that mildly malnourished, diseased, and stressed children, whose metabolism supports a rate of 6 ml oxygen/100 gm/min, develop normally to the age of 10 years but are unable to sustain a normal frontal function of adolescence, which requires an estimated metabolic rate of 7 to 9 ml oxygen/100 gm/min. According to Himwich,[59] the most recently developed area of the brain, that with the highest metabolic rate, is the most vulnerable to the energy deficits.

When teens have low supply or high demand, it is useless to tell them to solve their problems by organizing, initiating, or sustaining goal-directed behaviors. Those behaviors require high frontal function and too much energy. Although adolescents may function well at concrete levels, if they are forced to attempt frontal functions they are pushed into a rate that they cannot support, and their performance will deteriorate as the tension mounts.[55] When there is a BED, it is adverse. One tries to get rid of this adversity by increasing the energy supply (for example, by eating) or by decreasing the demand (by withdrawing, shifting to a simpler activity, or resolving the problem). Shifting to a simpler activity, such as shifting from writing a paper (9 ml/oxygen) to staring and kicking a table leg (4 ml oxygen), uses the motor cortex and gives the frontal cortex time and energy to recharge.

Previously it was assumed that all of the energy requirements of the brain had to be met by glucose, but now it is apparent that the brain can use ketone bodies as an alternative fuel. Even though ketone bodies can nourish the brain, they do not nourish the different areas of the brain in the same way.[60] It seems that the lower cortical layers consume many more ketone bodies than do the upper layers and that the amount consumed is somewhat dependent on how much is transported into the brain. The fact that the lower cortical layers can use ketones fits with the Munro hypothesis that the lower levels of brain function last longer in BED. Ketone bodies, however, cannot substitute entirely for the fuel of the brain, and some glucose is still required. The brain can still suffer if there is a lowering of blood sugar that lasts too long. The extent to which lack of nourishment lowers blood glucose is different with each person and depends on length of fasting, activity, and level of functioning.

Hunger does not affect neurological structures the way that malnutrition does. However, it may affect learning by decreasing the individual's receptivity to and ability to profit from new experiences. Read[61] states that changes in personality, emotionality, and behavior may interfere with the interpersonal relationships necessary for learning, and the effects of hunger probably play a part in bringing about these changes.

A study of Swedish children aged 7 to 17 years showed no difference in work performance, arithmetic test scores, or subjective reports of hunger or tiredness in children who consumed standard breakfasts of two calorie levels (400 kcal or 560 kcal) that were high in either carbohydrate or protein. However, breakfast intakes of less than 400 kcal adversely influenced performance.[62] Studies confirm the fact that adequate morning nutrition for children and adolescents in school improves attention, concentration, sociability, and scholastic attainment and reduces fatigue and distractibility.[61,63,64] Other data that do not support this may be in conflict because they measure different mental abilities and different sensitivities to nutrition.[65,66] However, the data do give some indications that short-term hunger caused by lack of breakfast may have some adverse effects on emotional behavior, arithmetic and reading ability, and physical work output.[67]

Pollitt and co-workers[68] studied the effect of skipping breakfast on the behavioral arousal in 34 9- to 11-year-old children. Their findings are potentially applicable to adolescents. They postulated that hunger (no breakfast) was a mild environmental stress affecting human performance. Plasma glucose, β-hydroxybutyrate (BOHB), lactate, and free fatty acids were measured before and after a 19-hour fast and were used as indicators of the extent of the stress. Stress was defined as the neurohormonal response required to maintain blood glucose and use fat as an alternative fuel source. The extent of the association of these metabolic variations with behavioral measures was determined. Fasting had an adverse effect on the accuracy of responses in problem solving conducted at 11 AM, before lunch, but it had a beneficial effect on immediate recall and short-term memory assessment. As expected, there were statistically significant differences for the BOHB, lactate, and free fatty acid values between noon values in the breakfast (BR) and no breakfast (NBR) conditions, but there was no statistically significant difference in noon blood glucose levels between the BR and

NBR groups. For the subjects with IQs below the median, the number of errors on one test increased from the BR to the NBR condition. Unexpectedly, though, in those subjects with IQs above the median, the number of errors dropped slightly from the BR to the NBR condition. The childrens' performances in the BR and NBR conditions on the other part of the Matching Family Figure Test (MFFT) and on the vigilance test were no different. On the memory test, there was a statistically significant difference in the last recall item of the series: the subjects in the NBR group performed better than those in the BR condition. Those subjects who had a large difference in blood glucose between the BR and the NBR conditions, as opposed to those who had low BR/NBR blood glucose differences, were more likely to increase the number of errors on both parts of the MFFT test from the BR to the NBR conditions. For these children with large differences in blood glucose, the fasting state constituted a considerable metabolic stress. These metabolic changes, although in no way pathological, are consistent with a relative elevation in adrenal corticosteroids and catecholamines and a relative decrease in plasma insulin levels.[69] Elevated catecholamine levels and cortisol, by their direct impact on the central nervous system, and reduced insulin, by altering neurotransmitter precursor availability in the central nervous system, could cause behavioral changes or simply be reflective of CNS changes correlated with the stress of short fasting.[68]

This study does not show a systematic causative advantage or disadvantage of the fasted state over the fed state, but it can be concluded that brief fasting does induce arousal changes that in turn have a qualitative effect over cognitive functions. These data suggest that brain function can no longer be assumed to be unaffected by subtle alterations in nutritional status and that cognitive operations may be influenced by between-meal timing. Much more information in this area is needed.[68]

Pharmacological Agents in Food

A variety of foods and drinks contain pharmacologically active substances that can induce behavioral changes in the adolescent. Caffeine is the most common example, but others include other methylxanthines (theobromine and theophylline), phenethylamine, and vasoactive amines.

Caffeine. By far the greatest consumption of caffeine in the United States is in the form of coffee. Coffee accounts for 75% of the caffeine consumption, tea is next with 15%, and the remaining 10% is from cola drinks, chocolate products, and medicines.[70] Even though the caffeine in this last category is a small percentage of the total caffeine consumption, it is significant in the teen's diet because the teenager is a heavy consumer of cola drinks. The largest consumers of soft drinks are boys 12 to 19 years of age, followed by men 20 to 34 years of age, and then girls 12 to 19 years of age. Teenage boys and girls drink almost three times as many soft drinks as do men and women 35 years and older, and a large percentage of those drinks are cola drinks.[71]

Substantial amounts of caffeine can be ingested from cola drinks, which contain about 3 mg/oz or about 36 mg in a 12-ounce can. Half of this caffeine is from the kola nut base, the other half is added in manufacturing. There are some soft drinks, in fact, that are not kola nut based but that still contain caffeine (for example, Mountain Dew). See Fig. 9-7 for the caffeine content of selected beverages and drugs. Chocolate, another popular item in the adolescent's diet, also contains caffeine and other xanthines. A cup of hot chocolate may contain as much as 40 mg of caffeine, and the standard 1-ounce chocolate bar has about 20 mg of caffeine.[70]

It is difficult to generalize about the effect of a given amount of caffeine on behavior, attitude, or mood, because it depends on the adolescent's usual caffeine consumption and knowledge of whether or not it is being administered. Two cups of aver-

age strength coffee (200 to 300 mg caffeine) can have mild physiological effects—an increase in general metabolism, peripheral vasodilatation except in the brain, and elevation of blood pressure. Caffeine has a diuretic action on the kidneys and stimulates gastric acid secretion, although this last effect may be less than that from other components in coffee.[72] It inhibits glucose metabolism, which results in elevated fatty acid levels as discussed in Chapter 6. Regular use of more than 350 mg caffeine (about 8 to 9 cans of cola drink) per day induces a physical dependence on caffeine. With a daily use of 600 mg, users may suffer from chronic insomnia, persistent anxiety, paranoia, depression, and stomach upset. Absence of caffeine also makes regular users feel both irritable and tired, and a severe headache can result.

Many children and adolescents are chronic consumers of caffeine, and the amount they consume (2 to 3 mg/kg/day for heavy drinkers) borders on the dose known to produce central nervous system stimulation in adults.[73] However, Elkins and co-workers[74] reported even higher intakes in some youth. They reported that an intake of 3 mg caffeine/kg/day was at the 50th percentile, and an intake of 11 mg/kg/day was at the 90th percentile of prepubertal boys studied.

The study also showed improved vigilance in normal children following caffeine ingestion, particularly at the high dose of 10 mg/kg/day. The low dose of 3 mg/kg/day had minimal or no acute behavioral effects. However, caffeine doses that improved vigilance performance also increased motor restlessness.

Both childrens' and parents' reports of insomnia, nervousness, stomachaches, and nausea were significantly higher during caffeine periods than during placebo periods. However, the effects were seen only in low caffeine users, not in the nine children who habitually consumed caffeine at high levels, approximately the dose used in this study.[74]

Other Substances. Phenylethylamine, another

pharmacological agent, is found in chocolate and has been reported to precipitate migraine headaches in some people.[75] However, the onset of a headache after chocolate ingestion in susceptible individuals probably is dependent on the presence of other factors such as stress, tyramine, alcohol, menstruation, and fasting.[76]

Vasoactive amines, which include epinephrine, norepinephrine, tyramine, dopamine, histamine, and 5-hydroxytryptamine, are also found in foods such as bananas (particularly the peel), tomatoes, avocados, pineapples, cheeses (particularly cheddar and Camembert), and certain wines. These are known to cause headaches in some individuals.[77]

Monosodium glutamate, a food additive, can act pharmacologically and may induce "Chinese restaurant" syndrome, consisting of severe headache, facial pressure, burning sensation, sweating, nausea, weakness, thirst, and chest and abdominal pain. L-glutamate is the culprit. It is also thought to be an important neurohumoral transmitter and a precursor of GABA, another neurotransmitter.[78]

PROPOSED THEORIES AND THERAPIES LINKING DIET TO BEHAVIOR

Orthomolecular Psychiatry or Megavitamin Therapy

In a 1973 report the American Psychiatric Association[79] rejected orthomolecular psychiatry on the basis that it is unsubstantiated by scientific evidence, uses questionable clinical methods, and yields results that are nonreproducible. This was also confirmed by the American Academy of Pediatrics,[80] which said that its use is not justified in children. Carefully controlled double-blind trials have been conducted to test megavitamin claims and the results have been negative.[81,82]

The term *megavitamin therapy* was coined in the early 1950s to describe a treatment for schizophrenia that employed large doses (3 to 30 gm/day, or 200 to 2000 times the RDA) of Vitamin B_3 (nicotinic acid or nicotinamide). Niacin was chosen because it is a nontoxic methyl acceptor, not because of its value as a nutrient.[83,84]

The advocates of megavitamin therapy received substantial support in 1968, when the practice of orthomolecular psychiatry was first proposed by Linus Pauling. Orthomolecular psychiatry supposes that optimal molecular concentrations of substances normally present in the body must be present in the mind for proper mental functioning and thus behavior.[85] Many of these substances are vitamins. Pauling claims that some people require larger quantities of some vitamins than do others for optimal mental functioning. *Orthomolecular psychiatry* takes a broader approach than megavitamin therapy and relies on several components, only one of which is large doses (10 to 500 times the RDA) of vitamins. Other components might be an antihypoglycemia diet, administration of trace minerals, or administration of hormones such as thyroid. In these situations large doses of vitamins, (for example, 100 mg to 6 gm daily of vitamin C, 5 to 500 mg daily of pyridoxine, and 25 to 900 mg daily of panthothenic acid) may also be used. Many critics feel that at these levels vitamins are really functioning as drugs.

Orthomolecular psychiatrists and physicians proclaim that their treatments are effective in a variety of mental and physical illnesses, including autism,[86] reading disabilities,[87] hyperactivity,[88] mental retardation,[89] and drug addiction.[90] However, none of these statements have been confirmed in well-controlled studies. Unfortunately, many molecular psychiatrists refuse to conduct well-controlled, double-blind experiments on the grounds that they would be withholding treatment that they know works. It is unacceptable to refuse to conduct proper experiments because one "knows" the efficacy of a particular regimen or because the *public* is willing to accept alternatives that have not been proven well. The *Journal of Orthomolecular Psychiatry,* formerly the *Journal of Schizophrenia,* published by the orthomolecular proponents, fails to adhere to the requirements of scientific protocol to promote the view of the journal.

Pauling feels that mental disease might be caused by suboptimal concentrations that could occur despite an "adequate" diet because some people, through evolutionary change, require more of particular vitamins. He concludes that since the vitamins of interest in psychiatry are water-soluble and reasonably nontoxic, administration of supermaximal doses might result in significant human health benefits and no harm. However, there are other considerations:

1. Is getting the maximal response from the system by giving large amounts of vitamins beneficial for the organism? There may be changes that result from the pharmacological effects that are unrelated to the action of vitamins.

2. The genetic variability of man may not be as great as Pauling implies.

3. There are still questions about the evolutionary alteration that presumably causes increased vitamin requirements.

4. Do large doses of vitamins taken orally really increase the brain levels of vitamins? There is considerable evidence that this is not the case and that the blood-brain barrier and other mechanisms maintain close control of brain levels of vitamins.[91]

5. Do vitamins have a role in the nervous system outside of their role as cofactors or coenzymes that catalyze metabolic steps? In other words, can large doses of vitamins have pharmacological effects?[92]

A very small number of people have been identified as having vitamin-dependency illnesses. Genetically, these disorders are *very rare* and less than 1000 cases have been described. These disorders are present from the moment of birth and produce clearly identified biochemical abnormalities. Although the vitamin-dependency diseases are very rare, the incidence of vitamin-insufficiency illnesses is not yet known. Even though it is likely they are more common than vitamin-dependency illnesses, they are probably still rare.[93]

Potential Toxicity. It may be that as more is learned about how the brain functions, the part that vitamins play, and the potential for persons to have greater than "normal" nutritional requirements for proper brain functioning, this therapy with vitamins may prove useful and clinically sound. However, our present concept of nutrient toxicity is very narrow and includes only short-term megadose effects. Even less is known about chronic nutrient toxicity where the effects develop slowly over time. Although the public seems to understand the undesirable effects of overconsumption of sugar, salt, or fat, it does not seem to understand that this can also pertain to vitamins and minerals. Very little is known about the toxic effects of minerals, but antagonisms do exist between minerals. Abnormally high levels of some trace elements can displace other elements. For example, increased copper interferes with iron and zinc metabolism. Since the presence or absence of one element may influence the role of a second and modify the requirement of still another, the diet with large doses of minerals may upset the body. Since there is no evidence of benefit and there is some potential for harm, the treatment of adolescents with megadoses of vitamins or minerals cannot be advocated.

Biochemical Individuality. Since the phrase "biochemical individuality" is often used in discussion of megavitamin therapy, it deserves exploration. The idea of biochemical individuality was first put forth by Dr. Roger Williams in 1946 and has since been elaborated on.[75] Williams states that human beings are individuals biochemically just as they are in other ways. For this reason, nutrient requirements are individualized. Some people thus may need much more of a nutrient than the general population, and others may need less. He goes on to say that the most commonly accepted line of demarcation between normal and abnormal in biological work is the 95% level. All values outside those possessed by 95% of the population may be regarded as deviant values. If 95% of the population is normal with respect to 1 measurable item, only 90.2% would be normal with respect to 2 measurable items, and only 60% would be normal with respect to 10 measurable items. The existence in every human being of a vast array of attributes that are potentially measurable makes it quite plausible that practically every human being is deviant in some respect.[94] In the majority of people, the abnormalities may be well enough concealed so that they are not revealed by clinical examination. Nevertheless they may easily have an important bearing on the susceptibility of the individual to disease throughout life.[75] That is the hypothesis for biochemical individuality.

Another part in the biochemical individuality argument is derived from numerous studies related to partial genetic blocks—inherited impaired capacities that allow metabolic reactions to take place but at a much slower pace. There are presumably all degrees of partial genetic blocks, and the enzyme systems within a body may vary widely in effectiveness.[95]

Williams' genetotrophic principle is as follows: "Every individual organism that has a distinctive genetic background has distinctive nutritional needs which must be met for optimal well being."[75] There may be unusually high nutritional needs for specific substances that are not provided adequately by the environment in which the organ or tissue resides. According to Williams, it theoretically should be possible to meet the needs of almost any developing organism. Even unusual needs can be met if they are known. Although it is admitted that from a practical standpoint supplying the needed environmental factors may be far from simple, the genetotrophic idea emphasizes the theoretical possibility that practically any human weakness, deformity, deficiency, or disease can be combated with some success by supplying the needed nutrients to the right locality at the right time. Inversely, almost any deformity or weakness can be created or accentuated by a lack of a crucial nutrient in a crucial tissue at a crucial time. Carried one step further, this principle would mean that any adolescent behavior could be modified by the nutritional environment of the brain tissue. There is no evidence to substantiate this.

Brozek[96] states that although severe nutritional stresses bring about a deterioration of behavior, the pattern of changes may be different in different people because of individual idiosyncracies. In some, for example, it affects primarily sensory functions, in others motor functions, and in still others personality. In young men maintained on a thiamin-free diet there were different personality changes such as hypochondriasis, depression, and hysteria depending on the individual resistance to the dietary stress. Even when the changes are qualitatively the same, the onset of the symptoms in the deficiency state may vary with the individual. The differential response can be interpreted, for the most part, in terms of a known intake of thiamin before a period of acute thiamin deficiency, but that does not account for all of the variation.[97] Other studies of energy intake, protein requirements, and vitamin needs also show wide variability. Brozek[97] concludes that the study of individual variability represents a difficult but intriguing field of research.

The fact that the RDA are established high enough to meet the needs of 95% of the population takes into account the fact that there is individual variation in requirements.

Sugar

Sugar is often claimed to be a causative agent in the diet of teens with behavioral problems. Perhaps sugar *should* receive scrutiny, since it makes up a large proportion of our diets. Researchers in Bogalusa, Louisiana, found that some 10-year-olds consumed as much as 48% of their calories from sucrose.[98]

Results of a study by Prinz, Roberts, and Hartman[99] suggest an effect of sucrose consumption on the behavior of hyperactive children. In 4- to 7-year-old hyperactive children, they found a significant positive association between consumption of sugar products, as noted by a 7-day food record, and playroom behavior. There was a significant relationship between sugar product consumption and destructive-aggressive and restless behavior. In the normal control group, destruction-aggression and restlessness were not associated with dietary variables but general activity was. This suggests that sugar may have some relationship to the behavior of both hyperactive and nonhyperactive children. Further study of this relationship and of whether the same observations can be made in adolescents is needed.

Kolata[100] reports that in another study Rapoport observed the activity of normal children and children whose parents were convinced that they were made hyperactive by sugar. Both groups of children were given a sugar or placebo-containing drink in a double-blind fashion. She found that none of the boys' activity increased after the sugar drink, and in fact their activity was slowed down by sugar. The normal boys showed a slowing effect 3 hours after ingesting sugar, while the "hyperactive" boys showed a slowing effect in 1 hour. Again there is cause for further study.

As was already discussed, consumption of carbohydrate increases the brain level of serotonin, but the behavioral result of this change is not known. Wurtman, quoted in Liebman and Moyer,[101] states that "since sugar causes insulin to be released more rapidly, it may have a greater effect on serotonin levels. At that time of day [breakfast] plasma levels tend to be low due to the overnight fast. Eating sugar for breakfast *could* have a particularly dramatic effect on brain composition and behavior." What connection this could have with behavior is still unknown, but there could be a connection between sugar consumption and the behavioral changes reported in some children and adolescents. Some postulate that the way in which sugar consumption may affect behavior is related to the way in which sensitive individuals metabolize sugar, but again there is no controlled study that supports this. Langseth and Dowd[102] administered a 5-hour glucose tolerance test to 261 hyperkinetic children (ages 7 to 9 years) and found that 74% had "abnormal" glucose tolerance curves. Half of the abnormal curves were low and flat, similar to those seen in individuals with hypoglycemia. However, this should be interpreted cautiously because there is controversy regarding the standards and significance of glucose tolerance testing in children and because these researchers did not include a nonhyperkinetic control group in their study. It is known that when blood glucose drops to a low point there is an adrenergic response by the body that triggers production of epinephrine and norepinephrine. Higher levels of these hormones can cause the type of behavior seen in hyperkinetic children.[69] But that does not allow us to make any further conclusions regarding the possibility of a behavioral response to sugar ingestion.

In pondering the question of sugar's effect on behavior, some researchers have looked at insulin in the brain. It has been found in rats that insulin is detectable in the brain. This has led to the question of why insulin is present in the brain, which supposedly is insulin insensitive. In further work, it was found that the brain insulin receptors are independent of circulating insulin levels. This raises the idea that insulin and its receptors in the nervous system are regulated differently and have different actions from those in the rest of the body. The researchers speculate that insulin may be a neurotransmitter and may have a different function in the central nervous system as compared with its role in other tissues.[103]

Another area to consider is the possible interaction between caffeine and sugar, which often occurs when adolescents drink cola soft drinks or sweetened coffee or tea. In some adolescents, this may mean a combination of two stimulating factors.

Food Additives and the Feingold Diet

In 1973 the allergist Ben Feingold[104,105] first proposed that a child's behavior, particularly hyperkinetic behavior, could be modified by eliminating artificial colors and flavors, the preservatives monosodium glutamate (MSG), butylated hydroxyanisole (BHA), and butylated hydroxytoluene (BHT), and salicylate-containing foods from the diet. He claimed dramatic results in 40% to 50% of the hyperkinetic children. Many studies have been performed to substantiate or disclaim Feingold's statement, which he based on anecdotal evidence. Several studies[106-111] have shown no significant results from the implementation of the Feingold diet in controlled double-blind studies. Others have shown small but significant improvement in behavior or learning in a small percentage (about 10%) of hyperactive youth. Those likely to respond are young children (preschoolers).[112-115]

Neurotransmitters have been studied for their role in hyperkinesis or hyperactivity.[116,117] There is no conclusive evidence that children with hyperkinesis have different metabolism of neurotransmitters.[118,119]

The Nutrition Foundation Advisory Committee panel and the Interagency Collaborative Group of the U.S. Department of Health, Education, and Welfare have made statements to the effect that the Feingold diet has no efficacy in the treatment of hyperactivity and that the role of artificial colors and flavors is unclear.[120,121] However, parents and families continue to claim fabulous results with the use of the diet, so the National Institutes of Health formed a panel to study the situation. Their report states that the diet seems to have a beneficial effect in a small percentage of children, and if the physician and family agree, the diet could be used as a first-treatment trial in the management of hyperkinesis.[122] More detailed discussion of nutrition in hyperkinesis can be found elsewhere.[123]

Placebo Effect. The placebo effect is an important consideration when evaluating the effectiveness of the Feingold diet or any other diet change on behavior.[124] Not only is there an effect from knowing that the dietary change might make a difference, but there also is an effect on behavior from the changed interactions between the child or adolescent and the family. Because implementation of a diet change may be complex and time consuming, there will likely be increased attention to food preparation and the dietary needs of the young person. If a teen has been behaving badly in a bid for more attention, the new diet can become the focus for increased positive attention, and the adolescent's behavior may improve. Parents, teachers, or counselors claim that the diet "works," when actually it is the interaction around the diet that has "worked." Another outcome of the diet is a change in the approach to the adolescent's bad behavior. Instead of assigning responsibility to the teen for choosing to be bad, the questioning concentrates on what the teen had to eat. The motivation for the behavior is transferred from the young person to the suspect food that made the teen behave inappropriately. This shift alone can have an effect on the teen's behavior.

In addition, if teens are involved in the dietary change to improve their behavior, they may begin to feel that through changing their diet they can take responsibility for their behavior and that they *can* change it. This could result in improved behavior regardless of the composition of the diet.

Food Allergies

Several chronic, frustrating problems of adolescence are being ascribed to food allergies. Most of these problems are chronic health problems that are difficult to solve, and many are related to behavior. The idea that these behaviors could be caused by food allergies is not new. Kahn,[125] for example, has used the phrase *allergic toxemia* to define the fatigue, pallor, and difficulty in concentration that occurs in patients with severe hay fever. Rowe[126] has coined the term *cerebral allergy* to describe the mental symptoms of allergies (for example, drowsiness; interference with concentration, thinking, and memory; confusion; depression; irritability; emotional instability; nervous tension; disturbed sleep; and muscular pain and stiffness, especially of the neck, shoulders, and back of the legs). Speer[127] has used the term *allergic tension fatigue syndrome* to describe a condition occurring in allergic children that consists of alternating symptoms of tension and excessive fatigue. These children sleep restlessly and often have nightmares and night sweats. Other symptoms are described below:

ALLERGIC TENSION FATIGUE SYNDROME*

Tension
  Motor (hyperkinesis)
    Overactivity
    Clumsiness
    Poor manual control
    Inability to relax
  Sensory (hyperesthesia)
    Irritability
    Insomnia
    Oversensitivity
    Photophobia
    Hypersensitivity to pain and noise

Fatigue
  Motor
    Fatigue
    Sluggishness
  Sensory
    Torpor
    Achiness

Associated Systemic Signs
  Almost always present
    Pallor
    Infraorbital circles
    Nasal stuffiness

Common
  Infraorbital edema
  Increased salivation
  Increased sweating
  Abdominal pain
  Headache
  Enuresis
  Musculoskeletal pains

Less Common Mental and Nervous Symptoms
  Mental depression
  Feeling of unreality
  Bizarre, irrational behavior
  Paranoid ideas
  Inability to concentrate
  Nervous tics

Speer[127] reported that eliminating particular foods, such as cow's milk, chocolate, colas, corn, wheat, and eggs, from the diet often resulted in a remarkable improvement in symptoms. Most of these symptoms are attributed to a delayed-onset food reaction in which the symptoms start 2 or more hours after the ingestion of foods. An immune basis for delayed-onset food allergy, if one exists, has yet to be defined.

These types of food sensitivity are not identified by skin testing or the radioallergosorbent test (RAST), since the majority do not appear to be IgE-mediated. There is a suggestion from studies that prostaglandins may be mediators of these food intolerances in some patients. It may be one of several immune reactions, or it may be caused by a nonimmune mechanism.[128] The term *allergy* has come to have a broad, vague definition that often makes its meaning unclear. Technically, an allergic reaction is the adverse consequence of a specific immune event, that is, of an interaction between an antigen and antibody or sensitized lymphocyte. Not all reactions involving food ingestion are truly allergic or mediated by an immune mechanism.[129] For instance, some foods contain substances with pharmacological action (see p. 207).

Several authors have reported improvement of behavioral disorders in children through manage-

---

*Modified from Frick, O.L.: Controversial concepts and techniques with emphasis on food allergy. In Bierman, C.W., and Pearlman, D.S., editors: Allergic diseases of infancy, childhood and adolescence, Philadelphia, 1980, W.B. Saunders Co.

ment of their food allergies,[130-132] but most of these studies are anecdotal and not well controlled. In one controlled double-blind test, it was shown that cognitive-emotional symptoms can be produced by exposure to allergens.[133] However, the issue of whether allergies can cause behavioral problems is still open to debate.

Environmental Toxicants

Lead. Environmental toxicants are being scrutinized for their possible effect on human behavior. This is justified because of the increasing number and concentration of these pollutants in our environment. Although this discussion will be limited to those environmental factors that are related to food and drink, many more toxicants exist in the air and water.

Weiss[134] defines a behavioral teratogen as a substance that interferes with brain chemistry and neuropharmacological development but fails to produce clear morphological abnormalities. The growing organism is more sensitive to these teratogens than the adult. Poisoning from food and drink can remain camouflaged for a long time because of diverse consumption patterns and highly individual susceptibilities that blur the relationship. Incipient toxicity is often marked by a collection of vague, subjective, nonspecific psychological and somatic complaints. Another confounding factor is that the nutritional status and diet of the individual can influence whether the individual is susceptible to toxicity.

Probably the most widely researched environmental pollutant that is known to affect behavior is lead, the presence of which has increased tremendously within the past 40 years. The largest source of lead exposure for adolescents is probably airborne lead from the combustion of leaded gasoline.

Silbergeld and Adler[135] demonstrated that even at very low concentration lead can penetrate the neuron and have an adverse effect on neuronal ion metabolism. Pathways mediating inhibition in the brain that use γ-aminobutyric acid (GABA) as a transmitter appear most sensitive to lead.

It also appears that a poor diet makes the child or teen more susceptible to lead intoxication. Nutritional status with respect to calories, fat, vitamin D, calcium, iron, and zinc is influential. A diet low in calories, high in fat, and low in calcium, zinc, and iron seems to increase lead absorption.[136] High intakes of calcium and iron have a protective effect.[137] Unfortunately, these are the same two minerals found to be low in the diets of teenagers.[47]

The effects of lead toxicity are well known and include vomiting, irritability, weight loss, weakness, headaches, abdominal pain, insomnia, and anorexia. More severe symptoms of extreme poisoning are anemia, kidney problems, peripheral neuritis, muscular incoordination, joint pains, and encephalopathy. Death eventually can result. Children with confirmed lead poisoning often have several psychological and neurological sequelae even after treatment. Children with elevated lead levels during their first three years of life had IQ abnormalities, fine motor coordination problems, and behavior problems when they were tested at 7 and 8 years of age.[138]

What are the effects of lead intake that does not result in confirmed lead poisoning? Some suspect that low-level lead consumption may lead to behavioral problems such as hyperactivity, impulsiveness, and short attention span. In another study the most sensitive measures of the effects of lead were verbal and auditory processing, attention, reaction time, and classroom behavior. The teachers in the study further reported increased distractibility, increased prevalence of daydreaming, lack of persistence, inability to follow directions, and lack of organization in children with high lead levels.[139]

Using chelation therapy, David and co-workers[140] showed an improvement in behavior in children 6 to 10½ years of age who also had elevated blood lead levels. The question of whether lead can damage the central nervous system of young children in the absence of the overt signs and symptoms of toxicity is an extremely controversial issue.

Could subclinical toxicity limit academic achievement and promote behavioral disorders?[134] It is difficult to distinguish the effects of environmental insult from lead from the effects of lack of stimulation and inheritance (parental IQ). La Porte and Talott[141] postulate that the effect of lead may not be evident on simple learning tasks but rather in the ability for complex thought and long-term memory.

Other Metals. Other metals in toxic doses may have behavioral effects. Symptoms that have been ascribed to metal toxicity are given in Table 8-4.

Hair Analysis. When referring to minerals or trace metals influencing behavior, one of the questionable methods being used to "diagnose" a metal toxicity or deficiency is hair analysis. Since there is little information on the role of minerals in behavior, except in the case of iron and lead,

Table 8-4. Symptoms that have been ascribed to metal toxicity

Symptoms	Aluminum	Antimony	Arsenic	Boron	Cadmium	Lead	Manganese	Mercury	Nickel	Selenium	Tellurium	Thallium	Tin	Vanadium
Anosmia			●		●									
Appetite loss		●						●			●			●
Convusions						●								
Depression				●						●				●
Disorientation				●								●		
Dizziness		●	●						●	●			●	
Dysarthria	●						●	●						
Fatigue, lethargy		●	●		●			●		●				
Headache		●						●						●
Incoordination, ataxia	●					●	●	●				●	●	
Insomnia									●					
Jitteriness, irritability		●		●										●
Mental retardation						●		●						
Paralysis	●													
Paresthesias		●	●					●					●	
Peripheral neuropathy			●			●		●						
Polyneuritis		●	●										●	
Psychiatric signs	●					●	●	●						●
Somnolence											●	●		
Tremor	●					●	●	●						●
Visual disturbances						●	●	●		●			●	●
Weakness			●	●		●	●	●	●	●				

Modified from Weiss, B.: Behavior as a common focus of toxicology and nutrition. In Miller, S., editor: Nutrition and behavior, Philadelphia, 1981, The Franklin Institute Press, p. 100.

where the information is accumulating, hair analysis to determine possible behavioral consequences is presumptive. Data regarding the normal levels of metals other than zinc in the hair of persons of different ages are also scarce, and standards are only beginning to be developed. Chapter 3 contains a full discussion of hair analysis.

IMPLICATIONS FOR COMMUNITY RESPONSIBILITY AND POLICY

Theories relating nutritional intake and body chemistry to behavior have potentially wide applications. Unfortunately, some of these applications will be inappropriate. For example, nutritional theories have been used as grounds for defense in criminal trials. In 1979 a former San Francisco city supervisor was tried for the murder of that city's mayor and another supervisor. The defense counsel described their client as suffering from manic-depressive illness and coping with intolerable pressures because of a heavily mortgaged house and the necessity of supporting his family on the income from work at a fast-food stand. The defense, which came to be known as the "Twinkie defense," centered around the client's penchant for gobbling down sugary foods—Twinkies, cakes, doughnuts, and candy bars. The defense claimed that this "junk food" exacerbated the client's depression and led to an imbalanced mental condition when he committed the murder. This case illustrates the potential for misuse of the growing knowledge of nutrition's effect on behavior. Nutrition is grasped at as a cause of inappropriate behavior because it seemingly is easy to isolate in the complex of factors influencing a person's behavior. However, it is just as simplistic and erroneous to say that a teen stole a car because he had a cola and doughnut for breakfast as it is to say that it is because the book he wanted from the library was checked out.

The cost/benefit ratio must also be considered when trying to modify behavior through dietary changes. At juvenile institutions that are currently using an orthomolecular approach for treatment of behavioral problems, the use of dietary supplements is costly. Because the treatment's effectiveness is questionable, its ultimate worth is debatable.

SUMMARY

Food and adequate diet are not, as some claim, panaceas that will solve juvenile delinquency, criminal behavior, and learning problems. Since food intake and diet can be manipulated and controlled, the internal biological system of an individual is seen as being much more easily changed than the external factors that lead to crime such as an unstimulating environment, family influence, unemployment, educational deficits, feelings of inadequacy, powerlessness, or revenge. Man's belief in the curative, protective, and magical properties of food is as old as civilization itself. The power of food thus makes people very susceptible and vulnerable to food faddism. Food has an emotional rather than intellectual value. Nutrition does play a large role in health and disease, both physical and mental, but even here nutrition is only one of many determinants of good health. Juvenile offenders have a difficult enough time with poor family relations, alcoholism, low self-esteem, and drug abuse without having the additional strain of poor nutrition and health. If eating habits can be improved in juvenile deliquents and if they are in good nutritional health, they may be in a better position to cope with other problems in their lives. There is insufficient evidence, however, to say that changing a teenager's diet will eliminate tendencies toward criminal behavior.

REFERENCES

1. Scrimshaw, N.S., and others: Protein metabolism of young men during university examinations, Am. J. Clin. Nutr. **18**:321, 1966.
2. Fisher, H.L., Brush, M.K., and Griminger, P.: Reassessment of amino acid requirements of young women on low

nitrogen diets. III. Isoleucine, threonine, phenylalanine and summation, Am. J. Clin. Nutr. **27:**130, 1974.

3. Growdon, J.H.: Neurotransmitter precursors in the diet: their use in the treatment of brain diseases. In Wurtman, R.J., and Wurtman, J.J., editors: Nutrition and the brain, vol. 3, New York, 1979, Raven Press.

4. Fernstrom, J.D., and Wurtman, R.J.: Brain serotonin content: increase following ingestion of carbohydrate diet, Science **174:**1023, 1971.

5. Fernstrom, J.D.: Effects of the diet on brain neurotransmitters, Metabolism **26:**207, 1977.

6. Cohen, E.L., and Wurtman, R.J.: Brain acetylcholine: control by dietary choline, Science **191:**561, 1976.

7. Fernstrom, J.D.: How food affects your brain, Nutr. Action **6**(12):5, 1979.

8. Sitaram, N., and others: Choline: selective enhancement of serial learning and encoding of low imagery words in man, Life Sci. **22:**1555, 1978.

9. Schmeck, H.M., Jr.: Nutrition, memory and depression, Nutr. Action **6**(12):12, 1979.

10. Fernstrom, J.D., and Wurtman, R.J.: Nutrition and the brain, Sci. Am. **230:**84, 1974.

11. Lytle, L.D., and others: Effects of long-term corn consumption on brain serotonin and the response to electric shock, Science **190:**692, 1975.

12. Hartmann, E.: L-Tryptophan: a rational hypnotic with clinical potential, Am. J. Psychiatry **134:**366, 1977.

13. Growdon, J.H., and Wurtman, R.J.: Dietary influences on the synthesis of neurotransmitters in the brain, Nutr. Rev. **37:**129, 1979.

14. Kantak, K.M., and others: Effects of dietary supplements and tryptophan-free diet on aggressive behavior in rats, Pharmacol. Biochem. Behav. **12:**173, 1980.

15. Holman, R.B., Elliott, E., and Barchas, J.D.: Neuroregulators and sleep mechanisms, Annu. Rev. Med. **87:**499, 1975.

16. Hartmann, E.: L-Tryptophan: effects on sleep, Monogr. Neural Sci. **3:**26, 1976.

17. Phillips, E., and others: Isocaloric diet changes and electroencephalographic sleep, Lancet **1:**723, 1975.

18. Porter, J.M., and Horne, J.A.: Bed-time food supplements and sleep: effects of different carbohydrate levels, Electroencephalogr. Clin. Neurophysiol. **51:**426, 1981.

19. Fernstrom, J.D., and Faller, D.V.: Neutral amino acids in the brain: changes in response to food ingestion, J. Neurochem. **30:**1351, 1978.

20. Gelenberg, A., and others: Tyrosine for the treatment of depression, Am. J. Psychiatry **137:**622, 1980.

21. Fernstrom, J.D.: Nutrition, brain function and behavior. In Miller, S.A., editor: Nutrition and behavior, Philadelphia, 1981, The Franklin Institute Press.

22. Zioudrou, C., and Klee, W.A.: Possible role of peptides derived from food proteins in brain function. In Wurtman, R.J., and Wurtman, J.J., editors: Nutrition and the brain, vol. 4, New York, 1979, Raven Press.

23. Worthington-Roberts, B.S.: Suboptimal nutrition and behavior. In Worthington-Roberts, B.S., editor: Contemporary developments in nutrition, St. Louis, 1981, The C.V. Mosby Co.

24. Levitsky, D.A., editor: Malnutrition, environment and behavior, Ithaca, N.Y., 1979, Cornell University Press.

25. Lloyd-Still, J.D., editor: Malnutrition and intellectual development, Littleton, Mass., 1976, Publishing Sciences Group.

26. Pollitt, E., and Thomson, C.: Protein-calorie malnutrition and behavior: a view from psychology. In Wurtman, R.J., and Wurtman, J.J., editors: Nutrition and the brain, vol. 2, New York, 1977, Raven Press.

27. Barnes, R.H.: Dual role of environmental deprivation and malnutrition in retarding intellectual development, Am. J. Clin. Nutr. **29:**912, 1976.

28. Hoorveg, J., and Stanfield, J.P.: Intellectual abilities and protein energy malnutrition: acute malnutrition vs. chronic undernutrition. In Brozek, J., editor: Behavioral effects of energy and protein deficits, U.S. Department of Health, Education, and Welfare, National Institutes of Health Publication 79-1906, 1979.

29. Ricciutti, H.N.: Malnutrition and human behavioral development. In Brozek, J., editor: Behavioral effects of energy and protein deficits, U.S. Department of Health, Education, and Welfare, National Institutes of Health Publication 79-1906, 1979.

30. Ramos-Galvan, R., and others: Aspectos sociales y epidemiologicos. In Humanismo y pediatra, Mexico City, 1968, Nestle Editorial Fund of the Mexican Academy of Pediatrics.

31. Winick, M., Meyer, K.K., and Harris, R.C.: Malnutrition and environmental enrichment by early adoption, Science **190:**1173, 1975.

32. Stein, Z., and others: Famine and human development: the Dutch hunger winter of 1944-45, London, 1975, Oxford University Press.

33. Graves, P.L.: Nutrition and infant behavior: a replication study in the Katmandu Valley, Nepal, Am. J. Clin. Nutr. **31:**541, 1978.

34. Lonsdale, D., and Shamberger, R.J.: Red cell transketolase as an indicator of nutritional deficiency, Am. J. Clin. Nutr. **33:**205, 1980.

35. Kinsman, R.A., and Hood, J.: Some behavioral effects of ascorbic acid deficiency, Am. J. Clin. Nutr. **24:**455, 1971.

36. Adam, K.: Lack of effect on mental efficiency of extra vitamin C, Am. J. Clin. Nutr. **34:**1712, 1981.

37. Nobbs, B.T.: Pyridoxal phosphate studies in clinical depression, Lancet **1:**405, 1974.

38. Kane, F.J.: Iatrogenic depression in women. In Fann, W.E., and others, editors: Phenomenology and treatment of depression, Jamaica, N.Y., 1977, Spectrum Publications, Inc.

39. Leibel, R.L.: Behavioral and biochemical correlates of iron deficiency, J. Am. Diet. Assoc. **71:**398, 1977.

40. Fairbanks, V.F., Fahey, G., and Beutler, E.: Clinical disorders of iron metabolism, New York, 1971, Grune & Stratton, Inc.

41. Symes, A.L., Missala, K., and Sourhes, T.L.: Iron and riboflavin-dependent metabolism of a monamine in the rat in vivo, Science **174:**153, 1971.

42. Finch, C.A., and others: Iron deficiency in the rat: physiological and biochemical studies of muscle dysfunction, J. Clin. Invest. **58:**447, 1976.

43. Voorhees, M.L., and others: Iron deficiency anemia and increased urinary norepinephrine excretion, J. Pediatr. **86:**542, 1975.

44. Webb, T.E., and Oski, F.A.: Iron deficiency anemia and scholastic achievements in young adolescents, J. Pediatr. **82:**827, 1973.

45. Leibel, R.L., Pollitt, E., and Greenfield, D.: Methodologic problems in the assessment of nutrition-behavior interaction: a study of effects of iron deficiency on cognitive function in children. In Miller, S.A., editor: Nutrition and behavior, Philadelphia, 1981, The Franklin Institute Press.

46. Massaro, T.F., and Widmayer, P.: The effect of iron deficiency on cognitive performance in the rat, Am. J. Clin. Nutr. **34:**864, 1981.

47. U.S. Department of Health, Education, and Welfare: Ten state nutrition survey, 1968-1970, Department of Health, Education, and Welfare Publication (HSM) 72-8132-8134, Washington, D.C., 1972.

48. Prasad, A.S., and others: Experimental zinc deficiency in humans, Ann. Intern. Med. **89:**483, 1978.

49. Antoniou, L.D., and others: Reversal of uremic impotence by zinc, Lancet **2:**895, 1977.

50. Henkin, R.I., and others: A syndrome of acute zinc loss: cerebellar dysfunction, mental changes, anorexia and taste and smell dysfunction, Arch. Neurol. **32:**745, 1975.

51. Caldwell, D.F., Oberleas, D., and Prasad, A.S.: Psychobiological changes in zinc deficiency. In Prasad, A.S., and Oberleas, D., editors: Trace elements in human health and disease, New York, 1976, Academic Press, Inc.

52. Gordon, E.F., Gordon, R.C., and Passal, D.B.: Zinc metabolism: basic clinical and behavioral aspects, J. Pediatr. **99:**341, 1981.

53. Lassen, N.A., Ingrar, D.H., and Skinhoj, E.: Brain function and blood flow, Sci. Am. **239:**62, 1978.

54. Sokoloff, L.: Influence of functional activity on cerebral glucose utilization. In Ingrar, D.H., and Lassen, N.A., editors: Brain work: the coupling of function, metabolism, and blood flow in the brain, New York, 1976, Academic Press, Inc.

55. Munro, N.: The brain energy model: a theory about nutrition and behavior, Paper presented at 62nd annual meeting of the American Dietetic Association, Las Vegas, Oct. 22-26, 1979.

56. Pribam, K., and Luria, A.R., editors: Psychophysiology of the frontal lobes, New York, 1973, Academic Press, Inc.

57. Norberg, K., Ljunggren, B., and Seisjo, B.K.: Cerebral metabolism in relation to function in insulin-induced hypoglycemia. In Ingram, D.H., and Lassen, N., editors: Brain work, Copenhagen, 1975, Munksgaard.

58. U.S. Department of Health, Education, and Welfare: Perspectives on human deprivation, Washington, D.C., 1968, U.S. Government Printing Office.

59. Himwich, H.E.: Historical review. In Himwich, W., editor: Developmental neurobiology, Springfield, Ill., 1970, Charles C Thomas, Publisher.

60. Hawkins, R.A., and Biebuyck, J.F.: Ketone bodies are selectively used by individual brain regions, Science **205:**325, 1979.

61. Read, M.S.: Malnutrition, hunger and behavior. II. Hunger, school feeding programs and behavior, J. Am. Diet. Assoc. **63:**386, 1972.

62. Arvedson, I., Sterky, G., and Tjernstrom, K.: Breakfast habits of Swedish schoolchildren, J. Am. Diet. Assoc. **55:**257, 1969.

63. Tuttle, W.W., and others: Effect on school boys of omitting breakfast: physiologic responses, attitudes and scholastic attainments, J. Am. Diet. Assoc. **30:**674, 1954.

64. Dwyer, J.T., and others: Effects of a school snack program on certain aspects of school performance, Fed. Proc. **31:**718, 1972.

65. Lieberman, H.M., and others: Evaluation of a ghetto school breakfast program, J. Am. Diet. Assoc. **68:**132, 1976.

66. Tisdall, F.F., and others: Canadian Red Cross school meal study, Can. Med. Assoc. J. **64:**477, 1951.

67. Pollitt, E., Gersovitz, M., and Gorgiulo, M.: Educational benefits of the United States school feeding program: a critical review of the literature, Am. J. Public Health **68:**477, 1978.

68. Pollitt, E., Leibel, R.L., and Greenfield, D.: Brief fasting, stress and cognition in children, Am. J. Clin. Nutr. **34:**1526, 1981.

69. Santiago, J.V., and others: Epinephrine, norepinephrine, glucagon and growth hormone release in association with physiological decrements in the plasma glucose concentration in normal and diabetic man, J. Clin. Endocrinol. Metab. **51**:877, 1980.

70. Gilbert, R.M.: Caffeine: overview and anthology. In Miller, S.A., editor: Nutrition and behavior, Philadelphia, 1981, The Franklin Institute Press.

71. Lebovit, C.: Who eats the sweets? Natl. Food Rev. p. 62, Sept. 1978.

72. Cohen, S., and Booth, G.H.: Gastric acid secretion and lower esophageal sphincter pressure in response to coffee and caffeine, N. Engl. J. Med. **293**:897, 1975.

73. Life Sciences Research Office: Evaluation of health aspects of caffeine as a food ingredient, Bethesda, Md., 1978, Bureau of Food, Food and Drug Administration, Federation of American Societies of Experimental Biology.

74. Elkins, R., and others: Acute effects of caffeine in normal prepubertal boys. In Miller, S.A., editor: Nutrition and behavior, Philadelphia, 1981, The Franklin Institute Press.

75. Williams, R.J.: Biochemical individuality: the basis for the genetotrophic concept, Austin, Tex., 1956, University of Texas Press.

76. Moffett, A.M., Swash, M., and Scott, D.F.: Effect of chocolate in migraine: a double-blind study, J. Neurol. Neurosurg. Psychiatry **37**:445, 1974.

77. Dalessio, D.J.: Dietary migraine, Am. Fam. Physician **6**:60, 1972.

78. Nemeroff, C.B.: Monosodium glutamate-induced neurotoxicity: review of the literature and call for further research. In Miller, S.A., editor: Nutrition and behavior, Philadelphia, 1981, The Franklin Institute Press.

79. Megavitamin and orthomolecular therapy in psychiatry: excerpts from a report of the American Psychiatric Task Force on Vitamin Therapy in Psychiatry, Nutr. Rev. **32**(suppl. 1):44, 1974.

80. Committee on Nutrition, American Academy of Pediatrics: Megavitamin therapy for childhood psychoses and learning disabilities, Pediatrics **58**:910, 1976.

81. Ban, T.A., and Lehman, H.E.: Nicotinic acid in the treatment of schizophrenias: Canadian Mental Health Association collaborative study—progress report II, Can. Psychiatry Assoc. J. **20**:103, 1975.

82. Kershner, J., and Hawke, W.: Megavitamins and learning disorders: a controlled double-blind experiment, J. Nutr. **109**:819, 1979.

83. Hoffer, A., and others: Treatment of schizophrenia with nicotinic acid and nicotinamide, J. Clin. Exp. Psychopathol. **18**:131, 1957.

84. Hoffer, A., and Osmond, H.: Nicotinamide adenine dinucleotide (NAD) as a treatment for schizophrenia, J. Psychopharmacol. **1**:78, 1966.

85. Pauling, L.: Orthomolecular psychiatry: varying the concentration of substances normally present in the human body may control mental disease, Science **160**:265, 1968.

86. Rimland, B., Callaway, E., and Dreyfus, P.: The effect of high doses of vitamin B$_6$ on autistic children: a double blind crossover study, Am. J. Psychiatry **135**:472, 1978.

87. Green, R.G.: Reading disability, Can. Med. Assoc. J. **100**:586, 1969.

88. Hoffer, A.: Hyperactivity, allergy and megavitamins, Can. Med. Assoc. J. **111**:906, 1974.

89. Carter, C.H.: Handbook of mental retardation syndromes, Springfield, Ill., 1970, Charles C Thomas, Publisher.

90. Libby, A.F., and Stone, I.: The Hypoascorbemia-kwashiorkor approach to drug addiction therapy, J. Orthomol. Psychiatry **6**:300, 1977.

91. Spector, R.: Vitamin homeostasis in the central nervous system, N. Engl. J. Med. **296**:1393, 1977.

92. Dreyfus, P.M.: The nutritional management of neurological disease. In Miller, S.A., editor: Nutrition and behavior, Philadelphia, 1981, The Franklin Institute Press.

93. Lipton, M.A., Mailman, R.B., and Nemeroff, C.B.: Vitamins, megavitamin therapy and the nervous system. In Wurtman, R.J., and Wurtman, J.J., editors: Nutrition and the brain, vol. 3, New York, 1979, Raven Press.

94. Keys, A.: The physiology of the individual as an approach to a more quantitative biology of man, Fed. Proc. **8**:523, 1949.

95. Blass, J.P., and Gibson, G.E.: Abnormality of a thiamine-requiring enzyme in four patients with Wernicke-Korsakoff syndrome, N. Engl. J. Med. **297**:1367, 1977.

96. Brozek, J.: Research on diet and behavior, J. Am. Diet. Assoc. **57**:321, 1970.

97. Brozek, J.: Psychological effects of thiamine restriction and deprivation in normal young men, Am. J. Clin. Nutr. **5**:109, 1957.

98. Frank, G.C.: Personal communication. In Liebman, B.F., and Moyer, G.: The case against sugar, Nutr. Action **7**(12):9, 1980.

99. Prinz, R.J., Roberts, W.A., and Hantman, E.: Dietary correlates of hyperactive behavior in children, J. Consult. Clin. Psychol. **48**:760, 1980.

100. Kolata, G.: Food affects human behavior, Science **218**:1209, 1982.

101. Liebman, B.F., and Moyer, G.: The case against sugar, Nutr. Action **7**(12):9, 1980.

102. Langseth, L., and Dowd, J.: Glucose tolerance and hyperkinesis, Food Cosmet. Toxicol. **16**:129, 1978.

103. Insulin and insulin-receptors in the brain, Nutr. Rev. **38:** 157, 1980.
104. Feingold, B.F.: Why your child is hyperactive, New York, 1974, Random House, Inc.
105. Feingold, B.F.: Hyperkinesis and learning disabilities linked to artificial food flavors and colors, Am. J. Nurs. **75:**797, 1975.
106. Harley, J.P., and others: Hyperkinesis and food additives: testing the Feingold hypothesis, Pediatrics **61:**818, 1978.
107. Harley, J.P., and Matthews, C.G.: Food additives and hypersensitivity in children. In Knights, R., and Bakker, D.J., editors: Treatment of hyperactive and learning-disordered children, Baltimore, 1980, University Park Press.
108. Goyette, C.H., and others: Effects of artificial colors on hyperkinetic children: a double-blind challenge study, Psychopharmacol. Bull. **14:**39, 1978.
109. Connors, C.K.: Food additives and hyperactivity, New York, 1980, Plenum Press.
110. Levy, F., and others: Hyperkinesis and diet: a double-blind crossover trial with tartrazine challenge, Med. J. Aust. **1:**61, 1978.
111. Mattes, J.A., and Gittelman, R.: Effects of artificial food colorings in children with hyperactive symptoms, Arch. Gen. Psychiatry **38:**714, 1981.
112. Conners, C.K., and others: Food additives and hyperkinesis: a controlled double-blind experiment, Pediatrics **58:**154, 1976.
113. Weiss, B., and others: Behavioral responses to artificial food colors, Science **207:**1481, 1980.
114. Swanson, J.M., and Kinsbourne, M.: Food dyes impair performance of hyperactive children in a laboratory learning test, Science **207:**1485, 1980.
115. Williams, J.I., and others: Relative effects of drugs and diet on hyperactive behaviors: an experimental study, Pediatrics **61:**811, 1978.
116. Tagliamonte, A., and others: Increase of brain tryptophan and stimulation of serotonin synthesis by salicylate, J. Neurochem. **20:**909, 1973.
117. Augustine, G.J., and Levitan, H.: Neurotransmitter release from a vertebrate neuromuscular synapse affected by a food dye, Science **207:**1489, 1980.
118. Khan, A.U., and Dekirmenjian, H.: Urinary excretion of catecholamine metabolites in hyperkinetic child syndrome, Am. J. Psychiatry **138:**108, 1981.
119. Ferguson, H.B., and others: Plasma-free and total tryptophan, blood serotonin, and the hyperactivity syndrome: no evidence for serotonin deficiency hypothesis, Biol. Psychiatry **16:**231, 1981.
120. National Advisory Committee on Hyperkinesis and Food Additives: Report to The Nutrition Foundation, New York, 1975, The Nutrition Foundation.
121. Interagency Collaborative Group on Hyperkinesis: First report of the preliminary findings and recommendations of the Interagency Collaborative Group on Hyperkinesis, 1976, U.S. Department of Health, Education, and Welfare.
122. Consensus on diets and hyperactivity, Science **215:**958, 1982.
123. Lucas, B.: Diet and hyperactivity. In Pipes, P., editor: Nutrition in infancy and childhood, ed. 2, St. Louis, 1981, The C.V. Mosby Co.
124. Brunner, R.L., Vorhees, C.V., and Butcher, R.E.: Food colors and behavior, Science **212:**578, 1981.
125. Kahn, I.S.: Pollen toxemia in children, JAMA **88:**241, 1927.
126. Rowe, A.H.: Allergic toxemia and fatigue, Ann. Allergy **8:**72, 1950.
127. Speer, F.: Allergic tension-fatigue syndrome, Pediatr. Clin. North Am. **1:**1029, 1954.
128. Frick, O.L.: Controversial concepts and techniques with emphasis on food allergy. In Bierman, C.W., and Pearlman, D.S., editors: Allergic diseases of infancy, childhood and adolescence, Philadelphia, 1980, W.B. Saunders Co.
129. Bierman, C.W., and Furukawa, C.T.: Food allergy, Pediatr. Rev. **3:**213, 1982.
130. Crook, W.G., and others: Systemic manifestations of allergy, Pediatrics **27:**790, 1961.
131. Kittler, F.J., and Baldwin, D.C.: Allergic factors in minimal brain dysfunction, Ann. Allergy **28:**203, 1970.
132. Rapp, D.J.: Food allergy treatment for hyperkinesis, J. Learn. Dis. **12:**42, 1979.
133. King, D.S.: Can allergic exposure provoke psychological symptoms? Biol. Psychiatry **16:**3, 1981.
134. Weiss, B.: Behavior as a common focus of toxicology and nutrition. In Miller, S.A., editor: Nutrition and behavior, Philadelphia, 1981, The Franklin Institute Press.
135. Silbergeld, E.K., and Adler, H.S.: Subcellular mechanisms of lead neurotoxicity, Brain Res. **148:**451, 1978.
136. Mahaffey, K.R.: Nutritional factors in lead poisoning, Nutr. Rev. **39:**353, 1981.
137. Levander, O.A.: Nutritional factors in relation to heavy metal toxicants, Fed. Proc. **5:**1683, 1977.
138. de la Burde, B., and Choate, M.S.: Early asymptomatic lead exposure and development at school age, J. Pediatr. **87:**638, 1975.
139. Needleman, H.L., and others: Deficits in psychologic and classroom performance of children with elevated dentine lead levels, N. Engl. J. Med. **300:**689, 1979.
140. David, O.J., and others: Lead and hyperactivity: behavioral response to chelation: a pilot study, Am. J. Psychiatry **133:**1155, 1976.
141. LaPorte, R.E., and Talott, E.E.: Effects of low levels of lead exposure on cognitive function: a review, Arch. Environ. Health **33:**236, 1978.

Chapter 9

Adolescence, Nutrition, and Pregnancy: Interrelationships

JANE MITCHELL REES
BONNIE WORTHINGTON-ROBERTS

Teenage pregnancy must be studied in light of the highly dynamic nature of adolescence. Both the psychological and physical status of the adolescent have implications for the course of any pregnancy that may occur. The interrelationships of factors in adolescent development and in reproduction have great clinical significance to all aspects of the pregnancy, including the nutritional aspect. Indeed, adolescents are changing so profoundly that pregnancy for the younger, less mature teen will be different than for the more mature adolescent.

Less mature teenagers will be more dependent on others and less able to act and make decisions on their own. They will be more narcissistic and less able to comprehend the needs of others. These teens will be less realistic, engage more in fantasy and wishful thinking, and have less insight into their own behaviors and motives. In general, younger teens will have fewer intellectual and physical skills to cope with any situation, especially a complex reproductive experience. Many of the difficulties related to pregnancy in adolescence stem from this immaturity. As development advances, a person is able to carry out reproduction and child rearing in a more normal, less problem-fraught way.

REPRODUCTION DURING ADOLESCENCE

Physical Development

As Chapter 1 describes, the female adolescent is rapidly changing in the physical sense. Many authorities have assumed the pregnant teenager to be in a state of rapid physical growth, with the growth of the fetus superimposed on the teen's own physical development.[1-5] Recently it has been pointed out that, since pregnancy can take place only after a certain state of sexual maturity has been reached, growth would have ceased or markedly slowed before the beginning of pregnancy or shortly thereafter[6] because of the high levels of ovarian hormones present at these periods. At the present time, data are not available to show whether the slow growth expected after the menarche[7,8] continues through and after pregnancy or stops during the course of pregnancy. A recent preliminary study found a lack of linear growth during the year in which adolescents experienced their first pregnancy. Measurements began at the first clinic visit. The results indicated that such a study would need to be extended for a longer period to demonstrate an absolute cessation or alteration in the expected growth pattern. It is possible that those who were closer to the onset of menarche and/or younger might indeed be found to increase in height.[9]

There may be a difference in the course of pregnancy for those in an earlier versus a later stage of physical development. It is probably rare that a young woman conceives soon after the onset of menses, since the initial cycles of teens are often anovulatory for 12 to 18 months.[10] Theoretically, those who have menstruated for several years may be more physically capable of successful reproduction than those who are closer to the age of menarche. Their bodies will have had more time for maturation and for storage of nutrients after rapid growth. Some authors[1,4,5] have hypothesized that a period of up to 4 years after the onset of menses is a high-risk period for pregnancy. A precise method for determining risk is to calculate the gynecological age, which represents the amount of time past the menarche of a particular woman, and to consider those of younger gynecological age to be at greater risk for adverse pregnancy course or outcome. The risk is suggested by knowledge that an organism is vulnerable in periods of physiological change.

An additional point about physical growth is that late maturation in the teenage girl may to some extent be related to suboptimal nutritional status.[11] If this is the case, these late maturers who conceive close to the onset of menses would be at higher risk than those who matured earlier and conceived about the same time after menarche.

Thus it is essential to consider both stage of adolescent physical development and chronological age in estimating reproductive risk and planning management strategies. In all circumstances the pregnant adolescent has recently experienced rapid linear growth. Because this growth draws on nutritional stores, it therefore increases the likelihood that pregnancy will be initiated under less than optimal nutritional conditions.

Fertility and Contraception

Indications are cited by Tanner[10] that the young woman of the 1970s and 1980s is fertile at a much younger age than in past generations. Chapter 1 discusses this point at more length. Similar studies of the age of sexual maturity in young men are not generally available, but it can be hypothesized that the same factors that lower the age of maturity in young women also affect young men. Most likely the age of full sexual drive has been lowered for both sexes. In addition, there are social and cultural reasons for the earlier onset and greater frequency of intercourse among teenagers, including changes in sexual mores and the influence of the news and entertainment media.[4,12]

Recent studies indicate that 7 out of 10 young women become sexually active as teenagers.[13] Although contraceptives are more readily available than in former years, teens often do not use them. Those who do attempt to prevent conception may do so ineffectively.[14,15] Thus the number of live births to teens under 19 years of age in 1977 was 570,609.[16] This can be compared to 189,188 live births to teens under 17 years of age in 1960.[17] Although part of this increase is due to the rise in number of teens as a percentage of the whole population, the number of teen pregnancies is considerable.

Psychological Development

Successfully carrying out a pregnancy requires a sense of responsibility that is difficult to possess before a person has become fully autonomous through the normal developmental process. The acceptance of responsibility by teens is related to their particular state of development and is therefore highly variable and difficult to predict.

The adolescent parent-to-be generally has neither developed a sexual identity in the full sense nor become accustomed to an adult sexual role.[18] A pregnancy will force the teenager to face this issue before she may be ready, causing her to experience disequilibrium. The necessity of accepting a role as parent is an additional stress for the individual in an immature state of development.

In addition, the very reasons for the immature

teenager's conception and maintenance of pregnancy may be rooted in a disturbed adolescence. She may attempt to manipulate others by self-destructive means, seek instant gratification, and show a lack of concern for the future.[19]

Some teens may seek close relationships that include sexual intimacy to deal with a personal loss of family members through death or separation.[20] Others may use pregnancy to build self-esteem or feel that the baby will fill unmet needs for love and a sense of family belonging.[19] Teens without either interest in school or skills to gain employment may look on parenthood as a way to obtain an independent role in life.[21] Less mature pregnant teens may lack ego strength to the extent that they actually fail to obtain the proper food and other resources needed to maintain a healthy pregnancy.[18]

In summary, there may be a number of reasons that must be acknowledged for a teenager choosing to keep a pregnancy. It is as Feinfeld and Speller[22] wrote in 1980, "To treat what we see as a problem, we must realize that this problem often seems the solution to the adolescent."

Prenatal Care

Teen pregnancies, although often unplanned, are not in the full sense unwanted pregnancies.[23,24] By the time the young woman is seen for prenatal care, she often either has an awareness of the possible alternatives to carrying out the pregnancy and has rejected them or has delayed facing the problem until abortion is not an option.[12] Although she may be ambivalent about this decision, she has committed herself and on that basis generally will declare that she is happy about the pregnancy. The outward psychological state of the teen may be positive, but there may be underlying negative feelings about the pregnancy. Negative feelings may surface in relation to physical symptoms, labor and delivery, and the need to maintain healthful habits for the sake of the unborn child. *Herein lies the difficulty for the clinician: the teen will be strong verbally in her commitment to the pregnant state but unwilling or unable to do those things necessary to successfully carry it out and rear a child.*

Teenagers often obtain prenatal care late in their pregnancy.[13,15,24] Some ignore the whole question for a time. They may not believe they are pregnant and wait some months before seeking a confirmation. It may be easy to overlook a missed period if conception occurs before the cycle has stabilized. Additional time may pass while the teenager is deciding whether or not to have an abortion. For these and other reasons, the teenager may be well into the second trimester before she seeks care.[13,24] Fig. 9-1 presents a comparison of initiation of prenatal care by different age groups.

Psychosocial Concerns

The Developing Body Image. Because pregnancy may intervene before body-image development has advanced, the feelings of the girl about her body may have a negative impact on her feelings about the pregnancy. Most teens are somewhat uncomfortable with the more mature figure that they acquire as they mature sexually. When the physical changes of pregnancy are superimposed in rapid fashion, it may be difficult for the teen to feel positive about herself physically. She will often think of herself as getting "fat." Young male partners and other peers may support the idea by teasing her; this is often a reflection of their own bodily concerns. The usual result is that the teen will have difficulty accepting the weight gain necessary for a healthy pregnancy.

Significant Others. The food choices and basic ideas about nutrition of a pregnant teenager often will be influenced by her partner, by friends or other peers, and by family members. The ideas these people hold about nutrition range from strict adherence to misguided philosophies gained from inappropriate sources, through reasonable knowledge of nutrition principles, to a complete lack of concern. If she continues to live at home, her mother may be taking full responsibility for food

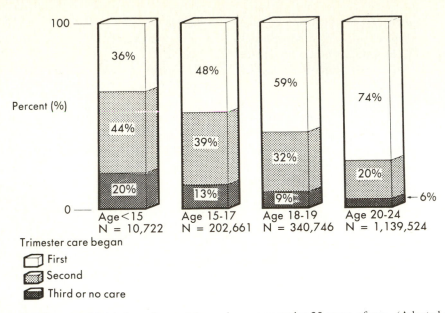

Fig. 9-1. Trimester of initiation of prenatal care in women under 25 years of age. (Adapted with permission from Teenage pregnancy: the problem that hasn't gone away, published by The Alan Guttmacher Institute, New York, 1981.)

planning, buying, and preparation. If she is establishing a home with her partner, he may demand that they have certain foods that he prefers without regard for their relationship to health.[25] If she spends much of her time with friends, eating will be part of their social activities. This may mean eating away from home, often in restaurants or fast-food outlets.

Income Level. As a general rule, a pregnant teenager is a person who does not or has not had sufficient income to support herself and a family. Even if she belongs to a high-income family, she often is not financially independent at the outset of her pregnancy. The problem of establishing economic stability is common and can affect the food available to the pregnant teen.

Stress. Teenagers outwardly react to the stress inherent in their pregnancy in many different ways, some of which affect nutrition. They may experience more nausea than is normal in preg-

nancy.[26] They may derive a sense of comfort from overeating or restrict their food intake as a way of denying their pregnancy. Less apparent results of stress in pregnancy are being investigated. In animal models the neuroendocrine adaptive reactions to stress have been shown to interfere with in utero cardiorespiratory processes to the detriment of fetuses.[27,28] In humans negative attitudes have been found to be associated with unfavorable outcomes of pregnancy in a study of 8000 women by Laukaran and van den Berg.[29] Although biochemical reactions of the human body to stress have not been fully elucidated, it is inevitable that the consequent change in hormonal balance will alter the normal metabolism to some degree. Stress may affect the utilization of nutrients and therefore the overall nutritional status of the pregnant teen. Typical examples of the types of potentially stressful psychosocial events in a teen pregnancy that can affect nutritional status are presented on a time line

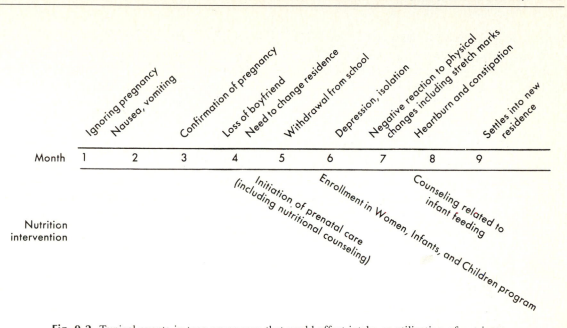

Fig. 9-2. Typical events in teen pregnancy that could affect intake or utilization of nutrients.

with the major milestones in the initiation of nutritional care in Fig. 9-2.

Influential Life-Style Variables

Substance Abuse. Much is known (or at least being asked) about the results of ingesting various nonnourishing substances during pregnancy. There is great concern for the vulnerable position of the fetus related to toxic substances that enter its environment. The effect of a particular substance is often tied to the nutritional status of a pregnant woman, whether because of the substance's interrelationships with nutrients and its effect on weight gain or because the substance is taken by mouth.

Drugs. Teenagers may be using ''hard'' drugs, controlled drugs obtained in illicit transactions on the street, or over-the-counter drugs such as vitamins or laxatives that are available without prescription.[30,31] Their use and effects during pregnancy have been reviewed by Hollingsworth, Erickson, and Doughty.[31] The dangers of narcotic use during pregnancy include increased fetal mor-

bidity and mortality related to respiratory distress and a possibility of central nervous system abnormalities.[31] At least one case has been reported where phencyclidine (''angel dust'') was suspected of causing fetal abnormalities, including behavioral, skeletal, and neuromuscular components.[32]

Caffeine. Attention has turned to the potential harm of caffeine during pregnancy. Although the evidence that it is teratogenic in humans is mainly circumstantial at this point, it has been shown to cause birth defects in rats.[33] Because of its inclusion in soft drinks, it is commonly ingested by teens, even those who do not drink coffee or tea. Although the exact role of caffeine during human pregnancy has not been determined, it appears wise for pregnant women to use this drug in moderation. The Food and Drug Administration made a recommendation to this effect in October 1980. The effects of caffeine on behavior are discussed in Chapter 8.

An important reason for focusing on the overuse of caffeine is that it appears to be transmitted via breast milk from mother to baby, setting up a cycle of hyperirritability.[34]

Smoking. A substantial number of individuals in the teenage population are known to be using cigarettes. In a study of 406 pregnant adolescent subjects, 43% of the young women were smokers.[31] Although the study did not pinpoint smoking as a causative factor in teenage problem pregnancies, others[35-37] have found an increased incidence of low birth weight and lower average maternal weight gain among women who smoke. Although smoking women do not appear to have a reduced energy intake compared with nonsmokers, one clinical trial has shown that supplemental protein and food energy increased birth weight of infants born to smokers.[38-41] Although the precise mechanism by which maternal smoking retards fetal growth is not clear and although there is some question as to whether the cause is in the smoking or the basic physiological makeup of the individual,[35] authorities have advocated cessation of cigarette smoking during pregnancy.[31,42]

Although evidence has not been produced to link marijuana use to adverse outcomes of pregnancy in humans, there is sufficient evidence of teratogenic potential based on animal studies that women who either are or could become pregnant are advised not to use the drug.[43] A recent review[31] has suggested the need for investigation of marijuana's link to chromosomal abnormalities, impairment of cell-mediated immunity, and possible damage to the immature hypothalamus. Cannabinoids are fat soluble and can be stored in the body. Portions of the drug cross the placenta. Therefore exposure to the fetus is possible even when marijuana is used only occasionally.[31]

Alcohol. Alcohol, commonly used throughout recorded history, has been conclusively linked to birth defects in recent years. Children born to alcoholic women may suffer growth and mental retardation, craniofacial abnormalities, and a variety of other developmental defects seen in fetal alcohol syndrome.[44,45] Social drinking (two drinks or more per day on a regular basis) has also been associated with intrauterine growth failure, increased risk of anomalies, behavioral decrements in the infant, increased risk of stillbirth and miscarriage, and decreased placental weight.[45,46] Although the effect of lower doses of alcohol is not conclusively proven, it is said that there is no safe amount for the pregnant woman, as the alcohol is known to cross the placenta and expose the fetus.

There appears to be some natural mechanism in pregnant women for limiting exposure to toxic substances. Women often report that they develop an aversion to alcohol, coffee, and cigarettes during pregnancy, a phenomenon also observed in pregnant animals.[47,48]

A study of the role of alcohol in the prepregnancy period was published in 1980.[49] Researchers found that heavy drinkers who ceased drinking during pregnancy delivered babies with a significantly smaller mean birth weight (258 gm [9.03 oz] less) than women who had not been heavy drinkers before conception.

The significance of alcohol abuse in a pregnant adolescent is easy to surmise from the previous data. Although most young women have not lived long enough to develop the classic picture of alcoholism, they may use alcohol in such excessive amounts that risk to their infants does exist. The teenager's use of alcohol, drugs, and tobacco is further discussed in Chapter 4.

Exercise and Rest. Teenagers who become pregnant commonly drop out of normal activities in which they previously engaged. They may become somewhat lethargic, as they no longer want to be seen roller skating or dancing and are physically less capable of carrying out these forms of exercise. Available data suggest that they spend a considerable amount of time watching television and sleeping.[50] Moderate exercise during pregnancy is generally beneficial in that it maintains good muscle tone, alleviates constipation, and allows for expenditure of extra food energy. Occasionally, however, a teen will be overzealous in exercising, either in a misguided attempt to "keep from getting fat" or in a self-destructive struggle to "keep up" with her usual life-style. Such exercise can be detrimental to her health. Maintenance of physical health of pregnant teens requires efficient use of nutrients for successful weight gain, and lack of rest may compromise this process. This situation would be of special concern if combined with other life-style hazards.

The Father's Role

Those teen fathers who stay involved with their partners throughout pregnancy can be very possessive of their role in the reproductive process. As part of this response, they may be curious about the genetic contribution of the male to the makeup of the infant. Apart from the known contribution to hair, eye color, and physique, research in animals has indicated that unknown factors in the genetic contribution of male partners may cause a trend toward unfavorable pregnancy outcomes even in low-risk females.[51] Work showing that the father's advanced age may be linked to the incidence of Down's syndrome, although recently criticized, further supports the relevant contribution of fathers to pregnancy course and outcome.[52] There also has been concern about possible reproductive hazards caused by the father's exposure to pollutants.[42]

NUTRITIONAL NEEDS OF PREGNANT ADOLESCENT

The rationale for the nutritional needs of pregnant women[17,53-56] and of adolescent pregnant women[1,4,24,55,57] has been reviewed frequently. The usual recommendations for adolescents are based on the RDA for that age group with added nutrient amounts that are recommended for all pregnant women. In the absence of more relevant recommendations, these figures are provided in Table 9-1 as approximate amounts of nutrients needed. As was pointed out in Chapter 3, the RDA is based on chronological age, which does not take into account the state of maturity of the teenager. The added amount for growth will not be necessary for women who are several years past the rapid-growing period.

For pregnant teens, the concept of gynecological age, as discussed earlier in this chapter, is an important consideration in determining their nutrient needs. Those young women closest to the onset of menses are probably in greatest need of additional nourishment. They are closest to the growing period and have not had time to store nutrients even if they have stopped growing. Because of rapid growth preceding sexual maturity, variable amounts of time between onset of menses (with slowing down of growth) and pregnancy, differing energy expenditure, and possible continuation of the maturation process during pregnancy, there is no means of calculating the nutritional needs of the pregnant teen in a precise manner.

Of additional relevance is the observation that many teens receive medical care in public health clinics,[24,58] where sophisticated biochemical studies of nutriture are not available. Clinicians in these settings do not have specific indicators of tissue nutrient levels for a particular individual. Recommendations thus will necessarily be made on the basis of less than accurate evidence of deficiencies and deviations from recommended amounts.

Experience with at-risk teens shows they are often unresponsive to suggestions about food choices that are phrased in terms of units of nutrients per day (such as gram of protein per day) or number of servings of a particular food per day. Many of them do not conceptualize their food intakes in this way. Traditional techniques of managing nutrition in pregnancy have been well described[59,60] and will be useful for the motivated and mature teens who respond to them. For the remainder, including those at highest risk, alternative approaches to nutritional guidance must be employed. In preparation for understanding these techniques, it is valuable to consider the nutritional needs of pregnant

Table 9-1. Recommended dietary allowances for pregnant adolescent females

Nutrient	Age (Reference Height)			
	11-14 yr (157 cm)		15-18 yr (163 cm)	
	Total RDA	RDA/cm	Total RDA	RDA/cm
Energy (kcal)	2500	15.9	2400	14.7
Protein (gm)	76	0.48	76	0.47
Calcium (mg)	1600	10.2	1600	9.8
Phosphorus (mg)	1600	10.2	1600	9.8
Iron (mg)	18*		18*	
Magnesium (mg)	450	2.9	450	2.7
Iodine (μg)	175	1.1	175	1.1
Zinc (mg)	20	0.13	20	0.12
Vitamin A (μg RE)	1000	6.4	1000	6.1
Vitamin D (μg)	15	0.09	15	0.09
Vitamin E (mg α-TE)	10	0.06	10	0.06
Ascorbic acid (mg)	70	0.45	80	0.49
Niacin (mg NE)	17	0.11	16	0.10
Riboflavin (mg)	1.6	0.01	1.6	0.01
Thiamin (mg)	1.5	0.01	1.5	0.01
Folacin (μg)	800	5.1	800	4.9
Vitamin B (mg)	2.4	0.02	2.6	0.02
Vitamin B_{12} (μg)	4	0.03	4	0.02

Modified from Food and Nutrition Board, National Academy of Sciences–National Research Council: Recommended dietary allowances, ed. 9, Washington, D.C., 1980.
*Supplemental iron recommended

teens by keeping in mind both the traditional principles of nutritional needs during pregnancy and the current common teenage dietary patterns. The food-related behaviors of teens who are at most risk will doubtless follow the trends of the 1980s. To summarize from Chapter 4, that will include eating fewer meals at home, eating more meals in fast-food franchises, and being less likely to follow an accustomed meal pattern. Teens will be apt to choose impulsively items from a narrow range of foods that are considered "prestigious" by their peer group, are readily available, or take little preparation.

Energy

Energy intake must be considered foremost among the nutritional needs of the pregnant teen because of its overall influence on nutritional status, protein utilization, and tissue synthesis. Except for those attempting to stay abnormally thin, teens appear to take in sufficient energy.[17,61] For example, the proportion of underweight subjects at the outset of pregnancy in two studies was 5% and 7%.[62,63]

Certain unique circumstances of pregnancy may interfere with the intake of food energy, however. Energy intake of pregnant teens in San Francisco was one of the nutritional components found to compare least favorably with the 1968 RDA.[64] Psychological stress, restriction of intake, nausea and vomiting, or strained economic resources of the young woman may affect the amount and utilization of food intake.

Hytten and Leitch[65] have presented data that

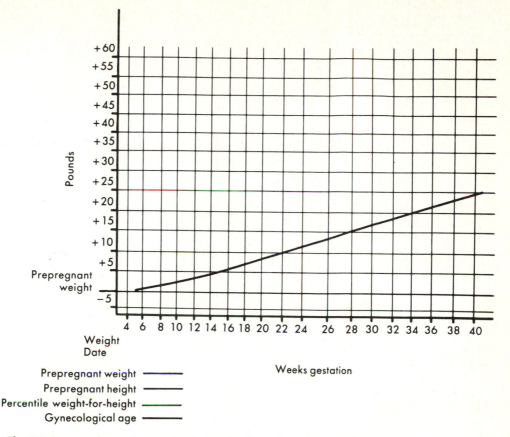

Fig. 9-3. Pattern of normal prenatal weight gain. (From Committee on Maternal Nutrition, Food and Nutrition Board, National Academy of Sciences–National Research Council: Maternal nutrition and the course of pregnancy, Washington, D.C., 1970, U.S. Government Printing Office.)

suggested the energy needs of a pregnant woman (as compared with a nonpregnant woman) are 300 kcal more per day during the last 30 weeks of pregnancy. If this guideline is used for the pregnant teen, it could be estimated that she needs this amount of energy added to her typical intake if her weight is appropriate for height at the time of conception. If she is above average weight-for-height or gaining weight at the time of conception, she will need a smaller increase. If she has been losing weight or is underweight, she will need to increase her energy intake by a greater amount. This as-

sumes that the young woman's energy output remains the same, which may or may not be the case. Thus the energy needs of the pregnant teen vary with the individual.

Guidance in arriving at an appropriate intake of energy comes from following the weight gain throughout pregnancy. The recommended pattern (Fig. 9-3), reflecting a gain of around 11.25 to 13.5 kg (25 to 30 lb), is a good guideline. However, it has not been specifically designed for teen pregnancy. Preliminary data show that the mean weight gain for a group of 80 pregnant adolescents

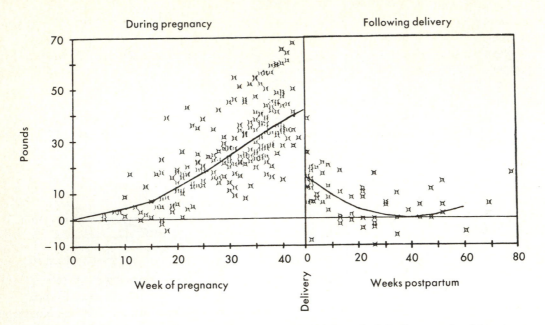

During pregnancy   Following delivery

Fig. 9-4. Weight changes with adolescent pregnancy. (From Meserole, L.P.: Patterns of weight gain and loss in pregnant and postpartum adolescents, master's thesis, Seattle, 1982, University of Washington.)

(Fig. 9-4) was higher than that reflected in the usual curve, suggesting the need for research to determine the optimal gain for teens.[9] Further discussion of this question begins on p. 232.

Protein

Protein is a nutrient of high priority in the diets of pregnant teens. It is, of course, essential for tissue formation. Most surveys in the United States indicate that protein is not lacking in the diets of adolescent female populations.[17,61] The protein intakes of two pregnant adolescent populations have been found to be favorable in comparison with recommended amounts.[62,64] However, because of low-income status or because concentrated carbohydrate and high-fat foods may be chosen over protein-rich foods, the amount of protein in the diets of individual pregnant teens may be marginal.

The exact amount of protein needed by the pregnant adolescent is difficult to pinpoint. This difficulty is partially accounted for by the difference between theoretical calculations and the results of balance studies.[66] It is certain that rich sources of animal or vegetable protein must be among the foods commonly eaten by the pregnant teen if she is to be adequately nourished. There must also be sufficient food energy to allow for utilization of the protein for tissue synthesis rather than as a source of needed energy.

Calcium

Calcium nutriture of the pregnant teen is especially important. She must both support normal growth and development of her fetus following her own growth spurt and maintain calcium stores. Lactation presents additional requirements that cannot be overlooked.

There is evidence that calcium is not consumed in optimal amounts by pregnant teens.[64] Young women who do not consume dairy products are in a special risk category with respect to calcium nutriture. Supplemental calcium will be necessary for any teenager whose calcium intake falls short of recommended amounts.

Iron

Iron has rightly received a great deal of attention regarding its role in the nutritional status of women of reproductive age. In the past young women in various surveys have reported inadequate iron intakes.[67] With the exception of meats, foods commonly eaten by teens generally are low in iron.

Iron deficiency of the degree that results in anemia has only sometimes been found in non-pregnant study populations, but a lack of stored iron is probably common.[1,68] Thus anemia may develop in pregnant teens as a result of the large amount of this mineral needed in pregnancy.[17,62,69] Because of the difficulty of obtaining iron from food sources, it is generally thought necessary to use iron supplements to provide for both the mother and the fetus.[1,2,17,64]

As larger amounts of iron are given, smaller percentages are absorbed. Excessive supplemental iron thus will not be used by the body.[70] Since pregnancy does increase the efficiency of absorption, supplements greater than 30 to 60 mg of elemental iron are unnecessary and may increase gastrointestinal discomfort in a way that discourages teens from taking the iron.[71] Compliance in taking supplements may be low in any case, so use of products providing multiple daily doses should also be discouraged.[64] When a pregnant teenager is found to be anemic or iron deficient, 50 mg elemental iron in addition to the approximately 60 mg present in prenatal supplements will provide sufficient iron because of the additional absorption efficiency of anemic individuals.

Folic Acid

Because of its role in the reproduction of cells, folic acid is an important nutrient in the diet of pregnant teens. Those who do not eat liver, lean beef, or green leafy vegetables will be at greatest risk for developing a deficiency.[72] In response to the immediate nature of the requirement for folic acid, a supplement is usually suggested for high-risk patients.[1,2,17,24]

Other Vitamins and Micronutrients

Other nutrients and vitamins must be considered as significant to overall nutritional status in teenage pregnancy. Although deficiencies that cause clinically observable symptoms are rare, there are indications that modern dietary trends are away from foods that provide such micronutrients as zinc and chromium (see Chapter 4). Various studies have shown certain of the vitamins are consumed in limited amounts by teens in general. Vitamin B_{12}, for example, is nearly absent from the diets of pregnant vegans, necessitating supplementation.[1] Although the risks of inadequacies of these nutrients to the teen and her infant are generally so low that they cannot be measured, the consequences of mild to moderate deficits could be great. By this reasoning, vitamins and micronutrients are needed for an optimal state of nutrition. This concern may be translated to pregnant teens by counseling them to include a wide variety of fresh and lightly processed foods in their diets.

Fiber

Highly processed foods, which make up a large part of the diet of teens who are at greatest risk nutritionally, are notably low in fiber content. Various studies have shown the importance of dietary fiber in promoting normal gastrointestinal motility and regular bowel movements.[73] This may be of special consequence to the pregnant teenager who has difficulty avoiding constipation in the latter part of pregnancy and after delivery.[54]

Summary

The teen will need to be supported in obtaining a diet made up of a variety of nutrient-rich foods if optimal nourishment is to be achieved. These foods should be eaten in a quantity conducive to supporting weight gain at the suggested rate. Sources of protein, calcium, folic acid, and iron are of particular importance. Fresh and lightly processed foods must be eaten to contribute other vitamins, trace minerals, and fiber.

PATTERNS OF WEIGHT GAIN IN PREGNANT TEENAGERS

The suggested weight gain of pregnant women has been on the order of 11.25 to 13.5 kg (25 to 30 lb) since the late 1960s.[24] There is no evidence, however, that this amount of weight gain is optimal for adolescents. Following the patient's progress in weight gain has become standard clinical practice in many health-care facilities. In fact, many patients are actively counseled to gain at the rate indicated by the curve seen in Fig. 9-3 so as to achieve a total gain in the suggested range if possible. It has been noted that some variation from this pattern is normal.[53] Data from Naeye[74] indicate gains as low as 9 kg (20 lb) and as high as 14.4 kg (32 lb) provide optimal support for pregnancy.

The total amount of weight gain during pregnancy has not usually been thought of as relating to prepregnant weight. For example, in one study of young women, mean weight gains for the "thin," "normal," and "obese" groups were nearly the same.[63] In another study of 18 pregnant teens, those weighing the least gained most, but the same correlation was not found in a larger group of 34 subjects.[64] Since these reports did not state whether the weight gains were achieved under the guidance of clinicians who were focusing attention on the gaining of weight according to the suggested rate, it is not clear whether results could be partially attributable to clinical counseling or whether the gains resulted from a natural process related to the normal course of pregnancy.

It has been suggested that women who are underweight at the time of conception should be encouraged to gain more weight than normal or overweight women.[53,74-76] This would allow for im-

Table 9-2. Approximate increments in weight of postmenarcheal women

Postmenarcheal Year	Pounds	Kilograms
1	10.12	4.6
2	6.16	2.8
3	2.42	1.1
4 and 5	1.76	0.8

Data from Frisch, R.E.: Hum. Biol. **48**:353, 1976.

provement of nutritional status—the need for which is indicated by the initial low weight-for-height proportion—and for continued nourishment during pregnancy. Another idea supporting higher than average weight gain is that the normal weight increment of the particular stage of adolescent development should be allowed in addition to the typical gestational gain.[75,77] Adding both increments to the normal recommended gain yields the suggested weight gain for the underweight adolescent female. The weight gain necessary for her to reach the "critical body mass" to support a normal pregnancy might be calculated as follows:

_____ To bring weight to normal for height
_____ For the 9-month postmenarcheal interval corresponding to gynecological age (Table 9-2)
_____ For the pregnancy
_____ Total

Although the importance of adequate weight gain has been well documented over a number of years, there is evidence that both the general public and clinics and practitioners still are not sufficiently aware of the implications.[78] Clinicians whose training preceded the reported experiences of the past decade need to study the collected research and incorporate the suggested principles into clinical care strategies.

One might think of measuring skinfolds to assure that the weight gain of the pregnant woman is made up of the ideal components (Fig. 9-5).

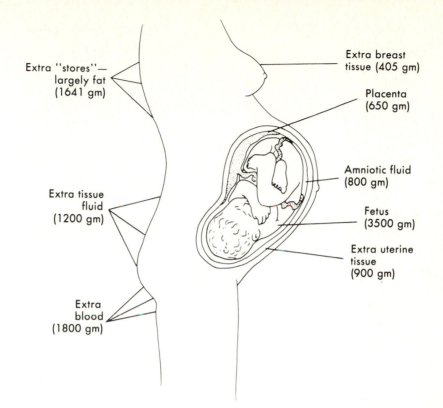

Extra "stores"—
largely fat
(1641 gm)

Extra tissue
fluid
(1200 gm)

Extra
blood
(1800 gm)

Extra breast
tissue (405 gm)

Placenta
(650 gm)

Amniotic fluid
(800 gm)

Fetus
(3500 gm)

Extra uterine
tissue
(900 gm)

Fig. 9-5. Distribution of extra maternal weight at the end of a normal 40-week pregnancy. (From Worthington-Roberts, B.S.: Contemporary developments in nutrition, 1981, St. Louis, The C.V. Mosby Co.)

(Chapter 3 discusses fatfold measurement techniques.) However, the inability to measure fat stored internally throughout the body must be taken into account when considering the accuracy of any such measurement. In addition, standards for assessment of such measurements in pregnancy are not available. The usefulness of a practical clinical procedure for monitoring fatfold changes during pregnancy, however, warrants the allocation of resources to support the research necessary for development of validated standards. One study[79] indicates the search might be fruitful. Skinfold changes during pregnancy at sites other than the triceps were, in the main, consistent with what

is known about changes in body composition. The exception was a rapid decrease in nonfat components of skinfolds close to the time of delivery and for about one week postpartum. These changes could not be accounted for.[79]

A sudden rapid weight gain in any pregnant woman is a probable sign of developing preeclampsia, which signifies the need for immediate comprehensive care. A gradual but excessive gain in weight by the pregnant teen is also of concern. Gains in weight of over 18 kg (40 lb) have been associated with significantly larger skinfolds in infants born of these pregnancies.[80] A teen who has become isolated from peers and family and turns to food for comfort or who has a cultural bias toward high maternal weights is likely to need intensive support from a clinician to keep her weight within suggested limits of gain.

Some teens will be extremely heavy at the time of conception. In a study of pregnant teens in Kentucky, 13% were classified as obese. Obese pregnant women have been found to have excessive wound infection, gestational diabetes, hypertensive disorders, and thromboembolism.[80-83] The question of appropriate weight management for obese teens has been under discussion in recent years. Evidence is now available that heavy women, including teens, produce infants of adequate size even if they gained a lower than average total amount of weight.[80,81] This follows the principle that high prepregnancy weight and high pregnancy gain are independent factors that positively influence the infant's birthweight.[84] Thus the optimal weight gain for an obese woman during pregnancy has been suggested to be from around 6.75 to 9 kg (15 to 20 lb).[74,84] The point has also been made that since there is no evidence that identifiable components of the weight gained in pregnancy per se represent dispensable deposits of fat, the gain for the obese pregnant woman should be the same as for the normal-weight woman.[85]

It seems clear that as long as the weight gain is within the range of 10.8 kg (24 lb) (plus or minus about 3.6 kg [8 lb]), the principle of meeting nutritional needs should take precedence over concerns about weight gain in the nutritional management of pregnancy in obese teens. The need for nutrients is universal, so the food intake should never be restricted to an amount that interferes with the teen consuming adequate sources of nutrients. An underlying reason for encouraging a reasonable food intake is that the young woman should avoid energy deficits severe enough to cause ketoacidosis.[85] Nor should the energy intake decrease to the point that nitrogen cannot be utilized for tissue synthesis.[64] For these reasons both obese and normal-weight young women who have gained a large amount of weight in the early months, perhaps

before coming for prenatal care, should be counseled to continue gaining weight at a very slow pace (about 0.22 kg/wk [0.5 lb/wk]) until the time of delivery. In fact, the amount of weight that an obese pregnant woman gains gradually in pregnancy will be a relatively small percentage of her total weight. Theoretically, the physiological disadvantage of this weight gain to the woman would not compare with the possible detriment of a semi-starvation regimen to the more vulnerable fetus. Nutritional guidance therefore should be devoted to helping the obese or rapid weight-gaining teen improve her food choices and control her weight gain rather than to restricting her overall intake to cause a cessation of weight gain.

In summary, it can be stated that a weight gain within the normal suggested range can generally be achieved by the pregnant adolescent with the guidance provided by a strong clinical program. The clinician can support a relatively greater gain for women who are underweight at conception and somewhat smaller gains for those who are heavy at the outset.

POSTPARTUM WEIGHT LOSS IN ADOLESCENTS

Although a great deal of work has been devoted to studying the weight gain patterns of pregnant women, the patterns of weight loss during and after delivery have not been well documented. For pregnant teens the question of return to normal weight is particularly pertinent. The knowledge that the weight gain is temporary can sometimes dispel the reluctance to accept weight gain during pregnancy. Generally, pregnant teens want to know specifically what to expect. Studies of the usual postpartum weight-loss patterns in teens would be very helpful.

In one study of adults, the weight at 6 to 8 weeks postpartum remained about 2.7 to 3.1 kg (6 to 7 lb) above the prepregnant weight.[79] In another study, 69% of Japanese women had returned to within 2 kg (4.4 lb) of their pregestational weight by 4 months postpartum.[86] It is not known in what number of these women lactation may have contributed to the loss of weight recorded.

Other factors that influence the normal process of weight loss after delivery are the teen's level of exercise and the type of birth control method she may decide to use. It is hoped that she will exercise at least as much postpartum as she did in the prepregnancy period to help adjust her weight. If she decides on oral contraceptives, she may gain 1.35 to 2.7 kg (3 to 6 lb) because of the metabolic effects of the hormones involved. Otherwise, the normal hormonal adjustments following delivery favor loss of the weight gained in pregnancy, providing it has been within normal limits.

A preliminary study of pregnant adolescents suggested that most teens can be expected to return to their prepregnant weight by about 40 weeks postpartum, and many sooner than that. However, the teens may then experience a gain in weight above their prepregnancy weight[9] (see Fig. 9-4). In fact, it is probably inappropriate for a young woman to attempt to return to a pregravida weight based on a fixed point in the past at an age where all women are gaining yearly in the process of maturation (see Table 9-2).

A final comment relates to the finding that reinitiation of the menstrual cycle can be delayed in women who are poorly nourished.[87] It thus should be of interest to note the resumption of periods in teens who showed signs of being poorly nourished before and/or during pregnancy (for example, prepregnancy underweight, low gynecological age, or late onset of menses). Coupling menstrual history with long-term weight gain and loss could become an important clinical method for identifying poorly nourished women in vulnerable groups.

COMPLICATIONS IN ADOLESCENT PREGNANCIES

Hazards to Mother

Given the complexity of pregnancy in the adolescent period and the multitude of both psycho-social and physical factors, it is logical to question how these young women fare during pregnancy. Complications often described for the mother during the gestational period[88] are listed below:

First and third trimester bleeding

Anemia

Difficult labor and delivery

Cephalopelvic disproportion

Hypertensive disorders including preeclampsia and eclampsia

Maternal mortality is also a problem, with the rate being two-and-one-half times greater for mothers under 15 years of age than for those 20 to 24 years of age from 1977 to 1978.[13] Apart from the physical sequelae, pregnancy often affects teenagers' psychological development, education, and acquisition of economic independence.[18] Clearly these developmental steps are difficult to complete in any case, and for some adolescents pregnancy is not a cause of failure but a coinciding event. Whatever situations were responsible for early pregnancy often remain unresolved, and many teenage girls have additional pregnancies before the adolescent years are over.[13,22]

Of those complications previously listed, the most common physical problem in teen pregnancies is preeclampsia. The disorder usually manifests itself in the third trimester by increased weight gain, fluid retention, high blood pressure, and proteinuria and does not appear to run a different course in pregnant teens than in older women.[53] It has been pointed out by some researchers[88] that it is a disease of first pregnancies. By and large, data support this observation. In addition, the harmful effects of preeclampsia (or more serious states of eclampsia) may be greater in teens. Damage to the cardiovascular and renal systems initiated with a first pregnancy early in life and exacerbated by insults such as other pregnancies can increase the risk of affected women demonstrating cardiovascular and renal problems with increasing age.[4] Factors that influence the well-being of the mother and implications for nutritional care are listed in Table 9-3. *Text continued on p. 240.*

Table 9-3. Review of factors affecting well-being of adolescent pregnant women and their infants

Factor	Effect	Mode of Effect	Implications for Nutritional Care
Impact on Adolescent Pregnant Women			
Economics	Economic situation is cited as single most important factor in determining outcome.[24]	Economics determine both type and amount of medical care and health of self and ancestors.	Mobilizing food resources is of highest priority.
Prenatal care	Quantity and quality of prenatal care are universally mentioned as affecting outcome[89-90]; advantages of care are evident when health complications in populations without care[91-97] are compared to those with care.[98-101]	There is debate as to whether incidence of preeclampsia can be decreased to that of adult populations[15,23,98,102]; otherwise, comprehensive care appears to reduce incidence of physical complications to that of adult populations.[23,98-100]	Care for adolescents should be comprehensive, including services of nutritionists and professionals in the psychosocial fields; teachers and others should encourage early prenatal care.
Age	Although difficult to study as sole uncontrolled variable,[6,88] it is generally acknowledged that, with possible exception of eclampsia and preeclampsia, adolescents are not at greater physical risk for complications than older mothers; psychosocial and economic factors, however, are more likely to have an impact.[15,23,58,90]	Hypothetically, physical effect may be greatest in women of low gynecological age[6,88,102,103]; studies assessing impact of low gynecological age have not looked at impact on physical complications to the mother,[102,103] but it was not predictive of development of preeclampsia in one study.[102]	Younger adolescents need greatest attention, as they are usually without traditional supports; those of low gynecological age are possibly at greatest biological risk.
Malnutrition	Although still debated, cause-and-effect relationship is still possible.[106-115]	Severe anemia is associated with high morbidity and mortality[105]; the following nutrients have been implicated in the disease process but not conclusively shown to cause toxemia: Calcium, iron, vitamin A (because they are consistently low in diets of young women)[69,107] Thiamin[108]	Effective techniques to encourage the consumption of nutrient-rich foods should be major component of prenatal counseling for adolescents.

Vitamin B$_6$[110]
Folic acid[11,116]
Excess dietary sodium[112,113]
Greater consumption of total fats and cholesterol[114]
Generalized malnutrition[62]
When mother is malnourished, fetus draws on mother's depleted stores, resulting in decreased energy and ability to support reproduction.

Impact on Infants

Maternal stress	Maternal stress is high in teen pregnancy[18,23,58,117]; there is no direct evidence this causes increased problems for the fetus, but outcomes are more favorable when teens have support of others.[18,23]	Stress may interfere with maintenance of satisfactory nutritional status[118] and intrauterine environment.[27-28]	Stress in pregnant teen's life must be considered in providing nutritional counseling; nutritionists and other clinicians must support pregnant teenage patients in stressful situations.
Maternal infections	The following are common infections concurrent with pregnancy: Viral infections—influenza, herpes, upper respiratory infections; Protozoan infections—toxoplasmosis; Sexually transmitted diseases—gonorrhea, syphilis, chlamydial infections. Depending on agent, effects on fetus range from no damage to mild complications (for example, increased susceptibility to disease) to severe damage (for example, prematurity, congenital anomalies, abortion, stillbirth).[116,119-121]	In addition to direct effect of agent, increased requirement for nutrients may create inadequacy for fetus.	Adolescents with infections during pregnancy are among priority patients for nutritional care; the goal is adequate nourishment to restore health and to meet requirements of pregnancy.

Continued.

Table 9-3. Review of factors affecting well-being of adolescent pregnant women and their infants—cont'd

Factor	Effect	Mode of Effect	Implications for Nutritional Care
Impact on Infants—cont'd			
Maternal malnutrition	Knowledge of role of specific nutritional deficiencies or excesses on development of problems in infant in human populations of developed countries is limited, although subjective evaluations suggest positive outcomes associated with well-nourished state. [54,122,123]	Correlation is known to exist between maternal hemoglobin level and infant birth weight[105]; it is suspected that anemia in mother augments maternal cardiac output to assure sufficient amount of inferior-quality blood is pumped to placenta to provide for fetus; with marginal malnutrition, both mother and infant will have less strength to establish bonding and feeding patterns[124]; severe malnutrition retards cellular growth[53,125-128]; nutritional supplementation of severely malnourished pregnant women reduces incidence of low birth weight but not necessarily anomalies[129]; supplementation in teen population did not significantly decrease incidence of low birth weight but significantly increased mean birth weight.[130]	Since nutrition and feeding can be controlled to assure a healthy fetal and infant environment, nutrition services are an important component of prenatal programs for adolescents; preparation for and follow-up of child-feeding practices by teen parents should be included.
Weight gain of mother	Prepregnant weight and weight gain are more important than either gynecological or chronological age in determining frequency of low–birth weight infants born to adolescents. [63,77,131]	Weight and height are clinically measurable evidence of nutritional status in societies with high standard of living where specific nutritional deficiencies are rare; evidence linking weight gain to infant birth weight is readily available[84,132,133]; inadequate weight gain is associated with increased incidence of low–birth weight infants and subsequent in-	Nutritional counseling for pregnant teens should place emphasis on adequate weight gain, especially for underweight patients.

Maternal age	Biological immaturity was initially suspected cause[17,92,102] of higher fetal complications and loss found in adolescent pregnancies[17,77,91,98,135-137], when psychological stress, economics, and other variables are controlled, age not shown responsible[58,97,124,138]; possible exceptions are rare teens who are pregnant at low gynecological age who have high frequency of low–birth weight infants[15,17,97,102,135], two studies of this were inconclusive, as gynecological age was not sole uncontrolled variable (for example, nutritional status was not controlled)[102,103]; effects of young age were not overcome by improved services in years between 1978 and 1981.[13,135]	
	crease in neonatal morbidity and mortality[102]; weight gain may have intergenerational effect (women small at birth are more likely to have small infants than women average or large at birth).[134] It has been suggested that structurally and functionally immature uterus has less than optimal vascular system and may react unfavorably to ovarian hormones[102]; possible biochemical evidence of nutritional risks is the competition for nutrients between immature gravida and fetus indicated by 2+ acetonuria found in 5% at age 10-14, 2% age 17-32 (fetal and neonatal death is 56% more frequent with 2+ acetonuria)[77]; psychological characteristics of ''premature parents'' such as unreasonable expectations for children and their parental abilities mediate unfavorable outcomes (for example, teen parents thought children would talk and be toilet trained by 6 months)[18,139,140]; failure to meet expectations contributes to infant morbidity and mortality.[18,139,140]	Gynecological age of adolescent patients may be predictor of biological risk to infants; support for developing realistic expectations and parenting skills in younger teens affects both psychological and biological consequences for the infant and must be built into prenatal and postnatal care protocols.
Prenatal care	Specialized comprehensive prenatal care is an important factor in decreasing adverse biological effects of teen pregnancy on the newborn*; nutrition services are integral part of such care.[4,90,91,142,144]	
	Comprehensive adolescent prenatal program reports 9% of infants versus 20.9% of those born to adolescents in general prenatal program weighed less than 2500 gm (5.5 lb).[90]	Pregnant teens should be high priority among vulnerable population groups when nutrition services are scarce.

*References 23, 58, 88, 99, 100, 141-143.

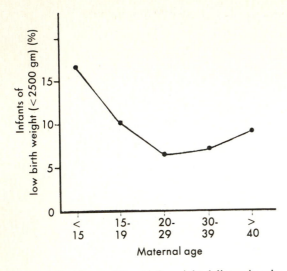

Fig. 9-6. Incidence of low birth weight delivery in relation to maternal age. (From Vital statistics of the United States, Public Health Service, National Center for Health Statistics, 1978.)

Hazards to Infant

Infants born to teenage mothers suffer a higher incidence of morbidity and mortality in the perinatal period than infants of older mothers. Problems seen in greater frequency in these infants are the following[4,88]:

Prematurity

Stillbirth

Low birth weight (appears to be the major hazard in adolescent pregnancy)

Perinatal and infant deaths

Physical deformities

Although it is difficult to compare the likelihood of these problems occurring in infants born to teens versus older women or to younger versus older teens, it is generally agreed that the problems occur in a considerable number of teen pregnancies. For example, the incidence of low birth weight is far greater when mothers are adolescents as seen in Fig. 9-6. Factors that increase risk to infants are summarized in Table 9-3.

ASSESSMENT AND MANAGEMENT OF NUTRITION FOR PREGNANT ADOLESCENTS

Assessment

In order that nutrition services can be provided efficiently and effectively, pregnant teenage patients should be screened for those physical risk factors most closely linked to poor outcomes. At this point, significant risk factors appear to be the following:

Low gynecological age

Low prepregnancy weight-for-height (or other significant evidence of malnutrition)

Low pregnancy weight gain

Infections during pregnancy

Excessive prepregnancy weight-for-height

Excessive pregnancy weight gain

Other risk factors gathered by history include the following:

Unhealthy life-style

Unfavorable reproductive history

Chronic diseases

Assessment of the pregnant teen follows more or less the general pattern for assessment of all pregnant women.[24,59,60,145] An assessment protocol is presented in the box on p. 241 as part of a plan for overall management of the pregnant teenager.

Strategies to Improve Nutrition for Teenage Pregnant Woman

The complex mix of social, emotional, and physical factors accompanying teenage pregnancy make it one of the most challenging situations in which nutritional counseling takes place. Issues that must be assessed and then addressed according to priorities demanded by the individual situation are summarized in the box on pp. 246-247. Above all, nutritional care of the pregnant teen cannot be isolated from its context. It must be coordinated with other members of the clinical team, as the same broad range of issues affects the work of all disciplines.

Protocol for Management of Normal Teenage Pregnancy

Initial Evaluation

Review intake material.
Review clinical data.
  Height and weight
  Arm muscle circumference
  Physical signs of health
  Expected delivery date
Review laboratory data.
  Hematocrit or hemoglobin
  Urinalysis
Begin to build relationship with the patient (and partner if available).
Assess intake patterns using dietary methodology best suited to patient and professional.
Make preliminary assessment of food resources and refer to supportive agencies if necessary.
Check for nausea and vomiting and suggest remedy.
Assess attitude toward weight gain.
Discuss supplemental vitamins and minerals.
Make initial plan that sets priorities for issues.
Come to agreement with patient about any initial changes and steps to take.

Follow-up Visit

Check on referrals to other agencies.
Discuss results of evaluation and suggest any changes necessary in dietary patterns (use printed materials *as appropriate*).
Do any further investigations necessary.
  Laboratory studies
    Protoporphyrin heme or serum ferritin ⎫
    Serum folate   ⎬ For specific diagnosis of anemia
    Serum albumin   ⎫
    Serum transferrin   ⎬ For suspected undernutrition
    Vitamin B_{12} For vegan
  Further probing of dietary habits if necessary
Use motivating audiovisuals.
Monitor weight gain and attitude of acceptance starting with patient's prepregnant weight status; discuss projected weight gain for following visit and total for gestation.
Assess and address issues (box on pp. 246-247) affecting nutritional status in order of priority for the individual.

Subsequent Visits

Monitor and support appropriate weight gain; include discussion of fitness and encourage habitual safe exercise.
Support upgrade in nutritional pattern in support of the woman and the developing infant; augment knowledge of principles of nutrition; continue to address issues affecting nutritional status.
Check for heartburn, small food-intake capacity, and elimination problems; suggest dietary interventions.

Final Visits

Discuss infant feeding if patient will keep infant.
Help patient to understand safe methods of managing weight following delivery.

When the partner of the young pregnant woman is available, he should be included in counseling sessions to build mutual nutritional support for the pregnancy. Specific outreach to the father can be beneficial. If he is employed or in school, an effort should be made to see him at least occasionally. This will be especially important if for some reason he is interfering with the young woman's ability to nourish herself. Sharing what is known about the father's contribution to the outcome of pregnancy helps some adolescent males become more interested in maintaining healthy living habits. (Where the term *pregnant teen* is used in this section, it should be kept in mind that both the young women and their partners will be included in counseling.)

To be effective, the clinician must work within the context of an individualized counseling relationship. The counselor will not "prescribe" but make suggestions and support the changing of teens' habits, usually in small increments, throughout the pregnancy.

The benefits of nutritional counseling will generally be seen in the long term rather than in a particular pregnancy. Prenatal care is one of the best opportunities to reach a vulnerable group of teens with nutrition information. Even if they seek care late in pregnancy and miss appointments, the contacts that are made will constitute the greatest input of health care during the adolescent period for most of these teens.

Helping pregnant adolescents to follow the suggested weight-gain curve can demonstrate dramatically in a few months the possibility of exerting control over eating and how that can affect weight status. There is great appeal in discussing the effects of various events on their bodies and on the growing fetus. Learning about the physiological needs of herself and the developing infant can be the impetus for upgrading the quality of the teen's diet to keep pace with the increase in energy intake needed to support adequate weight gain. Repeated counseling sessions to review those needs

may motivate a young woman to try new foods to obtain additional sources of nutrients. Attention to nutritional health in the prenatal period can become a model for taking responsibility for feeding a family. The young woman can gain experience in use of community resources to obtain food for herself and her family. To review, nutritional counseling in teenage prenatal care can accomplish the following:

1. Serve as a model for exerting control over what a person eats with visible results in terms of the weight-gain pattern and the quality of foods contributing to it.
2. Be an impetus for trying new foods.
3. Serve as a model for taking responsibility and using resources to feed a family.

Specific Counseling Issues

The problems pregnant teens face will change from month to month as they react to the physical changes and psychological aspects of pregnancy. These changes can affect the dietary intake. Some prominent issues that generally are important throughout the prenatal counseling period can be delineated.

Basic Nutrition Guidelines. Pregnant teens are at high risk of being individuals who do not care for themselves or attempt to control their physical environment. Imaginative individualized approaches will be necessary in planning nutritional care to meet their needs.

Once it has been established that the teen has access to adequate food, the goal will be to ensure that it is as high in quality as possible. If the young woman is not obtaining sufficient food energy to maintain a satisfactory rate of weight gain or if nutrient-rich foods are missing, plans for obtaining those foods will be the focus of counseling sessions. Talking with her about foods she likes and is familiar with is the starting point. Efforts should be made to find some source of all-important nutrients that the teen will eat regularly. When sources of certain nutrients are missing from the foods she normally eats, the attempt will be to find some source of those nutrients that she is willing to "add." When these goals are set realistically, there is a good probability of meeting them. Successfully adding a few new foods on a regular basis is much better than trying to get the girl to "meet the RDA" in all nutrients or to eat a certain number of servings of each type of food daily. Failure usually results if the goal is not based on the reality of the girl's actual food habits.

Because teenage eating habits often do not follow a traditional meal pattern, the clinician should be ready to suggest valuable foods that pregnant teens can choose in many places and at any time. Although establishing a more regular meal pattern may sound like a valuable goal, often it is not successful. As the counselor becomes more familiar with the patient's habits over time, suggestions can be more specific as to foods for particular times of day and for particular occasions.

A positive approach is more effective than a negative one that would put the clinician in the role of a disciplinarian and the teen in a position to rebel. This does not preclude labeling certain foods as ones that "don't give you what you need" or that "make you gain weight without giving you and your baby anything." For specialists in nutrition, counseling techniques can be quite detailed and related to specific nutrients. For clinicians whose time is limited to covering only the basics, primary points are the following:

Support for obtaining resources

Guidance in taking in food energy to permit appropriate weight gain

Counseling the inclusion of nutrient-rich foods

Dealing with issues that interfere with nourishment

Within the general population of pregnant teenagers, there will be certain ones who will be taking large amounts of supplemental nutrients. A family member, partner, or other acquaintance may have told them these supplements are necessary to have a healthy pregnancy, or they may have been taking them because they feel it will help them improve their performance in sports or keep them from feeling tired and run-down.

Counseling should follow the rule of assessing cultural dietary patterns, and the most harmful practices should be addressed first. The greatest harm would no doubt come from very high doses of the fat-soluble vitamins.[54] Thereafter, one would be concerned about high doses of the water-soluble vitamins, minerals, and micronutrients.[146] Evidence has long been available indicating that infants born to women taking large amounts of vitamin C may develop scurvy in the neonatal period.[147] If pregnant women insist on taking supplements, they should be counseled to modify the intake to a dosage no greater than two times the RDA.

One line of reasoning that can be used in a discussion of oversupplementation is that research cannot be done in humans to determine the effects of various levels of nutrients on the developing infant. Taking anything by mouth other than food or prescribed prenatal supplement is risky. This message can be coupled with educational campaigns devoted to avoidance of alcohol and drugs during pregnancy. These campaigns, unlike those related to smoking, appear to be quite widely accepted among pregnant teens.

Food Resources. It is of primary importance to realize that pregnant teens will often lack a stable food supply. This is caused in part by their tenuous status in separating themselves from their families and establishing residences together with partners. In any of a variety of living situations, the amount of money they can spend on food may be small. For example, there may be a high degree of disorganization in the living group, or the pregnant teen may be in competition for food with other members of the household. This is the reality on which all messages about food intake must be based.

The source, type, and amount of food available must be assessed, and suggestions then should be made for mobilization of all possible resources. Helping teens to successfully stretch limited funds, obtain supplemental foods, find foods they can keep in a room without refrigeration, and choose wisely when buying ready-prepared foods at a grocery or fast-food franchise become the standard focuses of the clinician serving this population. The total food knowledge and planning skill of the pregnant teen will generally need to be augmented.

Programs for pregnant women that supply food along with nutritional counseling[123,148] are especially effective resources for teens because they provide support in two most needed areas: (1) supplementation of resources and (2) guidance in the use of such resources. The design is appropriate to the cognitive development of the most vulnerable of teens, with abstract nutritional principles being reinforced in a concrete sense. The Supplemental Food Program for Women, Infants, and Children (WIC) is a valuable program of this type and serves adolescents and other high-risk groups.[148] As such, it channels resources in an effective manner to improve maternal and child health.

Weight Adjustment. The acceptance and management of a gradual weight increase that is not rapid or excessive is a major focus of much of the nutritional counseling of the pregnant teen. Although the need for this weight gain to be based on a nourishing dietary intake is an obvious goal, it will need to be articulated frequently. The teen should be asked how she feels about the ultimate weight gain in initial visits, and messages directed toward the cognitive and attitudinal aspects of weight gain should begin. Questions about ideal body type, fashions, and perception of peers and self yield information about personal body image. Cognitively, teens should be taught the components of the weight gain (see Fig. 9-5) and the role of weight gain in the development of the infant and for her own health in support of the pregnancy. Efforts will need to be directed toward assuring that pregnant teens can both emotionally accept a reasonable weight gain and intellectually under-

stand the process. Work toward changing their attitudes will often be necessary.

Effort should be made to counsel the pregnant teen who has given up active physical pursuits in exchange for a sedentary life-style. This change is a detriment (1) because a decreased energy output coupled with a increased need for nutrients can cause an excess weight gain and (2) because of the damage to the young woman's self-esteem and overall sense of well-being when she is not actively using her body. The nutritional counselor will want to provide information about reasonable fitness and conditioning, coordinating these suggestions with the exercises preparing her for labor and delivery. Although it has not been the nutritionist's traditional role to deal with physical fitness, it can be a very productive approach to discussing an overall healthful life-style that includes balancing nourishment with activity.

In certain ethnic groups there will be a tendency toward excessive gains that is supported by a cultural value attached to a full figure.[149] However, in the mainstream of American teen culture the value on slimness is pervasive. At the same time, body-image development is in a dynamic state. This will add to the adolescent's difficulty in accepting the recommended weight gain. "Talking through" the course of pregnancy can help to desensitize pregnant teens to the shock they feel as the scales climb. The ultimate weight goal can be discussed, and short-term goals can be set forth for the period of time between visits. Positive messages about the effects of appropriate gains on the pregnancy help teenagers to accept the gradual gains as the weeks go by. Because teens are very concerned about their own bodies, it should be repeated that the weight reflected on the scales is, for the most part, the weight being gained by the baby and the supporting tissue. The weight is not fat on her body as it would be if she were not pregnant. It is generally lost in a natural manner after delivery. Some teens will be interested in the physiological changes, including changes in hormone levels, that lead to postpartum weight loss.[150] Similarly, discussing the difficulty of losing excess weight can help the teen who is gaining more than she needs to bring her weight under better control.

In the postpartum period counseling revolves around the need to lose weight at a moderate rate. Teens should be encouraged to maintain a nourishing intake to replenish the losses of pregnancy and not to lose precipitously as result of a restricted intake. This is especially true in the situation where the girl may be breast-feeding and will need to be well nourished to support lactation.

Responsibility. Pregnant teens must take on responsibility (often for the first time) for their own nourishment and for that of others. Helping patients to understand and carry out this responsibility will be one of the main objectives of nutritional counseling.

Social, Emotional, and Economic Stress. Underlying all discussions with pregnant teens is the need to ascertain the degree of stress that they are under as a result of this tumultuous time in their lives. This stress must be taken into consideration in counseling them. Of prime importance is the decision they have to make to keep or relinquish their infant. Although the decision to give up a child is rare,[151] it may be considered when a supportive acquaintance or professional brings it up. The decision will determine whether messages about nutrition are directed toward a mother (or couple) bearing a child who will remain a part of her family or toward a woman who will only carry a child through its gestation. Because most teens are ambivalent about such a decision, it is important to word messages so they will not be judgmental of the apparent decision once it has been made. In some situations it will be important to leave the door open for change of mind. It is necessary to maintain communication with other members of the health-care team so as not to undermine their counseling efforts in this regard. Apart from the issue of relinquishment, many of the factors that potentially affect the nourishment of the teenager

and her unborn child are given in the box on pp. 246 and 247. These issues must be assessed and addressed in intervention strategies. The clinician will need to be sensitive to these issues in counseling the teen to achieve adequate nourishment.

Preparation for Infant Feeding. During the third trimester, pregnant teens need to gain an awareness of the responsibility for feeding the infant. They will often need to be taught the principles of infant feeding[152] and the skills necessary to adequately nourish their children. Bottle feeding versus breast feeding needs to be addressed in a manner appropriate for the level of maturity of the teen. Because of the psychological needs of the developing adolescent female herself, it is questionable as to whether she will be able to successfully maintain breast feeding.[117] Some clinicians consider it unwise to encourage most teens to nurse their infants. However, a number of young women will say they want to breast-feed and will need to be prepared. There are significant benefits even if they breast-feed only through the immediate postnatal period.[4]

Other aspects of infant feeding must also be addressed in the time available. Introduction of solid foods should receive some attention since overfeeding as a response to anxiety about parenting may adversely affect the infant. Consideration of issues related to safety and sanitation could also serve to protect the newborn later on. An effort should be made to strengthen the support family members and friends can lend to the management of feeding. A recent study of teenage parents suggests that postpartum services for them should contain very practical components geared toward helping them obtain housing, child care, employment, and food and not toward more theoretically based "counseling."[153]

Nausea, Heartburn, and Constipation. Nausea and vomiting, probably related to hormonal changes and a more acute sense of smell, can be quite disturbing to teens in the early weeks and up to the end of the first trimester of pregnancy.[26]

Issues in Adolescent Pregnancy that Influence Nutritional Well-Being

Acceptance of the Pregnancy

Desire to carry out successful pregnancy
Acceptance of responsibility (even if child is to be relinquished)
Clarification of identity as mother separate from her own mother
Realistic acceptance versus fantasy and idealization

Food Resources

Family meals (timing, quantity, quality, responsibility)
Self-reliance
School lunch
Fast-food outlets
Socially related eating
Food assistance (WIC program and others)
Mobilization of all resources

Body Image

Degree of acceptance of an adult body
Maturity in facing bodily changes throughout pregnancy

Living Situation

Acceptance by living partners and extended family
Role expectations of living partners
Financial support
Facilities and resources
Ethnic group (religious, cultural, and social patterns)
Emancipation versus dependency
Support system versus isolation

Relationship with the Father of Child

Presence or absence of father
Quality of relationship
Influence on decision making
Contribution to resources
Influence on mother's nutritional habits and general life-style
Understanding of physiological processes
Tolerance of physical changes in pregnancy and physical needs of mother and child
Influence on child feeding

Peer Relationships

Support from friends
Influence on nutritional knowledge and attitudes
Influence on general life-style

Nutritional State

Weight-for-height proportion
Maturational state
Tissue stores of nutrients
Reproductive and contraceptive history
Physical health
History of dietary patterns and nutritional status, including weight-losing schemes
Present eating habits
Complications of pregnancy (nausea and vomiting)
Substance use
Activity patterns
Need for intensive remediation

Prenatal Care

Initiation of and compliance with prenatal care
Dependability of supporting resources
Identification of risk factors

Nutritional Attitude and Knowledge

Prior attitude toward nutrition
Understanding of role of nutrition in pregnancy
Knowledge of foods as sources of nutrients and of nutrients needed by the body
Desire to obtain adequate nutrition
Ability to obtain adequate nutrition and to control food supply

Preparation for Child Feeding

Knowledge of child-feeding practices
Attitude and decisions about child feeding
Responsibility for feeding
Understanding the importance of the bonding process
Support from family and friends

Guidelines for alleviation of the symptoms include (1) eating small, frequent meals of dry foods, starting with a dry snack before getting up, (2) confining liquids to between meals, and (3) avoiding fatty foods and strong flavors or odors of any kind.[26,54] Medications probably do not help and can be harmful if not carefully tested and monitored.[26] If vomiting persists for either physical or psychological reasons, care should be taken to assure that the patient is continuously nourished and hydrated.

Heartburn and constipation, on the other hand, are discomforts of late pregnancy when the abdomen is filled by the enlarged uterus and growing fetus. Pressure on the stomach can cause a reflux of acidic material into the esophagus that results in a burning sensation near the heart (heartburn). Eating smaller and more frequent meals, elevating the head, and keeping clothing loose can decrease distress.[26] Pressure in the lower abdomen combined with lowered transit time contributes to constipation. Regular consumption of fiber-rich foods and large amounts of fluids can improve gastrointestinal function.[4,26,54] Greater physical activity should also aid the patient in dealing with this problem.[12] Approved stool softeners may be used in an effort to prevent constipation and to reduce risk of hemorrhoid discomfort.[63]

Substance Abuse. It is imperative that clinicians carefully investigate drug use by their patients and educate them about the potential danger of taking any drug without the advice of the attending obstetrician. It is often expedient for the clinician assessing nutritional status to study substance abuse habits with the patient's food habits. Several prenatal visits afford an opportunity to raise the teen's level of consciousness about the potential harm of drugs during future events (that is, breast feeding or future pregnancies). Use of narcotics, alcohol, and over-the-counter drugs should be completely discouraged. Patients should be counseled to moderate their use of alcohol and nicotine if they cannot be persuaded to avoid them completely. Be-

cause of the possible withdrawal symptoms,[154] teens should be advised to diminish gradually their use of caffeine. Fig. 9-7 provides a list of caffeine-containing substances. If a woman is planning to breast-feed, her pregnancy should be a period of retraining to avoid a cycle of hyperirritability between the mother and newborn infant caused by caffeine. Even if the teen is not planning to breast-feed, this retraining is especially important if the teen is one of those individuals who is more prone to irritability after using caffeine.[34] The bonding process between teens and their infants is a delicate matter and should not be hindered by factors that can be controlled such as overuse of caffeine.

Dietary Misinformation. The possibility that the pregnant teen is following some harmful practice is great enough that the clinician will need to probe the beliefs an individual holds and attempt to dispel those that are potential threats to her health. It is always difficult to counteract messages heard "on the street." Placing stress on the special situation of pregnancy is a strategy that may have sufficient appeal to teens to compete successfully with the influence of their own subculture.

Although the use of vegan diets is not as common as in the 1960s, this is one diet that is potentially harmful if the young woman has gained the wrong information. The person who is following a vegan pattern will need a clear understanding of protein complementation to support pregnancy and to feed a family.[155] In any situation where misinformation persists, helping the teen to understand the principles of nutrition by explaining the terms at their own intellectual level will be more effective than authoritarian stances in enabling the teen to change.

The Postpregnancy Period. During the final weeks of pregnancy or the postpartum period, teenage parents should be counseled about caring for themselves in the future months or years of their adolescence. Information can be provided about a number of issues, including educational opportunities, employment, housing, financial as-

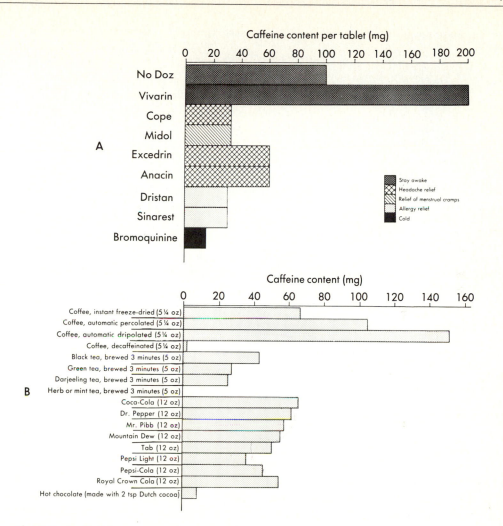

Fig. 9-7. A, Caffeine content of common over-the-counter medications. **B,** Caffeine content of common beverages. (From Worthington-Roberts, B.S.: JOGN Nurs. **12:**21, 1983.)

sistance, counseling services, legal assistance, and health maintenance. Maintenance of health involves attention to nutrition, and relevant concerns in this area should be addressed if teenage parents sever their contact with the team or individuals providing for their prenatal needs. If possible, teens should continue to receive specialized care following delivery. Clinically, it can be observed

that they are often more open to nutritional counseling once they experience the responsibility of nourishing their child full time. As seen in Fig. 9-8, they may be isolated and welcome contact with clinicians who anticipate and facilitate management of problems that are perhaps more detrimental to the ultimate welfare of their children than those of the prenatal period.[124]

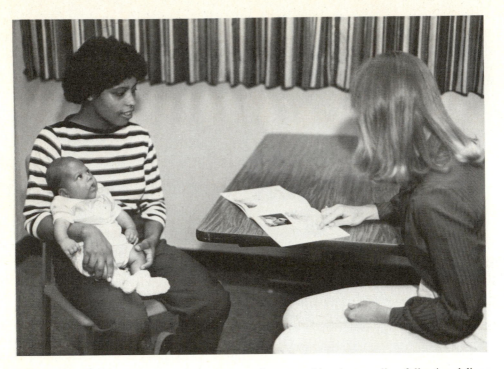

Fig. 9-8. Adolescent mothers may be more receptive to nutritional counseling following delivery than during the prenatal period.

The goal nutritionally should be to motivate teens to continue to upgrade their dietary practices so that optimal health can be established and maintained. Because another pregnancy may be anticipated for many young girls, arriving at a state of nutritional well-being might reduce risk of poor pregnancy outcome in the future. Guidance related to sensible weight reduction and rational approaches to augmenting body weight for the underweight girl should be provided. Correction of iron deficiency can be addressed as can other specific nutritional problems that may exist in a minority of teens after delivery. Community-based nutrition programs should consider these young women as high-priority patients for their services.[11]

A substantial number of adolescents may choose oral contraception.[13] Today's oral agents contain substantially lower levels of synthetic estrogens and progestogens than the original products of the 1960s, but side effects are still anticipated in a majority of users. Most side effects are merely annoying (for example, mild to moderate weight gain of 1.35 to 2.7 kg [3 to 6 lb], fluid retention, nausea, vomiting, emotional changes, facial pigmentation, slight loss of hair, and headaches). Evidence of folic acid and/or vitamin B_6 deficiency may also be found in some women. Individuals appear to differ in their physiological response to oral contraceptive agents. Adolescent girls should be informed about the potential side effects but advised that the problems are significant in only a minority of users. Information about food sources of folic acid and vitamin B_6 should be provided, and all girls should be encouraged to stop the pill at least 3 months before a planned pregnancy.

Guidance in infant feeding can be built on realistic responses to the developing child and therefore can be more meaningful than the theoretical discussions of the prenatal period. Continuing help in coordinating resources demonstrates the sincere interest of the nutritionist in the adolescent family. Teenage women or families who are not seen after delivery for child care and guidance in the same clinic as for prenatal care should be encouraged to establish an ongoing relationship with a clinical program of their choice for their own health and well-child care for their infants.

Counseling Techniques

A great deal of teens' attention is focused on themselves. Therefore an effective means of getting messages across to them is to tie the messages to their feelings about themselves. If counseling can be built around what will keep them "looking good" during their pregnancy, it has a good chance of being accepted. In addition, since most pregnant adolescents voluntarily elect to carry their pregnancies to term most verbalize a commitment to the unborn infant. Showing these girls how their own behaviors can affect the child thus can be effective.

Specific counseling techniques are listed below:
Use the team approach
Develop a one-to-one relationship
Address immediate needs
Include the significant other
Reinforce with auxiliary materials
Explore ethnic specificity
Use hands-on experience
   Role playing
   Demonstration and experience
   Sharing a meal
Provide supplemental food
Outreach to fathers
Make home visits

Many of these techniques are explored more completely in a section of Chapter 10. The use of nutrition education techniques (including print and audiovisual materials) in relation to pregnancy has been reviewed and discussed elsewhere.[156]

SUMMARY

The state of physical and psychological development affects and is affected by pregnancy in the adolescent years. Although questions remain about continued growth, nutritional needs, and the extent of biological immaturity as a risk factor, it is certain that the psychosocial and economic risks to the pregnant woman are great at this time. The nutritional needs of the teen can best be met by a weight gain close to that recommended that results from a consumption of foods with a high concentration and balance of nutrients. The recommended weight gain will be modified by the maturational stage and the prepregnant height-for-weight proportion.

As an integral part of health-care programs for pregnant teens, the nutritional consultant must be skillful in developing a relationship within which to counsel patients in the nutritional aspects of reproduction. To be effective the clinician must be flexible and employ innovative approaches. Counseling will need to extend to the postpartum period to have a real effect on the future of the parents and child.

REFERENCES

1. King, J.C., and Jacobson, H.N.: Nutrition and pregnancy in adolescence. In Zachler, J., and Brandstadt, W., editors: The teenage pregnant girl, Springfield, Ill., 1975, Charles C Thomas, Publisher.
2. Food and Nutrition Board, National Academy of Sciences–National Research Council: Recommended dietary allowances, ed. 9, Washington, D.C., 1980.
3. McGanity, W.J.: Nutrition in the adolescent. In Moghisse, K.S., and Evans, T.N., editors: Nutritional impacts on women throughout life with emphasis on reproduction, New York, 1977, Harper & Row, Publishers, Inc.
4. Worthington-Roberts, B.S.: Nutritional needs of the pregnant adolescent. In Worthington-Roberts, B.S.,

Vermeersch, J., and Williams, S.R., editors: Nutrition in pregnancy and lactation, ed. 2, St. Louis, 1981, The C.V. Mosby Co.

5. Marino, D.D., and King, J.C.: Nutrition concerns during adolescence, Pediatr. Clin. North Am. **27:**25, 1980.

6. Thompson, A.M.: Pregnancy in adolescence. In McKigney, J.I., and Munro, H.N., editors: Nutrient requirements in adolescence, Cambridge, Mass., 1976, The MIT Press.

7. Roche, A.F., and Davila, G.H.: Late adolescent growth in stature, Pediatrics **50:**874, 1972.

8. Fried, R.I., and Smith, E.: Postmenarcheal growth patterns, J. Pediatr. **61:**562, 1962.

9. Meserole, L.P., and others: Prenatal weight gain and postpartum weight loss patterns in adolescents, J. Adolesc. Health Care, Sept. 1983.

10. Tanner, J.M.: Fetus into man: physical growth from conception, Cambridge, Mass., 1978, Harvard University Press.

11. Wishik, S.M.: The implications of undernutrition during pubescence and adolescence on fertility. In Moghissi, R.S., and Evans, T.N., editors: Nutritional impacts on women throughout life with emphasis on reproduction, New York, 1977, Harper & Row, Publishers, Inc.

12. Hollingsworth, D.R.: The pregnant adolescent. In Kreutner, A.K., and Hollingsworth, D.R., editors: Adolescent obstetrics and gynecology, Chicago, 1978, Year Book Medical Publishers, Inc.

13. Teenage pregnancy: the problem that hasn't gone away, New York, 1981, The Alan Guttmacher Institute.

14. Kreutner, A.K.: Contraception. In Kreutner, A.K., and Hollingsworth, D.R., editors: Adolescent obstetrics and gynecology, Chicago, 1978, Year Book Medical Publishers, Inc.

15. Committee on Adolescence, American Academy of Pediatrics: Statement on teenage pregnancy, Pediatrics **63:**795, 1979.

16. U.S. Department of Health, Education, and Welfare: Teenage childbearing and abortion patterns, United States, 1977, Morbid. Mortal. Week. Rep. **29:**157, 1980.

17. Committee on Maternal Nutrition, Food and Nutrition Board, National Academy of Sciences–National Research Council: Maternal nutrition and the course of pregnancy, Washington, D.C., 1970, U.S. Government Printing Office.

18. Mercer, R.T.: When parents are premature. In Mercer, R.T., editor: Nursing care for parents at risk, Thorofare, N.J., 1977, Slack, Inc.

19. Youngs, D.D., and Niebyl, J.R.: Adolescent pregnancy and abortion, Med. Clin. North Am. **59:**1419, 1975.

20. Coddington, R.D.: Life events associated with adolescent pregnancies, J. Clin. Psychiatry **40:**180, 1979.

21. Curtis, F.L.: Observations of unwed pregnant adolescents, Am. J. Nurs. **74:**100, 1974.

22. Feinfeld, L.E., and Speller, M.L.: Children bearing children: adolescent pregnancy, Penn. Med., p. 16, July 1980.

23. Klerman, L.V.: Adolescent pregnancy: a new look at a continuing problem, Am. J. Public Health **70:**776, 1980.

24. Hollingsworth, D.R.: Prenatal care of the adolescent. In Kreutner, A.K., and Hollingsworth, D.R., editors: Adolescent obstetrics and gynecology, Chicago, 1978, Year Book Medical Publishers, Inc.

25. Yetley, E.A., and Roderuck, C.: Nutritional knowledge and health goals of young spouses, J. Am. Diet. Assoc. **77:**31, 1980.

26. Hollingsworth, D.R.: Common medical problems associated with adolescent pregnancy. In Kreutner, A.K., and Hollingsworth, D.R., editors: Adolescent obstetrics and gynecology, Chicago, 1978, Year Book Medical Publishers, Inc.

27. Myers, R.E.: Maternal psychological stress and fetal asphyxia: a study in the monkey, Am. J. Obstet. Gynecol. **122:**47, 1975.

28. Rosenfeld, C.R., and West, J.: Circulatory response to systemic infusion of norepinephrine in the pregnant ewe, Am. J. Obstet. Gynecol. **127:**376, 1977.

29. Laukaran, V.H., and van den Berg, B.J.: The relationship of maternal attitude to pregnancy outcomes and obstetric complications, Am. J. Obstet. Gynecol. **136:**374, 1980.

30. Block, J.R., and Goodman, N.: Illicit drug use and consumption of alcohol, tobacco, and over-the-counter medicine among adolescents, Int. J. Addict. **13:**933, 1978.

31. Hollingsworth, D.R., Erickson, A.J., and Doughty, G.H.: Drugs and adolescent pregnancy. In Kreutner, A.K., and Hollingsworth, D.R., editors: Adolescent obstetrics and gynecology, Chicago, 1978, Year Book Medical Publishers, Inc.

32. Golden, N.L., Sokol, R.J., and Rubin, I.L.: Angel dust: possible effects on the fetus, Pediatrics **65:**18, 1980.

33. Caffeine, Federal Register **45:**69817, Oct. 21, 1980.

34. Stephenson, P.E.: Physiologic and psychotropic effects of caffeine on man, J. Am. Diet. Assoc. **71:**240, 1977.

35. Hickey, R.J., Clelland, R.C., and Bowers, E.J.: Maternal smoking, birth weight, infant death, and the self-selection problem, Am. J. Obstet. Gynecol. **131:**805, 1978.

36. Meyer, M.B., and Tonascia, J.A.: Maternal smoking, pregnancy complications, and perinatal mortality, Am. J. Obstet. Gynecol. **128:**494, 1977.

37. Garn, J.M., Shaw, H.A., and McCabe, K.D.: Effect of maternal smoking on weight and weight gain between pregnancies, Am. J. Clin. Nutr. **31:**1302, 1978.

38. Jacobs, D.R., and Gottenborg, S.: Smoking and weight: the Minnesota Lipid Research Clinic, Am. J. Public Health, **71:**391, 1981.

39. Haworth, J.C., and others: Fetal growth retardation in cigarette-smoking mothers is not due to decreased maternal food intake, Am. J. Obstet. Gynecol. **137**:719, 1980.

40. Haworth, J.C., and others: Relation of maternal cigarette smoking, obesity and energy consumption to infant size, Am. J. Obstet. Gynecol. **138**:1185, 1980.

41. Rush, D., Stein, Z., and Susser, M.: A randomized controlled trial of prenatal nutritional supplementation in New York City, Pediatrics **65**:683, 1980.

42. Longo, L.D.: Environmental pollution and pregnancy: risks and uncertainties for the fetus and infant, Am. J. Obstet. Gynecol. **137**:162, 1980.

43. Committee on Drugs, American Academy of Pediatrics: Effects of marijuana on man, Pediatrics **56**:134, 1979.

44. Hanson, J.W., Jones, K.L., and Smith, D.W.: Fetal alcohol syndrome: experience with 41 patients, JAMA **235**:1458, 1976.

45. Streissguth, A.P., and others: Teratogenic effects of alcohol in human and laboratory animals, Science **209**:353, 1980.

46. Streissguth, A.P., and others: Effects of maternal alcohol, nicotine, and caffeine use during pregnancy on infant mental and motor development at eight months, Alcohol. Clin. Exper. Res. **4**:152, 1980.

47. Trumbleson, M.E.: Fetal alcohol syndrome in Sinclair (S-1) miniature swine. Paper presented before National Institute on Alcohol Abuse and Alcoholism Fetal Alcohol Syndrome Workshop, San Diego, Feb. 1977.

48. Elton, R.H., and others: Changes in ethanol consumption by pregnant pigtailed macaques, J. Stud. Alcohol **30**:2181, 1977.

49. Little, R.E., and others: Decreased birth weight in infants of alcoholic women who abstained during pregnancy, J. Pediatr. **96**:974, 1980.

50. Blackburn, M.L., and Calloway, D.H.: Energy expenditure and pregnant adolescents. In Protein requirements of pregnant teenagers, Final report to National Institutes of Health, Division of Research Grants, Grant no. H.D. 05246, 1973.

51. Sackett, J.: A non-human primate model for studying causes, effects and poor pregnancy outcomes. In Friedman, S.L., and Sigman, M., editors: Preterm birth and psychological development, New York, 1981, Academic Press, Inc.

52. Regal, R.R., and others: A search for evidence for a paternal age effect independent of maternal age effect in birth certificate reports of Down's syndrome in New York State, Am. J. Epidemiol. **112**:650, 1980.

53. Vermeersch, J.: Physiological basis of nutritional needs. In Worthington-Roberts, B.S., Vermeersch, J., and Williams, S.R., editors: Nutrition in pregnancy and lactation, ed. 2, St. Louis, 1981, The C.V. Mosby Co.

54. Worthington-Roberts, B.S.: Nutritional issues related to pregnancy. In Worthington-Roberts, B.S., editor: Contemporary developments in nutrition, St. Louis, 1981, The C.V. Mosby Co.

55. Committee on Nutrition of the Mother and Preschool Child, Food and Nutrition Board, National Academy of Sciences–National Research Council: Nutrition services in prenatal care, Washington, D.C., 1981, National Academy Press.

56. Metcoff, J., and others: Maternal nutritional status and fetal outcome, Am. J. Clin. Nutr. **34**(suppl. 4):708, 1981.

57. Heald, F., and Jacobson, M.S.: Nutritional needs of the pregnant adolescent, Pediatr. Ann. **9**:95, 1980.

58. Hollingsworth, D.R., and Kreutner, A.K.: Teenage pregnancy: solutions are evolving, N. Engl. J. Med. **303**:516, 1980.

59. Nutrition during pregnancy and lactation, Sacramento, 1975, California Department of Health.

60. Williams, S.R.: Nutritional guidance in prenatal care. In Worthington-Roberts, B.S., Vermeersch, J., and Williams, S.R., editors: Nutrition in pregnancy and lactation, ed. 2, St. Louis, 1981, The C.V. Mosby Co.

61. U.S. Department of Health, Education, and Welfare: Ten state nutrition survey, 1968-1970, Department of Health, Education, and Welfare Publication (HSM) 72-8130, Atlanta, 1972, Centers for Disease Control.

62. Kaminetzky, H.A., and others: The effect of nutrition in teenage gravidas on pregnancy and the status of the neonate, Am. J. Obstet. Gynecol. **115**:639, 1973.

63. Hollingsworth, D.R.: Pregnancy complicated by chronic medical problems. In Kreutner, A.K., and Hollingsworth, D.R., editors: Adolescent obstetrics and gynecology, Chicago, 1978, Year Book Medical Publishers, Inc.

64. King, J.C., and others: Assessment of nutritional status of teenage pregnant girls. I. Nutrient intake and pregnancy, Am. J. Clin. Nutr. **25**:916, 1972.

65. Hytten, F.E., and Leitch, I.: The physiology of human pregnancy, ed. 2, Oxford, 1971, Blackwell Scientific Publications, Ltd.

66. King, J.C., Calloway, D.H., and Margen, S.: Nitrogen retention, total body K and weight gain in teenage pregnant girls, J. Nutr. **103**:772, 1973.

67. Bowering, J., Sanchez, A.M., and Irwin, M.I.: A conspectus of research on iron requirements of man, J. Nutr. **106**:985, 1976.

68. Monsen, E.R., Kuhn, I.N., and Finch, C.A.: Iron status of menstruating women, Am. J. Clin. Nutr. **20**:842, 1967.

69. McGanity, W.J., and others: Pregnancy in the adolescent. I. Preliminary summary of health status, Am. J. Obstet. Gynecol. **103**:773, 1969.

70. Rees, J.M., and Monsen, E.R.: Absorption of fortification iron by the rat: comparison of type and level of iron incorporated into mixed grain cereal, J. Agric. Food Chem. **21**:913, 1973.

71. Council on Foods and Nutrition, American Medical Association: Iron deficiency in the United States, JAMA **203**:61, 1968.

72. Kitay, D.A.: Folic acid deficiency in pregnancy, Am. J. Obstet. Gynecol. **104**:1067, 1969.

73. Worthington-Roberts, B.S.: Dietary fiber. In Worthington-Roberts, B.S., editor: Contemporary developments in nutrition, St. Louis, 1981, The C.V. Mosby Co.

74. Naeye, R.L.: Weight gain and the outcome of pregnancy, Am. J. Obstet. Gynecol. **135**:3, 1979.

75. Rosso, P., and Lederman, S.A.: Nutrition in the pregnant adolescent. In Winick, M., editor: Adolescent nutrition, New York, 1982, John Wiley & Sons, Inc.

76. Edwards, L.E., and others: Pregnancy in the underweight woman: course, outcome and growth patterns of the infant, Am. J. Obstet. Gynecol. **135**:297, 1979.

77. Naeye, R.L.: Teenaged and pre-teenaged pregnancies: consequences of the fetal-maternal competition for nutrients, Pediatrics **67**:146, 1981.

78. Pomerance, J., and others: Attitudes toward weight gain in pregnancy, West. J. Med. **133**:289, 1980.

79. Taggart, N.R., and others: Changes in skinfolds during pregnancy, Br. J. Nutr. **21**:439, 1967.

80. Udall, J.N., and others: Interaction of maternal and neonatal obesity, Pediatrics **62**:17, 1978.

81. Edwards, L.E., and others: Pregnancy in the massively obese: course, outcome, and obesity prognosis of the infant, Am. J. Obstet. Gynecol. **131**:479, 1978.

82. Harrison, G.G., Udall, J.N., and Morrow, G.: Maternal obesity, weight gain in pregnancy, and infant birth-weight, Am. J. Obstet. Gynecol. **136**:411, 1980.

83. Cohen, A.W., and Gabbe, S.G.: Obstetrical problems in the obese patient. In Stunkard, A.J., editor: Obesity, Philadelphia, 1980, W.B. Saunders Co.

84. Eastman, N.J., and Jackson, E.: Weight relationship in pregnancy. I. The bearing of maternal weight gain and pre-pregnancy weight on birth weight in full term pregnancies, Obstet. Gynecol. Surv. **23**:1003, 1968.

85. Corruccini, C.G.: Nutritional management of obese pregnant women, Sacramento, 1977, Maternal and Child Health Branch, California Department of Health.

86. Kawakami, S., and others: Alteration of maternal body weight in pregnancy and postpartum, Keio J. Med. **26**:53, 1977.

87. Delgado, H., and others: Nutrition, lactation, and postpartum amenorrhea, Am. J. Clin. Nutr. **31**:322, 1978.

88. Hollingsworth, D.R., and Kreutner, A.K.: Outcome of adolescent pregnancy. In Kreutner, A.K., and Hollingsworth, D.R., editors: Adolescent obstetrics and gynecology, Chicago, 1978, Year Book Medical Publishers, Inc.

89. McAnarney, E.R., and others: Obstetric, neonatal, and psychosocial outcome of pregnant adolescents, Pediatrics **61**:199, 1978.

90. Felice, M.E., and others: The young pregnant teenager: impact of comprehensive prenatal care, J. Adolesc. Health Care **1**:193, 1981.

91. Coates, J.B.: Obstetrics in the very young adolescent, Am. J. Obstet. Gynecol. **108**:68, 1970.

92. Battaglia, F.C., Frazier, T.M., and Hellegers, A.E.: Obstetric and pediatric complications of juvenile pregnancy, Pediatrics **32**:902, 1963.

93. Marchetti, A.A., and Manaker, J.S.: Pregnancy and the adolescent, Am. J. Obstet. Gynecol. **50**:1013, 1950.

94. Aznar, R., and Bennett, A.E.: Pregnancy in adolescent girls, Am. J. Obstet. Gynecol. **81**:934, 1961.

95. Poliakoff, R.: Pregnancy in the young primigravida, Am. J. Obstet. Gynecol. **76**:746, 1958.

96. Grant, J.A., and Heald, F.P.: Complications of adolescent pregnancy: survey of the literature on fetal outcome in adolescence, Clin. Pediatr. **11**:567, 1972.

97. Duenhoelter, J.H., Jimenez, J.M., and Baumann, G.: Pregnancy performance of patients under fifteen years of age, Obstet. Gynecol. **46**:49, 1975.

98. Dwyer, J.F.: Teenage pregnancy, Am. J. Obstet. Gynecol. **118**:373, 1974.

99. Sarrel, P.M., and Klerman, L.V.: The young unwed mother: obstetric results of a program of comprehensive care, Am. J. Obstet. Gynecol. **103**:575, 1969.

100. Youngs, D.D., and others: Experience with an adolescent pregnancy program, Obstet. Gynecol. **50**:212, 1977.

101. Briggs, R.M., and others: Pregnancy in the young adolescent, Am. J. Obstet. Gynecol. **84**:436, 1962.

102. Zlatnik, F.J., and Burmeister, L.F.: Low "gynecologic age": an obstetric risk factor, Am. J. Obstet. Gynecol. **128**:183, 1977.

103. Coruh, M., and Topal, I.: Pregnancy and pregnancy outcome in Ankara (Gecekondu) adolescents, J. Adolesc. Health Care **1**:232, 1981.

104. Gatenby, P.B., and Lillre, R.S.: Clinical analysis of 1000 cases of severe megaloblastic anemia of pregnancy, Br. Med. J. **2**:1111, 1960.

105. Yusufji, D., Mathan, V.I., and Baker, S.J.: Iron, folate and B_{12} nutrition in pregnancy: a study of 100 women from Southern India., Bull. WHO **48**:15, 1973.

106. Lu, J.Y., and others: Intakes of vitamins and minerals by pregnant women with selected clinical symptoms, J. Am. Diet. Assoc. **78**:477, 1981.

107. Smith, E., O'Connell, M.J., and Zackler, J.: Food habits of pregnant teenagers and their potential relation to pregnancy outcome. Public Health Rep. **84:**213, 1969.

108. Chaudhuri, S.K., and others: Relationship between toxemia of pregnancy and thiamine deficiency, J. Obstet. Gynaecol. Br. Comm. **76:**123, 1969.

109. Chaudhuri, S.K.: Correlation of toxemia with anemia of pregnancy, Am. J. Obstet. Gynecol. **106:**255, 1970.

110. Brophy, M.H., and Siiteri, P.K.: Pyridoxal phosphate and hypertensive disorders of pregnancy, Am. J. Obstet. Gynecol. **121:**1075, 1975.

111. Hibbard, B.M.: The role of folic acid in pregnancy, J. Obstet. Gynaecol. Brit. Comm. **79:**159, 1964.

112. Chesley, C.C.: Sodium retention and pre-eclampsia, Am. J. Obstet. Gynecol. **95:**127, 1966.

113. Mengert, W.F., and Tacchi, D.A.: Pregnancy toxemia and sodium chloride, Am. J. Obstet. Gynecol. **81:**601, 1961.

114. Chung, R., and others: Diet-related toxemia in pregnancy. I. Fat, fatty acid and cholesterol, Am. J. Clin. Nutr. **32:**1902, 1979.

115. Williams, C., and others: Protein, amino acid and caloric intakes of selected pregnant women, J. Am. Diet. Assoc. **78:**28, 1981.

116. Plotkin, S.A.: Routes of fetal infection and mechanisms, Am. J. Dis. Child. **129:**444, 1975.

117. Levkoff, A.H.: Biologic, emotional and intellectual risks in teenage mothers and their babies. In Kreutner, A.K., and Hollinsworth, D.R., editors: Adolescent obstetrics and gynecology, Chicago, 1978, Year Book Medical Publishers, Inc.

118. Shills, M.E.: Food and nutrition relating to work, exercise and environmental stress. In Goodheart, R.S., and Shills, M.E., editors: Modern nutrition in health and disease, Philadelphia, 1980, Lea & Febiger.

119. Sever, J.L., and others: Infection and low birthweight in an industrialized society, Am. J. Dis. Child. **129:**557, 1975.

120. Stiehm, A.R.: Fetal defense mechanisms, Am. J. Dis. Child. **129:**438, 1975.

121. Alford, C.A., Stagno, S., and Reynolds, D.W.: Diagnosis of chronic perinatal infections, Am. J. Dis. Child. **129:**455, 1975.

122. Burke, B.S., and others: The influence of nutrition upon the condition of the infant at birth, J. Nutr. **26:**569, 1943.

123. Primrose, T., and Higgins, A.: A study of human antepartum nutrition, J. Reprod. Med. **7:**257, 1971.

124. Merritt, T.A., Lawrence, R.A., and Naeye, R.L.: The infants of adolescent mothers, Pediatr. Ann. **9:**100, 1980.

125. Winick, M.: Fetal malnutrition, Clin. Obstet. Gynecol. **13:**526, 1970.

126. Naeye, R.L., Blanc, W., and Paul, C.: Effects of maternal nutrition on the human fetus, Pediatrics **52:**494, 1973.

127. Habicht, J., and others: Relation of maternal supplementary feeding during pregnancy to birthweight and other sociobiological factors. In Winick, M., editor: Nutrition and fetal development, New York, 1974, John Wiley & Sons, Inc.

128. Lechtig, A., and others: Influence of maternal nutrition on birth weight, Am. J. Clin. Nutr. **28:**1223, 1975.

129. Lechtig, A., and others: Maternal nutrition and fetal growth in developing countries, Am. J. Dis. Child. **129:**553, 1975.

130. Paige, D.M., and others: Nutritional supplementation of pregnant adolescents, J. Adolesc. Health Care **1:**261, 1981.

131. Marinoff, S.C., and Schonholz, D.H.: Adolescent pregnancy, Pediatr. Clin. North Am. **19:**759, 1972.

132. Niswander, K.R., and others: Weight gained during pregnancy and prepregnancy weight, Obstet. Gynecol. **33:**482, 1969.

133. Gormican, A., Valentine, J., and Satter, E.: Relationships of maternal weight gain, prepregnancy weight, and infant birthweight, J. Am. Diet. Assoc. **88:**662, 1981.

134. Hackman, E., and Emmanuel, I.: Influence of maternal birthweight on infant birthweight: intergenerational effect, doctoral dissertation, Seattle, 1981, University of Washington.

135. Eisner, V., and others: The risk of low birthweight, Am. J. Public Health **69:**887, 1979.

136. Dott, A.B., and Fort, A.T.: Medical and social factors affecting early teenage pregnancy, Am. J. Obstet. Gynecol. **125:**532, 1976.

137. Symonds, E.M.: The prevention of prematurity, Practitioner **221:**839, 1978.

138. Hutchins, F.L., Kendall, N., and Rubino, J.: Experience with teenage pregnancy, Obstet. Gynecol. **54:**1, 1979.

139. Baldwin, W., and Cain, V.S.: The children of teenage parents, Fam. Plann. Perspect. **12:**34, 1980.

140. de Lissovoy, V.: Child care by adolescent parents, Child. Today **2:**22, 1973.

141. Klaus, H., Meurer, J., and Sullivan, A.: Teenage pregnancy: multidisciplinary treatment and teaching, J. Med. Educ. **48:**1027, 1973.

142. Adolescent reproductive care, statement of policy issued by the Executive Board, American College of Obstetricians and Gynecologists, Chicago, 1979.

143. Pregnancy and the unmarried girl, WHO Chron. **30:**108, 1976.

144. Task Force on Adolescent Pregnancy: Adolescent perinatal health: a guidebook for service, Chicago, 1979, American College of Obstetricians and Gynecologists.

145. Christakis, G., editor: Nutritional assessment in health programs, Am. J. Public Health **63**(suppl.):1, 1973.

146. Hill, E.P., and Longo, L.D.: Dynamics of maternal-fetal nutrient transfer, Fed. Proc. **39:**239, 1980.

147. Cochrane, W.: Overnutrition in prenatal and neonatal life, Can. Med. Assoc. J. **93**:893, 1965.
148. Berkenfield, J., and Schwarts, J.B.: Nutrition intervention in the community: the ''WIC'' program, N. Engl. J. Med. **302**:579, 1980.
149. Calderon-Elizondo, N.: Psychosocial variables of the health belief model and obesity, master's thesis, Seattle, 1978, University of Washington.
150. Dwyer, J.T., and others: Management of weight in pregnancy, Postgrad. Med. **48**:208, 1970.
151. Bracken, M.B., Klerman, L.V., and Bracken, M.: Abortion, adoption, or motherhood: an empirical study of decision-making during pregnancy, Am. J. Obstet. Gynecol. **130**:251, 1978.
152. Pipes, P.: Infant feeding and nutrition. In Pipes, P., editor: Nutrition in infancy and childhood, ed. 2, St. Louis, 1981, The C.V. Mosby Co.
153. Cannon-Bonventre, K., and Kahn, J.: Interviews with adolescent parents, Child. Today **8**:17, 1979.
154. Greden, J.F., and others: Caffeine-withdrawal headache: a clinical profile, Psychosomatics **21**:411, 1980.
155. Trahms, C.M.: Vegetarianism as a way of life. In Worthington-Roberts, B.S., editor: Contemporary developments in nutrition, St. Louis, 1981, The C.V. Mosby Co.
156. Rees, J.M., and Worthington-Roberts, B.S.: Establishing a nutritional environment supportive of reproduction: nutrition education issues. In Worthington-Roberts, B.S., Vermeersch, J., and Williams, S.R., editors: Nutrition in pregnancy and lactation, ed. 2, St. Louis, 1981, The C.V. Mosby Co.

Chapter 10

Nutritional Counseling for Adolescents

JANE MITCHELL REES

In recent years attention in the field of nutrition has turned toward the necessity of working in an interdisciplinary fashion and of incorporating knowledge of the social sciences into the practice of nutrition.[1,2] The need is very apparent in relation to nutritional counseling of adolescents.[3] Nutritional counseling, as distinguished from the broader scope of nutrition education activities or more specific dietary teaching techniques (see Chapter 3), is based on a continuing reciprocal relationship between counselor and client. The mutual goal for the relationship is improvement of the client's nutritional well-being. This relationship has been characterized as one of *mutual participation,* as opposed to *activity-passivity* seen in acute care or *guidance-cooperation,* which usually is used with younger children.[4]

The way in which a message is presented is as important as the message itself with the adolescent population. Nutritionists who wish to facilitate change in the nourishment patterns of teenagers must be able to communicate with them in such a way as to make them want to change. The challenge of the situation has to do in part with the stage of development,[5,6] with cognitive styles changing from concrete to abstract, and with control passing from authority figures to the teen. Adolescents have not experienced the consequences of their long-term behaviors as adults have. They have not yet developed an awareness of their own vulnerability and mortality, which can act as a motivation for learning to care for themselves. As pointed out in previous chapters, they will be very open to the influence of the media, friends, and other peers. Outside a hospital setting, they are free agents and will make changes in their dietary habits only if they think it is worth the effort and can visualize a way to change.

NATURE OF COUNSELING PROCESS

The counseling process has ben described by de Schweinitz and de Schweinitz[7] as being a specialized conversation that has a specific purpose and takes place within a relationship.[6,8] The professional will be primarily responsible for guiding the process so that the mutual goals are met. It can never be a unilateral responsibility, however, but must be shared by the client. In fact, the professional will need to help clients feel a responsibility for contributing if they do not do so spontaneously.[7] In these conversations the purposes will be to obtain information about the client, to provide information to the client, and to stimulate the client to take action.

Within the conversations of counseling, it is important to recognize that exchanges can be divided into *the content,* the information exchanged, and *the process,* the way the exchange takes place.[9,10] The content that is brought forth for discussion by clients consists of what they want to talk about, what they say their habits are, and, in some situations, irrelevant material used to avoid focusing on problems. It ultimately will be the responsibility of the counselor to guide the client in presenting material that contributes to the overall goals of counseling. The counselor will also be responsible for bringing in content that is suited to the client's needs in terms of quantity, type, and level.[7]

The process on the clients' part is made up of such aspects as their attitude toward the discussion, the way they express themselves, and their emotional response to the counseling session. The counselor's demeanor (beginning from the first meeting with the client in the waiting room or at the bedside), verbal and nonverbal reinforcement of the client's responses, and overall guidance of the session constitute the counselor's contributions to the process. Examples of the content of a nutritional counseling session would include information from the client about his or her eating habits and recommendations from the counselor about changes that need to be made. The process would include the way the client described his or her eating patterns and the kind of approach the counselor took in securing the information and in suggesting changes following an evaluation.

It is important to recognize both the content and process of counseling exchanges because to assess the results of a therapeutic relationship, each must be examined for appropriateness. There are times in initial nutrition interviews when the approach of the clinician is overly authoritarian to the degree that even though relevant information is given and received, a working relationship becomes impossible. On the other extreme is the relationship that builds rapport on irrelevancies but fails to approach difficult issues such as steps for making dietary changes.

Obtaining and providing information are relatively common processes, and it is easy to conceive of how this is done in counseling.[11] Stimulating a client to take action by means of a conversation, however, is a much more complex process to visualize and to accomplish than that of obtaining information. The following are descriptions of accomplishments in counseling that lead to change on the part of the client.

Increasing Self-Awareness

As a counselor and a client discuss the client's behavior, the client must focus more clearly on his or her motives and actions. The actions and the reasons for doing them become more apparent to the individual through this discussion. As teenagers learn to assess themselves with the counselor, they can begin to do it for themselves without the counselor's help.[11,12] Increasing self-awareness will take varying amounts of time for different individuals. The older adolescent with greater powers of abstract thinking will often be able to learn more rapidly. However, certain people whose problems are rooted in a lack of self-awareness will have great difficulty in focusing on themselves and will appear resistant to doing so. Overweight teenagers, for example, have often ignored motives and habits related to eating. Helping them to acquire self-discerning ability will take great skill on the part of the counselor.

Realizing Existence of Alternatives

For adolescents who have had few life experiences and have grown up in families that have followed stereotyped patterns of behavior, it will seem that there are no alternatives to their traditional responses to a given situation. Counseling offers an opportunity to explore the existence of alternative responses in a relatively low-risk situation.[12,13] Realizing that such alternatives are possible can be valuable in and of itself and is often the first step to making any changes.

EXAMPLE: A teenager who has a chronic disease that necessitates a sodium restriction, who "loves salty foods," and who has been taught to eat them by a family that traditionally eats many such foods can learn that there are other tastes that are enjoyable and satisfying.

Problem Solving

There are many ways of demonstrating effective problem solving in a counseling relationship.[11,12] Even arriving at a satisfactory time for a clinic appointment in a crowded schedule can loom as an insoluble problem to one who has not developed methods for solving problems. The counselor, working together with the adolescent, first will provide a model and then will support the adolescent in taking responsibility for solving problems. Although the teenagers then must put this process into action in the outside world, the opportunity to learn under the guidance of a counselor will often enable teens to develop a technique that they had not learned in their own environment.

EXAMPLE: A teenage athlete has not solved the problem of obtaining food as part of a training schedule. The nutritional counselor guides a process that includes facing and assessing the problem, listing alternatives, and discussing the merits and means of implementing those alternatives. Making a decision about the alternative to put into practice completes the process. Follow-up in counseling provides repeated opportunities for solving the problems that arise in carrying out the plan.

Experiencing Positive Communication Style

Relationships with others are a major component of many of the problems that develop around nutrition for the adolescent. Examples include eating disorders, where distorted relationships with family and peers are contributing factors to the disorders themselves, and nourishment in chronic disease, where the adolescent must maintain peer relationships although being unable to fully participate in social eating situations. Because communication is important in establishing relationships, the opportunity to experience a positive communication style within counseling contributes to the patient's ability to improve relationships in his or her own environment.

EXAMPLE: Bulimic teens tend to be vague, to gloss over problems, or to hesitate in making definitive statements, especially related to themselves. They often benefit from straightforward communication with the counselor, as they then are helped to discuss their problems. In time they begin to feel more comfortable with such a style, and with support they can begin to adapt it in relationship with others.

Experiencing Control Over One's Life

For the adolescent, much of life appears to be "given" and not open to control by the individual. This occurs to a detrimental degree in families where children have not been allowed to develop independence. Such children often are incapable of making decisions for themselves by the time they are adolescents. The notion that certain situations are controllable and that a particular individual can begin to exert control can be introduced and demonstrated within a counseling relationship.[11]

EXAMPLE: Buttressed by the support of the respected clinician, a teenager who is offered tempting foods by family and friends can learn that it is permissible to refuse such foods. He or she can rehearse positive techniques for doing so and go out to practice them in daily life. Discussing successes and failures over time provides reinforcement for progress in taking an active versus a passive role. A model within counseling for taking control occurs when the counselor requires the client to establish his or her own short-term goals.

Building Self-Esteem

In many cases adolescents who develop problems have not experienced esteem-building relationships. By respecting a client as a valuable individual, the clinician contributes to that person's self-esteem. Demonstrations of this respect include eliciting teenagers' ideas, treating them as individuals and not as children of their parents, expecting them to be capable of taking responsibility for themselves, and showing them professional courtesy.[14] As they are treated respectfully, they will begin to have greater respect for themselves. Goals for their progress will be established realistically so that they achieve success. As successes accrue, self-esteem improves.

EXAMPLE: The pregnant adolescent female frequently suffers from low self-esteem. Nutritional counseling in which she is respected and in which she is enabled to make positive changes in her nutritional intake improves her feelings about herself. Reinforcement by the counselor for taking responsibility for herself and her unborn child increases these positive feelings.

In all aspects of counseling just described, clients must think for themselves to actually integrate the accomplishments into their own experience. If the counselor merely provides the answer, the process will only be effective for a minority of highly motivated people. On the other hand, when clients are facilitated in realizing options or solving problems, they can gain new skills that enable them to make lasting changes.[14]

SPECIALIZED COUNSELING FOR ADOLESCENTS

Treating Adolescents as Independent Individuals

Even before children reach adolescence, they will be capable of getting much of their own food for themselves. They will not always be given the responsibility by their parents nor will they always act responsibly, but in many situations they will have access to food. Nutritional counseling therefore will need to be based on one-to-one relationships with individual adolescents, who then are facilitated in taking the responsibility to manage food to nourish themselves. In a clinical relationship an adolescent should be treated as an individual with an understanding of the factors that at times lead him or her to behave in a less than mature fashion.[5,14-16]

The usual confidentiality issues between clinicians and clients are complicated by the need to communicate with parents. It is best to clearly inform clients that information from them will not be passed on to parents or other authorities unless it discloses the possibility that they might harm themselves or another.[14,15] Likewise, information from parents will not be passed on to clients. The

counselor therefore will hold information that increases his or her knowledge of a situation without directly quoting or using it openly with the other parties involved.

There will be a difference in the approach to teenagers depending on whether they are in early, middle, or late adolescence. Those in the early stage will need greater guidance and support, as they are learning to take responsibility and to change habits. The more mature adolescent will need to be given freedom to act independently with less direction. The development of those in the middle will be less predictable. They must be assessed carefully to determine the appropriate degree of direction or encouragement of autonomy suitable in counseling the individual.

An issue that needs to be considered carefully in counseling adolescents is that of sexuality. Because of newly developing sexual feelings, some teenagers may become very anxious in the presence of a member of the opposite sex, even when that person is a professional. They may feel a great attraction to the counselor. Counselors must be observant for the signs that this reaction is occurring and take precautions to avoid problems. Meeting in a public place that does not allow closeness and being careful to communicate in a style that could only be construed as businesslike are two examples. It may be necessary to include others in counseling sessions with some teens to avoid a feeling of intimacy. Other members of the health-care team or receptionists who know the client can usefully serve in this capacity.

Including Significant Others

One of the challenging situations in dealing with teenage clients is that of incorporating others into the therapeutic process. This must be done in a manner that does not jeopardize the relationship between the adolescent and the therapist, yet gains the cooperation of others, keeps them informed, and allows them to share in the process of change.[14,15]

Parents often finance therapy and may be reluc

tant to continue if they are not satisfied with the results. Some will be anxious to be involved as much as possible, although others will want to be excluded. The counselor will need to ascertain their attitudes, judge the need for communication with them based on their contribution toward treatment goals, and coordinate the contact.[14] In some situations it may be necessary to use the telephone to keep in touch, but in other cases it will be necessary to work intensely with the parents.

Some parents will be eager to turn responsibility over to their teenager, but others will need help in doing this. All will need to arrive at a balance of being interested and supportive of their children, while at the same time allowing them the freedom to take responsibility and to gain independence. In the meantime, counseling will be devoted to enabling adolescents to take responsibility for their own health.[17]

Parents who intrude on and downgrade their teens and treat them as less than mature individuals have a very negative effect on their teenagers. Through modeling and even very direct messages from counselors, they can learn more positive approaches. Other parents may be very positive and supportive. They will need to be informed and shown how to best help their children to accomplish specific goals related to nourishing themselves.[18] Family conferences, where all members take part in discussions with the counselor or health-care team about results of evaluation or progress in meeting goals, are a valuable technique for maintaining communication.

Pregnant teens may live with their families at home and maintain a close relationship with a mother figure. Alternatively, they may live with a partner or husband. It is important to maintain contact with the significant person in either case. If it is a partner or husband, it is appropriate to counsel the couple together at each visit. At times it will be apparent that one partner is overdependent on the other, and in those situations remarks addressed directly to each one will help demonstrate the need for each to take independent responsibility for his

or her actions so that collectively they can provide what is necessary.

When the significant person is a mother, it is generally best to see the client separately to foster the independence desirable for a young woman to take on the responsibility inherently required in her position. The nutritionist will want to stimulate the mother's interest and support for her daughter's nutritional well-being but guide her into a noninterfering mode of providing that support. A close friend or a relative other than the mother sometimes will want to "follow" a client through the pregnancy. There may be self-serving motives in this behavior that can interfere with the client developing an independent sense of responsibility. The friend, like the mother, should be seen separately from the client and should be presumed to be a support to the client. The client remains the focus of the counseling relationship.

Counseling Environment

Environment is very important to teenagers. They also are usually "action oriented."[11] Nutritional counseling can be more effective if the counselor incorporates stimulating environments and activities. Appealing graphics can be used in clinic, office, and hospital settings. If the counseling is set within an institution, anxiety about the impersonal nature of the location can be offset by using components of the facilities that adolescents will find interesting. Participating in certain more adult experiences can sometimes improve self-esteem. Alternative settings such as the outdoors (Fig. 10-1), a coffee shop, or lounge can be used to great advantage. In some instances it will be possible to develop an environment suited to teens that is based on their own youthful culture.[19]

FACILITATING CHANGE INVOLVES WHOLE PERSON

Three aspects of a teenager's personality must be considered in the therapeutic process[20]: the cognitive or intellectual, the affective or emotional,

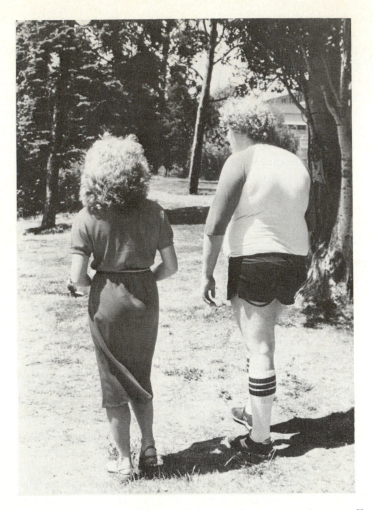

Fig. 10-1. Nutritional counseling in out-of-doors environment can be very effective.

and the behavioral. Some teens will be motivated most strongly by intellectual processes, suppressing the emotional and ignoring the behavioral. Others will be ruled by their emotions instead of using their intellectual potential to solve problems. Another group will ignore both intellect and emotions to the degree that their responses to the events of life are mainly behavioral. It is the function of counseling to help bring these three aspects of their lives into better balance. For each nutritional-counseling situation, the cognitive, affective, and behavioral aspects must be considered.

Assessment of nutritional problems is discussed in Chapter 3. If the initial evaluation of a situation reveals the need for counseling, more in-depth measures may be required to define the behavioral and affective components of the problem. These measures can be standardized tests such as the locus-of-control scale,[21] questionnaires,[22] in-depth probing by the counselor, or exchange of information with professionals of other disciplines who have assessed the individual.

Following an assessment, teenagers who are highly motivated to make use of new information can be treated on a relatively short-term basis. Those whose attitudes and behaviors appear to mitigate against their using information will require long-term attention directed toward changing attitudes and behavioral patterns.

Those with long-standing nutritional problems generally fall into the latter category. This contributes to the complex nature of nutritional counseling.

Strategies Directed Toward Enhancing Cognitive Skills

Following evaluation, new information will need to be presented in language teens understand and at a level that is appropriate to their overall functioning.[11] Information they have already received will often need to be presented in new ways, and misinformation will need to be replaced.

In certain situations specific dietary prescriptions will be used. Planned diets have a large cognitive component, but they require that clients have both an attitude of readiness and sufficient control over their behavior that they can change from previous patterns to carry the diet out. If a specific diet is used, with purely cognitive material being exchanged, follow-up will reveal whether or not additional attention must be devoted to attitudinal and behavioral components to enable the client to comply. The expectation that merely explaining a diet and the rationale behind its use will lead to a successful change of food intake is generally unrealistic.[18]

Cognitive material usually will be woven into messages and directed toward behaviors.[11] For example, when the goal is weight management, one of the types of information the client will need

relates to the high energy value of fats. Information about fat and fat-containing foods can be accompanied by strategies mutually designed by the counselor and the client for eliminating unnecessary fats from the diet. A series of successfully completed components of this type will lead to effective weight management.

A judicious use can be made of printed or audiovisual material to carry out the informing process. The goals will always be to help the client to retain information mentally rather than be dependent on media such as written material. Only information that is readily in the mind is reliable in the multitude of situations in which teenagers deal with food.

Strategies Directed Toward Affective Changes

The need to help teens examine and change both their attitudes and the underlying reasons for their behavior to facilitate their use of nutrition information is the aspect of nutritional counseling that may be least appreciated. This is reflected by the approaches described in the literature.[18,23] However, if the counselor is going to help a rebellious diabetic teen to carry out a diet, or an obese teen to stop using food to cope with stresses, or an immature teen to take responsibility for nourishing her unborn child, sophisticated facilitating techniques will need to be used. Even when a team of professionals is available to work with the individual and certain counselors are dealing with the emotional aspects of a health problem, nutritional counselors will be greatly hampered if they are unable to approach the affective component in their counseling. Those who are unable or unskilled in dealing with the emotional aspects of counseling will need to contain their efforts to working with more straightforward problems where only information dissemination is necessary. Supportive counseling directed toward the affective aspects of the individual should be the basis of all techniques used in nutritional therapy. Positive support for controlling food habits can diffuse the rebellious attitude of diabetic teenagers. For example, being helped to identify their motives as attempts to hurt others by damaging themselves can lead to a revision of their motivation.

Similarly, the attitude that "change is impossible" on the part of the obese adolescent can be turned to the realization that anyone can make changes when a counselor helps the teenager take on that view. Feelings of inadequacy that have led to depending on food for comfort can be examined and more appropriate feelings about the self adopted. Ego-building experiences in counseling can foster an attitude of responsibility in a pregnant teen who as a result can be helped to adopt a more selfless stance in relation to nourishing her child. Thus improvement of nutritional health can occur within the specialized conversation of the counseling relationship, much of which is directed toward the affective aspects of personality.

Strategies Directed Toward Behavioral Change

The most effective strategy for facilitating behavioral change will be to focus on small increments of change over a period of time, with the counselor providing support during the period when the changes are being put into practice.[18] The counselor will supply information and stimulation as needed, attending to all aspects, including the cognitive and affective aspects, of the individual's personality. A knowledge of human behavior[3,7] and the concepts of learning theory,[24] communication theory,[25] and behavior modification[20,26-28] are essential for nutritional counseling. A skilled counselor will utilize any of a variety of techniques, choosing those to which the particular individual responds well.

Outside of a purely research-oriented setting, behavior modification techniques can be effectively tailored for the individual and applied within the supportive relationship of counseling.[18,29] They not only will be applied in the sense of a specific treatment modality but will be incorporated into all counseling work. Perhaps the most important technique is the knowledgeable use of reinforcers. Counselors themselves will be agents of reinforcement; the family or hospital staff will provide reinforcement; and finally, clients will be helped to provide reinforcement for themselves.

Auxiliary techniques such as assertiveness and social skills training,[30] movement or dance therapy, and group therapy may be of value in facilitating behavioral change. These broaden the scope of coping mechanisms for individuals, allowing them to deemphasize inappropriate use of food. Mediated experiences such as audiovisual or written material have limited use in the area of stimulating actual behavior change except in the most highly motivated, intelligent client.

TECHNIQUES OF COUNSELING

Specific techniques used in interviewing and counseling have been described by social workers, psychologists, and psychiatrists.[8-10,31,32]

Goal Setting

Goal setting is one of the pivotal techniques in counseling. There are *process goals* that the counselor generally will be responsible for establishing and meeting. These create therapeutic conditions that enable the client to change. Maintaining an effective relationship is an example of a process goal. *Outcome goals*, both long and short term, are directly related to the individual client's problems. The responsibility for establishing these goals will be shared by the client and the counselor, although the counselor will guide the client. Effective goal-setting technique can be inferred from the checklist developed by Hackney and Cormier and presented in the box on p. 265. Various phases of goal setting will be interspersed throughout a counseling session. By the end of the session the goals thus are clarified. Mutual decisions are a necessity with adolescents. For example, the teens must help decide how often they will be involved in coun-

Goal-Setting Checklist

1. The counselor asked the client to identify some of the conditions surrounding the occurrence of the client's problem (*When* do you feel _____?).

           Yes   No   N.A.

2. The counselor asked the client to identify some of the consequences resulting from the client's behavior (What happens when you _____?).

           Yes   No   N.A.

3. The counselor asked the client to state how he would like to change his behavior (How would you like for things to be different?).

           Yes   No   N.A.

4. The counselor and client decided *together* upon counseling goals.

           Yes   No   N.A.

5. The goals set in the interview were specific and observable.

           Yes   No   N.A.

6. The counselor asked the client to orally state a commitment to work for goal achievement.

           Yes   No   N.A.

7. If the client appeared resistant or unconcerned about achieving change, the counselor discussed this with the client.

           Yes   No   N.A.

8. The counselor asked the client to specify at least one action step he or she might take toward his goal.

           Yes   No   N.A.

9. The counselor suggested alternatives available to the client.

           Yes   No   N.A.

10. The counselor helped the client to develop action steps for goal attainment.

            Yes   No   N.A.

11. Action steps designated by counselor and client were specific and realistic in scope.

            Yes   No   N.A.

12. The counselor provided an opportunity within the interview for the client to practice or rehearse the action step.

            Yes   No   N.A.

13. The counselor provided feedback to the client concerning the execution of the action step.

            Yes   No   N.A.

14. The counselor encouraged the client to observe and evaluate the progress and outcomes of action steps taken outside the interview.

            Yes   No   N.A.

From Harold Hackney, L. Sherilyn Cormier, Counseling strategies and objectives, 2nd ed., © 1979, pp. 160-162. Reprinted by permission of Prentice-Hall, Inc., Englewood Cliffs, N.J.

seling and what changes they will make between sessions.

Open-Ended Questions

The use of open-ended questions will allow clients to express themselves and bring up subjects that they think are important (**C,** counselor; **A,** adolescent; **M,** mother).

EXAMPLE

C: How did it go last week—with the diet plan?

as opposed to

C: Did you follow the diet plan we made last week?

Positive Regard

Counselors should maintain a positive regard for clients to demonstrate that they are valued as human beings. They should be accepting and nonjudgmental even when they disagree with the client.[6,15] They should control their own reactions so as not to bring their personal feelings into counseling, but at the same time they must show a genuine active interest in the client. The positive objective stance on the part of the counselor allows the client to feel secure in the counseling relationship.[10]

EXAMPLE: An immature adolescent expresses superficial guilt over poor food choices in the past week. The counselor responds objectively, asking what they can do together to enable the client to improve.

A: I really blew it (giggles). I had potato chips, cake . . . (more giggles).
C: So you had a rough time last week. What can we plan so that it will go better for you next time?

Timing

As a part of the responsibility for managing counseling, timing is an important concept. Timing includes planning for and accomplishing a reasonable amount of work at each session, closing the session on time, and organizing follow-up visits.[7,33] With practice an instinct develops for the therapeutic hour, and a pattern becomes set: an introductory checking in, a middle covering the main topics, and a closing that includes agreement on future plans.[7,9,10] During the main body of the session, timing takes on the dimension of knowing when to bring up a particular issue or to use a particular technique.

EXAMPLE: In an opening chat the client talks about school. Within this discussion, the counselor finds an opening to ask what the teenager usually eats at school.

Selection of Material

The counselor, as manager of the session, selects the material that will be focused on to move the session toward fulfilling the objective. This is accomplished by responding to those statements the client makes that the counselor feels are most appropriate to the purpose of the discussion.[33]

EXAMPLE: The teenager is describing the events of the past week.

A: My dog died Thursday. We had him since I was eight. Everybody was really sad.
C: Hmm.
A: We buried him under the apple tree. My sister brought some flowers. I really had trouble going to school Friday.
C: Did you? What other ways did it affect you?
A: Well, I ate a lot. I know I gained weight.

Verbal and Nonverbal Reinforcement

Restating or repeating the client's own responses and use of verbal or nonverbal reinforcers for continuing can help the patient contribute his or her thoughts in counseling sessions.[10]

EXAMPLE

A: Actually, last night I was thinking about why I can't stay on my diet.
C: (Nods.)
A: It seems like I've had diabetes forever.
C: Hmm.
A: It messes up everything I want to do. Just when I can get out of the house because I'm old enough.
C: It seems like it messes up everything.
A: Yeah. I get so tired of it. That's why I have trouble with my diet.

Active Listening

The practice of active listening is basic to the counseling process.[8-10,32] Although the client is talking, the counselor will be sifting through what is said for clues concerning how best to reach that client to facilitate positive change. The counselor will intermittently use techniques for drawing the patient out or any one of the other counseling techniques described here. The counselor not only will be hearing what the client has said in the usual sense but will be engaged in the process of managing the interview. For beginning counselors it may be almost as though two trains of thought are necessary, but eventually the process of listening to content and planning the process are one operation. Meanwhile, the face, eyes, voice, body, and gestures of the counselor are communicating to the client the attitude of the counselor.[9] The physical aspects of the counselor constitute another part of active listening. The therapeutic use of the self lies at the heart of the counseling process.[34]

EXAMPLE: The counselor sits with an open and relaxed but alert posture and maintains eye contact. The client begins anxiously but calms as she realizes that she has the counselor's full attention. The client is reporting events of the last week that would contribute to weight control.

A: I got my bike fixed like we talked about last week.
C: Wonderful!
A: My friend and I rode to the shopping center. We went to Clark's. I found this wonderful pink sweater.
C: (Thinks: "This doesn't seem a useful track." Says nothing but looks interested, encouraging A to continue.)
A: Anyway, on the way home, we rode the long way up to the school.
C: Great! (Thinks: "This is more productive." Leans forward a bit and speaks to emphasize the encouragement to continue with this topic.) How did you enjoy the ride?

Therapeutic Use of Silence

Therapeutic use of silence allows clients time to feel a responsibility for carrying on the session, to formulate thoughts, and to express themselves even if they must take more than a usual amount of time about it. This is important for teens who may not often have an opportunity to express themselves.[14] The silences should not be so long that they cause anxiety on the part of the teen. The greatest anxiety, however, usually lies with the counselor, who may ask questions or talk excessively in an effort to fill up empty spaces.

EXAMPLE

C: How did things go last week?
A: Well I had a little trouble. . . .
C: (Attentive, silent.)
A: I . . . didn't feel like eating. . . .
C: (Attentive, silent.)
A: Except for ice cream . . . I felt like eating ice cream.

Observation

Because a counselor will see clients for only a short portion of their lives, it is especially important to use observation as a way of learning more about them.[3,12] How they respond to different people or different topics as they arise in discussion is important information. Facial expressions, body language, gestures, and tone of voice all will be observable even within confined settings.[15]

EXAMPLE: As the counselor introduces herself in the waiting area, she describes how she and 15-year-old John will need some time to talk about the changes he will have to make in his food habits as part of his treatment for a newly diagnosed chronic disease. Then she and the mother will have a chance to talk.

C: So we'll see you in a bit.
M: Well, all right. (Seems anxious and reluctant to separate.) I'll keep your coat for you, John. How long do you think it will be?

The counselor observes that while John is surprised to be seeing a professional on his own, he is obviously pleased and ready, whereas the mother is anxious and fostering dependency. It will be important to help this family see that John is to take responsibility for his food choices.

Reflection of Feelings

Feelings can become a focus when the counselor reflects feelings expressed either verbally or nonverbally by the patient.[9] The counselor can shape the session by highlighting or downplaying the feelings that the client expresses.

EXAMPLE

A: I didn't do very well this week.

C: You feel pretty discouraged right now.

Interpretive Statements

Interpretive statements can be carefully used to help a person gain new insight. Examples would be statements from the counselor to ascribe a motive for behavior or to conceptualize a problem following a number of comments leading up to this conclusion by the client. The reason for caution is that such statements must not be made in an attempt to manipulate the client but to clarify and emphasize conclusions he or she has already come to but has not expressed clearly, thus indicating that the final synthesis has not been strongly realized. The best method of knowing if such a statement is on target is by the response of the client. If it is positive, the chances are that it fits directly into his or her train of thought. If the client rejects the interpretation, it either does not fit, or the client is not ready to face that particular interpretation.

EXAMPLE

A: My mother is really getting on my nerves. She bugs me all the time about something—my room, homework, practicing piano. She is always telling me what to eat.

C: She won't let you lead your own life.

A: Yeah, that's right.

Confrontation

Confrontation is a very active technique in counseling that again is generally used sparingly. However, if the usual efforts at helping clients come to grips with issues have failed, it may be necessary to point out incongruencies in their discussions or between what they say and how they behave as a way of enabling them to see things more clearly. This can be done objectively in one sentence without accusation or judgment.[9] The most common use in nutritional counseling is with clients who describe how they want to change their eating patterns and then bring up a number of reasons why other things they want get in the way.

EXAMPLE

A: I really want to do it [lose weight] this time. I've got to before spring, but all the foods I like have so many calories, and I don't really have time to exercise.

C: You say you're going to lose weight, but you like only foods that are high in calories. How is that going to work?

Overcoming Time Limitations

For a variety of reasons nutritional counselors may need to overcome the limitations of time in seeing their clients. This will require developing great skill in assessing the client's situation, determining which issues should be the major focus, and counseling effectively within the time available. A knowledge of human behavior in general and of teens in particular will be as important as a basic knowledge of nutrition. Such knowledge will be invaluable in carrying out these processes. The most important point is that goals will have to be set realistically in relation to the amount of time available. It has been pointed out that nutritional counselors should not allow themselves to be put in the position of trying to change long-standing behavior in a one-time inteview.[18] It may be necessary to be very assertive in changing referral patterns if nutritionists find themselves in this position. In situations such as teenage pregnancy, the entire health-care team will have severely limited time because the clients often initiate prenatal care late and because there are a multitude of issues that need attention. As with all teens, they will also tend to miss appointments. Meeting immediate needs will be a function of all team members.

EXAMPLE: During the initial interview, the nutritionist learns that a pregnant teenager and her partner live in a household that resents them to the extent that they do not allow them access to food. A discussion of nourishing foods they can keep in their room or car and eat immediately after buying is the first priority, outweighing other items of clinical protocol.

Ethnic Specificity

Acknowledging ethnic specificity is an important aspect of nutritional counseling because food patterns are so closely aligned with culture.[3] Especially when teenagers have health problems or are pregnant, they may turn to beliefs and customs of their families or of other segments of their society. Nutritional counselors can prepare themselves to some degree by studying various cultural food patterns, but to find out the exact practices of any individual, the counselor will need to explore the subject with the client. The counseling technique is to use prior knowledge of ethnic food practices as background but to make no assumptions about a particular client. In a meaningful dialogue, the counselor gains client-specific information on which to base advice about changing or maintaining established patterns.

EXAMPLE

C: What are the foods you have heard about that a person shouldn't eat when they are pregnant?

Teaching Aids

There is no magic in the use of teaching aids that can eliminate the need for an effective counseling relationship with teenagers, but if such materials are employed properly they can enhance the potency of messages delivered by clinicians. Materials should be designed specifically for the intended audience, using language, graphics, and messages that appeal directly to them.[35]

Items that are suitable for one subgroup of the teenage population may not be suitable for another. Each should be tested in an informal manner if formal evaluation is not possible. Informal evaluation refers to observing the reactions of the adolescents and discussing the materials with them.

A "mediated" experience[36] is probably of most value in the affective area, especially in changing attitudes. An audiovisual presentation can create a mood, provide a model,[37] or set situations in a new perspective. This enables a client to adopt new attitudes in a relatively short period of time, whereas many counseling sessions might be necessary to provide that same new vision. The amount of cognitive material the average adolescent can retain from audiovisual experiences with either print or graphic media will be small. Clear, concise messages presented interestingly will be most effective. The amount of information should be limited to enhance learning. Supportive counseling will be necessary in follow-up sessions to reinforce messages presented and to use these messages to facilitate behavior change.

Hands-On Experience

As has been pointed out many times, teens are usually action-oriented people. Therefore opportunities for them to try something rather than simply talking about it can be very effective learning experiences for them. It thus is worth the time it takes from the busy schedule to plan hands-on experiences. Using recipes, learning measurement, trying new foods, and engaging in various forms of exercise are good examples. "Keep things moving" is a useful rule with most teens. Sharing a meal would be especially appropriate in a pregnancy, diabetic, or other specialized clinic. There are many ways this can be organized: a breakfast group before clinic, a lunch group, or a group during break. The nutritionist can provide the food, introduce some new foods, or use supplemental foods. Patients can be responsible from time to time for planning, preparing, or bringing food. Valuable new experiences can be built into such a setting when sociability, food preparation, and discussion of nutrient content of the food are emphasized.

Role Playing

Role playing can also be helpful. Practicing assertiveness or social skills with a counselor can increase an adolescent's confidence in using the techniques in real-life situations. In a program for pregnant adolescents, role playing has been used as an active teaching device.[38] Teens may trade places with the nutritionist, solidifying their knowledge of nourishing behaviors in pregnancy by counseling a "patient." Making food choices, dealing with physical complaints such as nausea, selecting foods from an array when "shopping," and being assertive in obtaining food through an agency or relative are topics that would fit well into a role-playing format.

Demonstration-experience is a variation on role-playing. In this case a new food is prepared by the nutritionist with teens assisting and eventually demonstrating for others.

Groups

Meeting in groups with several adolescents at one time to discuss nutrition is one way to save some valuable time in the clinical setting. Group meetings are appealing because support can develop among members that can prove effective in helping them to upgrade the care they take of themselves. Indeed, if this is the only way a teen will have access to nutritional care, groups or classes should be organized. There are limitations in the kind of material that can be presented in the group setting, and it will be of a more general nature than the material used in individualized counseling. Groups thus should not be substituted for individual sessions when they can be provided.

Groups will need to be led by professionals who have had experience with group process, especially when discussion among the participants is part of the experience. Guiding discussions to assure that they are a learning experience requires skill, as the most vocal persons in the group may be the least dependable in terms of the knowledge they possess and the stability of their personalities. Under the right conditions, the group can be an important teaching tool by which to reach adolescents with nutrition messages.

Home Visits

Certain programs serving teens regularly plan home visits to their clients. Home visits demonstrate real concern on the part of professionals who will make the effort to get out of their own environment and into that of the client. The professional can learn more about the client, the facilities available, the responsibility the client takes for controlling his or her environment, and the style of life he or she leads. On the other hand, the home visit will not be welcomed by every client. Some will consider it intrusive and resist efforts on the part of the professional to visit them at home. The relationship between professional and client that allows for home visits generally will be effective because the visits are evidence of a mutual trust.

Counseling Termination

The termination of a counseling relationship requires a specialized sense of timing. The patient will need to be prepared far ahead of the final visit.[9,31] The preparation should fit the needs of the client. There are a number of reasons why termination may be necessary other than having reached a time when all goals related to a change in food habits have been met. Lack of further monetary resources and the client's moving or leaving a hospital setting are possible factors. For whatever reason, the client will now have to continue alone without the support of the counselor. Termination should allow the client time to discuss this in advance and experience the separation gradually. Many times the counselor will want to leave the way open for further appropriate contact or make a referral to another professional if the client should need counseling in the future.[9]

HEALTH-CARE TEAM

Adolescent health care is one of the most demanding of clinical problems. As such, it fits into

Table 10-1. Suggested members of health-care team to guide adolescents in issues arising in pregnancy

Issues	Discipline					
	Obstetrician	Adolescent Medical Specialist	Nurse	Nutritionist	Social Worker	Psychologist
General health and planning of continuous care		X	X	X		
Complications of pregnancy	X	X	X	X		
Labor and delivery preparation	X	X	X			
School program					X	X
Economic resources			X		X	
Substance abuse (cessation and education)		X	X	X	X	X
Psychological adjustment and stress	X	X	X	X	X	X
Developmental delay			X		X	X
Infant-care education		X	X	X		
Relinquishment counseling			X		X	X
Nutritional care		X	X	X		
Education		X	X	X		
Resource coordination			X	X	X	
Family or marital conflict					X	X

the category of situations best handled as a team effort. Any one professional will generally not possess the skill to meet all the patient's needs. For example, Table 10-1 lists some of the types of issues that will arise throughout the course of teenage pregnancies with a suggested list of professionals to guide the patient in managing those issues. This does not mean that certain problems are the responsibility of any one profession to the exclusion of others. Each professional can support the messages and guidance provided by others. Conferences where patient care is discussed by the team will aid in the coordination of care and increase the efficiency of the team in keeping abreast of the patient's progress in relation to various problems. Nutritionists and professionals who are in positions to influence program planning will do well to support the concept of development of clinical teams to care for adolescents.

Work with a team requires specialized skill.[39,40]

Team members bring their backgrounds, both professional and personal, with them. Fig. 10-2 depicts the various attributes of the individual professional that determine how that person will carry out a role on a team. The structure of the team, which may be any one of those in Fig. 10-3, will affect their work in a very basic fashion. Structure determines communication patterns between professionals and between professionals and clients.[41] Interrelationships between team members are complex and must be carefully developed by clinicians who are highly motivated to work together. The reward will be seen in improved comprehensive care for clients with complex problems.

DEVELOPING SKILL IN COUNSELING

A counselor's background, including race, sex, and socioeconomic status, will better prepare him or her for relationships with certain people than

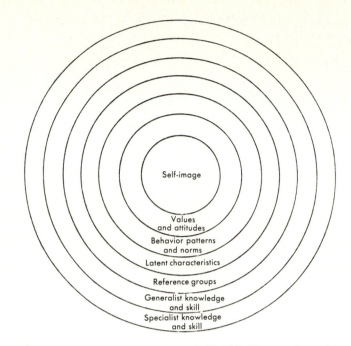

Self-image

Values
and attitudes

Behavior patterns
and norms

Latent characteristics

Reference groups

Generalist knowledge
and skill

Specialist knowledge
and skill

Fig. 10-2. Cross section of a team member. (From Brill, N.I.: Teamwork: working together in the human services, Philadelphia, 1976, J.B. Lippincott Co.)

others.[14,31] To serve a broader group of clients, counselors will need to increase their knowledge of people outside of their own particular circles. With more experience they will be able to form effective relationships with a greater variety of people.

For counselors who will serve adolescents, it is important to remember that they will bring their feelings about this turbulent stage in their own lives as a background to their work.[12] If, for example, they experienced a weight problem during adolescence, they will probably have very strong feelings related to the weight concerns of their clients. It is important to face such feelings and control the influence they have on a counseling relationship. Backgrounds can lead to understanding and empathy but should not lead to prejudice and intrusion.[13] Related to a weight-management problem, if the counselor "dealt with it by strong will-power," he or she must overcome any impatience with clients who are not as strong or the urge to

superimpose a "tower-of-strength" style on an adolescent for whom that style does not fit. The more self-awareness the counselor has, the more able he or she will be to overcome any personal problems or background that could interfere with a counseling relationship. Health-care professionals must often overcome a lack of training in counseling techniques. When they find themselves in situations demanding such skills, they will need to plan self-improvement. Some of the common pitfalls that indicate a need for improved skills are listed below:

Setting inappropriate goals

Communicating in overly authoritarian style

Losing the client's attention

Being deterred by the client's defenses

Losing control and therefore losing credibility

Being confused over the direction counseling
    should take

Failing to treat the client as an individual

Structure	Communication pathways	Best serves

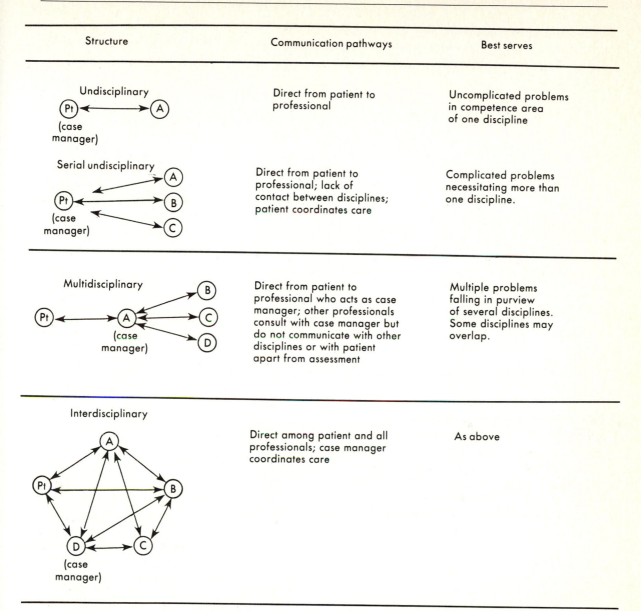

Structure	Communication pathways	Best serves
Undisciplinary	Direct from patient to professional	Uncomplicated problems in competence area of one discipline
Serial undisciplinary	Direct from patient to professional; lack of contact between disciplines; patient coordinates care	Complicated problems necessitating more than one discipline.
Multidisciplinary	Direct from patient to professional who acts as case manager; other professionals consult with case manager but do not communicate with other disciplines or with patient apart from assessment	Multiple problems falling in purview of several disciplines. Some disciplines may overlap.
Interdisciplinary	Direct among patient and all professionals; case manager coordinates care	As above

Fig. 10-3. Structure of health-care teams. *Pt,* Patient. *A, B, C, D,* Health-care specialists of various disciplines.

By constantly improving skills, a counselor will be more effective in a greater variety of settings. Resources for improving counseling skills are listed below:

Classes[42]
Workshops[33]
Experience[33]
Observation of others[33]
Working with other disciplines[33]
Reading[32]
Self-monitoring
   Video or audio[43]
   Client surveys[44]
Feedback from colleagues[6]
Assessing clinical outcome[45]
Self-assessment[46]

SUMMARY

In the field of nutrition a body of knowledge has accumulated relating to the physiological aspects of nutritional problems. However, apart from acute care in a hospital setting, nutritionists cannot "treat the client" to improve a physiological state. Nutritional care depends on providing information appropriate to a specific situation and in most cases on facilitating the client's use of it. This often requires that the client change long-standing behavior patterns. Adolescents will generally not be able to change their behavior until the reasons for the original adoption of those behaviors have changed. Studying problems, exploring alternative ways to conceptualize and deal with situations, solving problems, learning about communication, and forming relationships are necessary components of counseling directed toward enabling teenagers to make lasting changes that will improve their nutritional health. To accomplish these goals, nutritional counselors must make sophisticated use of counseling techniques developed in the social sciences. Herein lies the challenge of nutritional counseling: the requirement that techniques related to both the physiological and psychological aspects of life be used.

REFERENCES

1. Wardlaw, J.M.: Preparing the nutrition education professional for the 1980's, J. Nutr. Educ. **13**:6, 1981.
2. Olson, C.M., and Gillespie, A.H.: Proceedings of the workshop on nutrition education research: introduction, J. Nutr. Educ. **13**(suppl. 1):1, 1981.
3. Hammar, S.L.: The role of the nutritionist in an adolescent clinic, Children **13**:217, 1966.
4. Silber, T.J.: Physician–adolescent patient relationship, Clin. Pediatr. **19**:50, 1980.
5. Daniel, W.A.: Adolescents in health and disease, St. Louis, 1977, The C.V. Mosby Co.
6. Bjorksten, O.J.: Basic principles of counseling for the physician. In Kreutner, A.K., and Hollingsworth, D.R., editors: Adolescent obstetrics and gynecology, Chicago, 1978, Year Book Medical Publishers, Inc.
7. De Schweinitz, E., and De Schweinitz, K.: Interviewing in the social services, London, 1962, National Council of Social Services.
8. Rogers, C.R.: A counseling approach to human problems, Am. J. Nurs. **56**:994, 1956.
9. Hackney, H., and Cormier, L.S.: Counseling strategies and objectives, Englewood Cliffs, N.J., 1979, Prentice-Hall, Inc.
10. MacKinnon, R.A., and Michels, R.: The psychiatric interview in clinical practice, Philadelphia, 1971, W.B. Saunders Co.
11. Igoe, J.B.: Health counseling and teaching. In Howe, J., editor: Nursing care of adolescents, New York, 1980, McGraw-Hill Book Co.
12. Luckey, E.B., and Rich, J.: The counseling process and the counselor. In Semmens, J.P., and Krantz, K.E., editors: The adolescent experience: a counseling guide to social and sexual behavior, New York, 1970, Macmillan Publishing Co., Inc.
13. May, R.: The art of counseling, Nashville, Tenn., 1977, Abingdon Press.
14. Hammar, S.L., and Holterman, V.: Interviewing and counseling adolescent patients, Clin. Pediatr. **9**:47, 1970.
15. Smith, M.S.: An approach to the adolescent for the primary care physician, J. Fam. Pract. **8**:63, 1979.
16. Kimball, A.J., and Campbell, M.M.: Psychologic aspects of adolescent patient health care, Clin. Pediatr. **18**:15, 1979.
17. Hammar, S.L., Campbell, M.M., and Huffine, C.W.: Measures of adolescent anxiety responses to medical examinations, Adolescence **3**:161, 1968.
18. Zifferblatt, S.M., and Wilbur, C.S.: Dietary counseling: some realistic expectations and guidelines, J. Am. Diet. Assoc. **70**:591, 1977.
19. Frankle, R.T., and others: The door: a center of alternatives—the nutritionist in a free clinic for adolescents, J. Am. Diet. Assoc. **63**:269, 1973.

20. Maier, H.W.: Three theories of child development, New York, 1978, Harper & Row, Publishers, Inc.

21. Nowicki, S., and Strickland, B.R.: A locus of control scale for children, J. Consult. Clin. Psychol. **40:**148, 1973.

22. Wright, L.: Assessing the psychosomatic status children, J. Clin. Child Psychol. p. 94, Summer 1978.

23. McNutt, K.W., and Steinberg, L.H.: Persons with diet-related diseases, J. Nutr. Educ. **12**(suppl. 1):131, 1980.

24. Sears, R.R.: A theoretical framework for personality and social behavior, Am. Psychol. **6:**476, 1951.

25. Alexander, J.K.: What can nutrition educators learn from communication theories? J. Nutr. Educ. **13**(suppl. 1):27, 1981.

26. Coates, T.J.: Eating: a psychological dilemma, J. Nutr. Educ. **13**(suppl. 1):34, 1981.

27. Deibert, A.N., and Harmon, A.J.: New tools for changing behavior, Champaign, Ill., 1973, Research Press.

28. Hochbaum, G.M.: Strategies and their rationale for changing people's eating habits, J. Nutr. Educ. **13**(suppl. 1):59, 1981.

29. Wilson, G.T.: Behavior modification and the treatment of obesity. In Stunkard, A.J., editor: Obesity, Philadelphia, 1980, W.B. Saunders Co.

30. Gross, A.M., and Johnson, W.G.: The diabetes assertiveness test: a measure of social coping skills in pre-adolescent diabetics, Diabetes Educ. p. 26, Summer 1981.

31. Weiner, I.B.: Individual psychotherapy. In Weiner, I.B., editor: Clinical methods in psychology, New York, 1976, John Wiley & Sons, Inc.

32. Bruch, H.: Learning psychotherapy, Cambridge, Mass., 1974, Harvard University Press.

33. Zaro, J.S., and others: A guide for beginning psychotherapists, New York, 1979, Cambridge University Press.

34. Eggert, L.L.: The therapeutic process with adolescents experiencing psychosocial stress. In Longo, D., and Williams, R., editors: Clinical practice in psychosocial nursing: assessment and intervention, New York, 1977, Appleton-Century-Crofts.

35. Rees, J.M., and Worthington-Roberts, B.S.: Establishing a nutritional environment supportive of reproduction: nutrition education issues. In Worthington-Roberts, B.S., Vermeersch, J., and Williams, S.R., editors: Nutrition in pregnancy and lactation, ed. 2, St. Louis, 1981, The C.V. Mosby Co.

36. Simonson, M.: Liking and learning go hand in hand, Audiovisual Instruction p. 18, March 1978.

37. Wager, W.: Media selection in the affective domain: a further interpretation of Dale's cone of experience for cognitive and affective learning, Educ. Tech. p. 9, July 1975.

38. Pawlik, D., and Barkoukis, H.: Adolescent obstetric clinics, Nutr. News **41:**6, 1978.

39. Brill, N.I.: Teamwork: working together in the human services, Philadelphia, 1976, J.B. Lippincott Co.

40. Ducanis, A.J., and Golin, A.K.: The interdisciplinary health care team: a handbook, Germantown, Md., 1979, Aspen Systems Corp.

41. Leconte, J., and Rees, J.M.: Interdisciplinary team function: a model for training, Unpublished paper, Seattle, 1983, University of Washington.

42. Morgan, M.K., and Irby, D.M.: Evaluating clinical competence in the health professions, St. Louis, 1978, The C.V. Mosby Co.

43. Danish, S.J., and others: The anatomy of a dietetic counseling interview, J. Am. Diet. Assoc. **75:**626, 1979.

44. Campbell, M.M., and Flewelling, R.: Patient evaluation of an interdisciplinary adolescent clinic, Unpublished paper, Seattle, 1978, University of Washington.

45. Kaufman, M., editor: Preliminary guide to quality assurance in ambulatory nutrition care, Rockville, Md., 1981, Department of Health and Human Services.

46. Fuhrmann, B.S., and Weissbeurg, M.J.: Self-assessment. In Morgan, M.K., and Irby, D.N., editors: Evaluating clinical competence in the health professions, St. Louis, 1978, The C.V. Mosby Co.

Appendix A

Table A-1. Prediction of adult height using skeletal age*

Directions

1. Obtain skeletal age by wrist x-ray using the standards of Greulich & Pyle**
2. Find x for equation in table under skeletal age, using:
   Row A if skeletal age is within 1 year of chronological age;
   Row B if skeletal age is 1-2 years below chronological age, and
   Row C if skeletal age is 1-2 years advanced beyond chronological age.
3. Solve equation:

$$\text{Adult height} = \frac{\text{present height}}{x}$$

Skeletal Age	9-0	9-3	9-6	9-9	10-0	10-3	10-6	10-9	11-0	11-3	11-6	11-9	12-0	12-3	12-6	12-9	13-0	13-3	13-6	13-9
Males A.	.752	.761	.769	.777	.784	.791	.795	.800	.804	.812	.818	.827	.834	.843	.853	.863	.876	.890	.902	.914
Males B.	.786	.794	.800	.807	.812	.816	.819	.821	.823	.827	.832	.839	.845	.852	.860	.869	.880	—	—	—
Males C.	.720	.728	.734	.741	.747	.753	.758	.763	.767	.776	.786	.800	.809	.818	.828	.839	.850	.863	.875	.890
Females A.	.827	.836	.844	.853	.862	.874	.884	.896	.906	.910	.914	.918	.922	.932	.941	.950	.958	.967	.974	.978
Females B.	.841	.851	.858	.866	.874	.884	.896	.907	.918	.922	.926	.929	.932	.942	.949	.957	.964	.971	.977	.981
Females C.	.790	.800	.809	.819	.828	.841	.856	.870	.883	.887	.891	.897	.901	.913	.924	.935	.945	.955	.963	.968

Skeletal Age	14-0	14-3	14-6	14-9	15-0	15-3	15-6	15-9	16-0	16-3	16-6	16-9	17-0	17-3	17-6	17-9	18-0	18-3	18-6
Males A.	.927	.938	.948	.958	.968	.973	.976	.980	.982	.985	.987	.989	.991	.993	.994	.995	.996	.998	1.0
Males B.	—	—	—	—	—	—	—	—	—	—	—	—	—	—	—	—	—	—	—
Males C.	.905	.918	.930	.943	.958	.967	.971	.976	.980	.983	.985	.988	.990	—	—	—	—	—	—
Females A.	.980	.983	.986	.988	.990	.991	.993	.994	.996	.996	.997	.998	.999	.999	1.0				
Females B.	.983	.986	.989	.992	.994	.995	.996	.997	.998	.999	.999	.999	1.0						
Females C.	.972	.977	.980	.983	.986	.988	.990	.992	.993	.994	.995	.997	.998	.999	.999				

From Friedman, I.M. and Goldberg, E.: Pediatr. Clin. North Am. 27:193, 1980.
*Modified from Bayley, N., and Pinneau, S.R.: Tables for predicting adult height from skeletal age: Revised for use with the Greulich-Pyle hand standards. J. Pediat. 40:423-441, 1952.
**Greulich, W.W., and Pyle, S.I.: Radiographic atlas of skeletal development of the hand and wrist. Stanford, Calif., Stanford University Press, 1950.

Appendix B

Courtesy of Ross Laboratories, Columbus, Ohio.

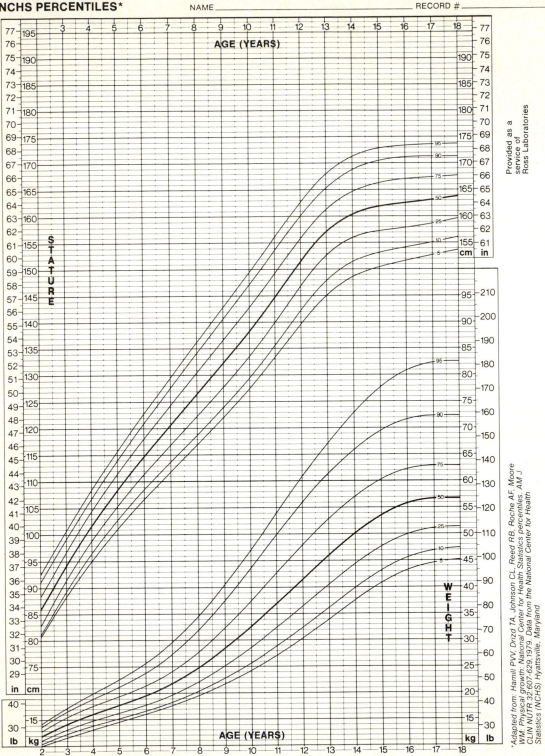

Provided as a
service of
Ross Laboratories

*Adapted from: Hamill PVV, Drizd TA, Johnson CL, Reed RB, Roche AF, Moore WM. Physical growth: National Center for Health Statistics percentiles. AM J CLIN NUTR 32:607-629,1979. Data from the National Center for Health Statistics (NCHS) Hyattsville, Maryland

© 1980 ROSS LABORATORIES

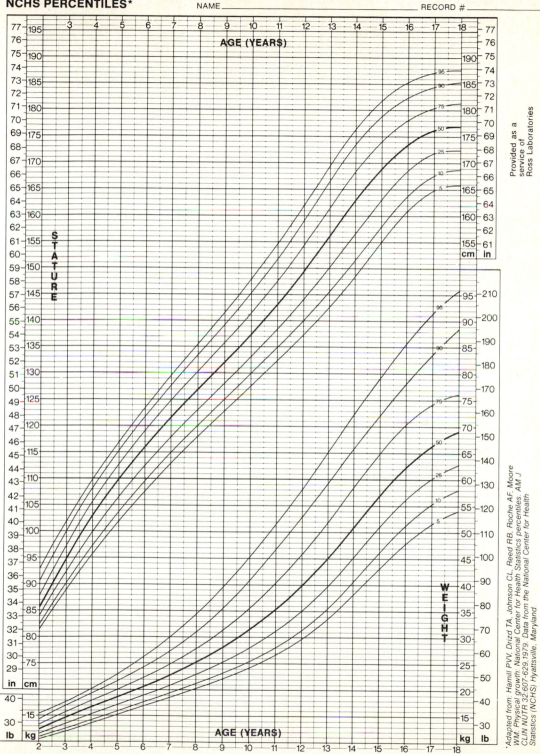

AGE (YEARS)

STATURE

AGE (YEARS)

WEIGHT

Provided as a
service of
Ross Laboratories

*Adapted from: Hamill PVV, Drizd TA, Johnson CL, Reed RB, Roche AF, Moore
WM. Physical growth: National Center for Health Statistics percentiles. AM J
CLIN NUTR 32:607-629,1979. Data from the National Center for Health
Statistics (NCHS) Hyattsville, Maryland

© 1980 ROSS LABORATORIES

Appendix C

Table C-1. Height in centimeters of youths aged 12-18 years by sex and quarter-year age group: average age, sample size, estimated population size, mean, standard deviation, standard error of the mean, and selected percentiles, United States, 1966-70

Sex and Age	Aver-age Age	n	N	$\overline{X}$	s	$s_{\overline{x}}$	5th	10th	25th	50th	75th	90th	95th
Male							**In Centimeters**						
12 years	12.10	43	144	151.1	8.18	1.44	138.6	141.2	146.1	150.5	153.9	159.9	163.8
12 1/4 years	12.24	150	465	150.2	7.87	0.65	138.3	140.1	144.1	149.5	155.9	161.0	162.7
12 1/2 years	12.50	187	577	151.5	8.33	0.87	138.0	140.4	145.9	152.6	156.8	161.2	165.1
12 3/4 years	12.76	184	589	154.3	7.48	0.62	142.3	146.1	149.6	153.7	158.0	164.4	167.6
13 years	12.99	165	520	154.7	9.37	0.67	136.9	143.0	148.1	155.4	161.4	166.6	170.3
13 1/4 years	13.25	154	511	158.9	8.55	0.82	146.2	148.5	153.0	157.8	164.9	171.1	174.4
13 1/2 years	13.49	162	524	159.7	9.11	1.06	144.7	148.2	153.3	158.8	165.3	173.2	176.1
13 3/4 years	13.75	158	478	161.4	8.44	0.68	148.1	149.9	155.8	161.8	167.5	173.1	174.6
14 years	14.00	135	465	164.0	7.90	0.69	151.4	153.2	157.8	164.2	169.8	173.6	177.0
14 1/4 years	14.26	159	503	165.4	10.01	1.15	148.5	152.5	157.9	165.1	172.7	178.5	182.1
14 1/2 years	14.50	155	487	167.5	7.96	0.79	153.5	156.6	161.5	169.4	173.0	176.5	178.7
14 3/4 years	14.76	151	467	167.1	8.46	0.99	152.7	155.2	162.3	167.7	173.5	176.5	180.8
15 years	15.00	155	489	169.4	7.59	0.59	156.3	158.7	163.7	169.4	174.8	178.1	181.4
15 1/4 years	15.25	169	511	171.4	7.57	0.62	159.2	160.8	166.5	171.7	176.5	180.5	183.1
15 1/2 years	15.50	159	493	171.2	6.89	0.43	159.8	162.8	166.8	171.2	174.7	179.5	185.0
15 3/4 years	15.75	150	461	171.9	7.04	0.70	159.1	163.9	167.6	172.6	176.1	181.0	183.0
16 years	16.01	134	456	172.9	6.13	0.53	161.5	164.5	170.1	173.7	177.0	179.6	181.3
16 1/4 years	16.24	157	541	174.5	7.33	0.82	162.4	163.9	170.4	175.1	178.8	184.0	186.5
16 1/2 years	16.50	135	413	174.3	6.56	0.44	165.1	166.8	170.5	173.9	178.4	182.4	184.5
16 3/4 years	16.75	122	401	174.7	6.78	0.66	164.6	166.1	169.8	174.4	179.6	183.1	185.4
17 years	17.00	136	479	175.1	6.94	0.61	163.2	166.4	170.5	175.6	179.7	183.7	186.3
17 1/4 years	17.26	125	435	176.4	6.97	0.71	162.6	167.5	172.1	176.7	181.3	184.3	188.0
17 1/2 years	17.50	111	396	175.4	7.15	0.89	162.9	165.8	170.3	175.2	180.1	185.4	187.8
17 3/4 years	17.75	113	409	175.1	7.32	0.77	162.7	167.2	170.3	175.3	179.7	184.7	189.3
18 years	17.97	76	275	176.0	6.46	0.63	165.7	167.3	171.3	175.8	180.4	185.3	186.4

From National Center for Health Statistics: Height and weight of youths 12-17 years, United States. In Vital and health statistics, series 11, no. 124, Health Services and Mental Health Administration, Washington, D.C., 1973, U.S. Government Printing Office. NOTE: n = sample size; N = estimated number of youths in population in thousands; $\overline{X}$ = mean; s = standard deviation; $s_{\overline{x}}$ = standard error of the mean.

Sex and Age	Average Age	n	N	$\overline{X}$	s	$s_{\overline{x}}$	Percentile						
							5th	10th	25th	50th	75th	90th	95th
Female							In Centimeters						
12 years	12.10	42	153	154.5	7.05	1.38	142.2	145.9	150.8	153.8	157.3	167.0	167.9
12 1/4 years	12.27	142	520	153.8	7.20	0.64	141.0	143.6	149.5	153.9	158.5	162.5	165.6
12 1/2 years	12.50	140	511	155.6	7.69	0.60	141.8	145.4	151.7	155.5	160.4	164.6	168.3
12 3/4 years	12.75	147	517	156.0	6.82	0.57	143.6	147.5	151.8	156.3	160.5	164.5	166.6
13 years	13.01	166	578	157.1	7.30	0.43	143.8	148.3	152.5	157.3	162.7	166.7	169.2
13 1/4 years	13.25	144	461	158.1	7.54	0.73	145.3	146.8	152.6	158.6	163.4	167.7	169.5
13 1/2 years	13.50	146	500	159.2	6.08	0.42	149.6	152.1	155.2	158.8	163.3	167.7	170.2
13 3/4 years	13.76	148	499	159.3	6.67	0.56	147.5	149.5	155.2	159.9	164.2	167.5	169.4
14 years	14.01	138	452	159.8	6.59	0.53	149.1	151.5	155.9	160.3	164.1	167.2	170.5
14 1/4 years	14.25	159	510	161.3	6.00	0.62	150.8	153.4	157.6	161.2	164.7	168.4	170.8
14 1/2 years	14.51	137	415	161.2	6.66	0.63	150.3	152.6	157.1	161.2	165.4	170.3	172.2
14 3/4 years	14.76	130	457	162.5	6.43	0.69	153.6	154.7	157.7	162.9	167.2	170.0	174.1
15 years	14.99	133	449	161.3	5.73	0.53	151.7	154.6	157.5	160.7	164.8	169.4	171.4
15 1/4 years	15.25	135	479	162.2	6.68	0.58	151.3	153.2	157.3	163.2	166.7	170.3	171.8
15 1/2 years	15.51	114	433	161.8	7.27	0.92	151.8	153.2	156.4	161.3	167.4	171.1	173.5
15 3/4 years	15.75	136	526	162.9	7.19	0.84	150.8	152.8	158.1	163.3	167.8	170.7	175.1
16 years	16.01	141	474	161.9	6.38	0.71	152.4	153.6	157.5	161.6	166.6	169.8	172.2
16 1/4 years	16.24	138	491	163.6	6.17	0.51	152.7	155.8	160.2	164.8	166.8	170.7	173.6
16 1/2 years	16.50	112	341	161.5	6.51	0.70	151.3	153.0	157.2	161.8	166.1	170.2	172.2
16 3/4 years	16.76	135	450	162.9	6.52	0.52	151.5	154.0	158.6	162.8	167.3	171.7	173.0
17 years	17.00	135	477	163.0	6.48	0.71	151.5	154.5	158.9	163.4	167.0	171.1	173.3
17 1/4 years	17.24	125	461	162.7	6.62	0.52	151.5	153.8	157.8	164.2	166.9	171.3	173.6
17 1/2 years	17.51	111	415	162.9	6.02	0.59	152.7	155.7	158.4	162.6	168.1	171.4	172.8
17 3/4 years	17.75	90	325	162.9	5.90	0.87	152.4	154.4	158.3	163.1	167.4	169.9	171.7
18 years	17.97	79	306	163.0	6.77	0.74	152.5	154.6	158.2	162.5	167.6	171.4	175.3

Appendix D

Table D-1. Weight in kilograms of youths aged 12 years at last birthday by sex and height group in centimeters; sample size, estimated population size, mean, standard deviation, standard error of the mean, and selected percentiles, United States, 1966-70

Sex and Height	n	N	$\overline{X}$	s	$s_{\overline{x}}$	Percentile 5th	10th	25th	50th	75th	90th	95th
Male						In Kilograms						
Under 130 cm	5	15	*	*	*	*	*	*	*	*	*	*
130.0-134.9 cm	4	8	*	*	*	*	*	*	*	*	*	*
135.0-139.9 cm	34	111	32.50	3.741	0.727	26.6	27.6	30.2	31.6	34.7	37.7	39.4
140.0-144.9 cm	80	241	34.28	3.635	0.601	28.1	30.0	31.8	34.1	36.5	38.6	40.7
145.0-149.9 cm	123	386	39.27	6.243	0.615	32.1	33.2	35.7	38.2	40.9	46.1	52.5
150.0-154.9 cm	156	513	42.90	6.314	0.480	34.9	36.1	38.2	42.1	46.0	51.6	56.3
155.0-159.9 cm	135	432	47.35	7.551	0.769	38.3	39.4	41.9	46.2	50.5	57.4	61.9
160.0-164.9 cm	65	201	50.82	8.735	1.388	42.1	42.7	44.9	48.4	56.0	61.1	67.1
165.0-169.9 cm	29	88	55.75	8.811	2.031	43.3	46.4	49.0	54.4	59.9	68.3	76.6
170.0-174.9 cm	8	21	62.37	4.503	1.993	54.0	58.1	60.1	61.0	66.0	69.1	69.5
175.0-179.9 cm	3	10	*	*	*	*	*	*	*	*	*	*
180.0-184.9 cm	1	2	*	*	*	*	*	*	*	*	*	*
185.0-189.9 cm	—	—	—	—	—	—	—	—	—	—	—	—
190.0-194.9 cm	—	—	—	—	—	—	—	—	—	—	—	—
195.0 cm. and over	—	—	—	—	—	—	—	—	—	—	—	—

NOTE: n = sample size; N = estimated number of youths in population in thousands; $\overline{X}$ = mean; s = standard deviation; $s_{\overline{x}}$ = standard error of the mean.

From National Center for Health Statistics: Height and weight of youths 12-17 years, United States. In Vital and health statistics, series 11, no. 124, Health Services and Mental Health Administration, Washington, D.C., 1973, U.S. Government Printing Office.

Sex and Height	n	N	$\overline{X}$	s	$s_{\overline{x}}$	Percentile						
						5th	10th	25th	50th	75th	90th	95th
Female								In Kilograms				
Under 130 cm	—	—	—	—	—	—	—	—	—	—	—	—
130.0-134.9 cm	3	10	*	*	*	*	*	*	*	*	*	*
135.0-139.9 cm	12	44	29.41	3.372	0.914	25.0	25.0	26.4	28.9	32.1	34.1	34.2
140.0-144.9 cm	32	116	38.30	7.314	1.194	28.8	30.6	33.3	36.8	41.4	49.2	55.1
145.0-149.9 cm	72	258	39.78	6.205	0.975	31.8	32.8	35.5	38.5	42.8	48.3	50.6
150.0-154.9 cm	147	517	44.00	7.421	0.677	34.4	35.8	38.9	42.8	47.4	52.9	57.4
155.0-159.9 cm	144	525	48.74	8.369	0.714	37.9	39.2	43.0	46.8	53.8	60.7	63.5
160.0-164.9 cm	95	336	53.06	8.010	0.658	42.5	43.9	47.2	51.1	57.2	65.6	69.6
165.0-169.9 cm	31	117	54.89	7.022	1.384	43.9	47.1	50.4	53.1	59.7	64.5	71.3
170.0-174.9 cm	11	42	63.66	14.501	6.214	48.7	50.1	50.8	56.7	82.2	86.0	86.1
175.0-179.9 cm	—	—	—	—	—	—	—	—	—	—	—	—
180.0-184.9 cm	—	—	—	—	—	—	—	—	—	—	—	—
185.0-189.9 cm	—	—	—	—	—	—	—	—	—	—	—	—
190.0-194.9 cm	—	—	—	—	—	—	—	—	—	—	—	—
195.0 cm. and over	—	—	—	—	—	—	—	—	—	—	—	—

Table D-2. Weight in kilograms of youths aged 13 years at last birthday by sex and height group in centimeters: sample size, estimated population size, mean, standard deviation, standard error of the mean, and selected percentiles, United States, 1966-70

Sex and Height	n	N	$\overline{X}$	s	$s_{\overline{x}}$	Percentile						
						5th	10th	25th	50th	75th	90th	95th
Male						In Kilograms						
Under 130 cm	—	—	—	—	—	—	—	—	—	—	—	—
130.0-134.9 cm	2	5	*	*	*	*	*	*	*	*	*	*
135.0-139.9 cm	6	25	32.62	5.624	7.716	27.2	27.6	28.9	31.0	34.9	43.1	43.2
140.0-144.9 cm	18	56	36.54	5.852	1.607	30.0	30.5	32.1	36.1	39.2	41.7	53.2
145.0-149.9 cm	65	204	39.03	5.270	0.662	32.4	33.9	36.1	37.9	41.2	44.5	46.4
150.0-154.9 cm	99	312	42.58	6.724	0.865	34.8	36.2	37.9	41.0	45.5	49.4	61.0
155.0-159.9 cm	131	421	47.27	7.482	0.717	37.8	39.2	41.7	45.8	51.1	58.7	61.7
160.0-164.9 cm	125	393	53.01	9.324	0.916	41.5	43.7	46.9	50.4	58.2	64.4	72.5
165.0-169.9 cm	91	285	55.92	8.560	0.833	46.3	47.5	49.3	53.6	59.4	69.0	75.0
170.0-174.9 cm	63	215	62.01	10.362	1.033	51.2	51.6	53.7	60.1	67.0	76.0	85.0
175.0-179.9 cm	19	68	67.92	12.085	3.428	56.3	57.9	60.1	63.3	70.3	88.3	89.0
180.0-184.9 cm	5	15	*	*	*	*	*	*	*	*	*	*
185.0-189.9 cm	—	—	—	—	—	—	—	—	—	—	—	—
190.0-194.9 cm	—	—	—	—	—	—	—	—	—	—	—	—
195.0 cm. and over	—	—	—	—	—	—	—	—	—	—	—	—
Female												
Under 130 cm	—	—	—	—	—	—	—	—	—	—	—	—
130.0-134.9 cm	1	3	*	*	*	*	*	*	*	*	*	*
135.0-139.9 cm	—	—	—	—	—	—	—	—	—	—	—	—
140.0-144.9 cm	15	51	37.13	7.317	2.259	26.6	27.5	30.5	36.7	40.1	44.5	56.1
145.0-149.9 cm	47	165	42.23	6.880	0.888	34.7	35.6	38.2	40.5	44.2	53.6	57.6
150.0-154.9 cm	98	329	44.32	7.029	0.787	35.6	36.5	39.2	42.9	47.3	53.7	57.9
155.0-159.9 cm	152	499	49.75	8.757	0.699	39.1	39.9	43.8	48.4	53.8	61.0	65.9
160.0-164.9 cm	156	515	53.16	8.399	0.522	41.2	43.9	47.7	52.2	57.0	63.8	68.5
165.0-169.9 cm	86	284	58.17	9.125	0.921	46.2	47.4	52.2	58.1	61.5	69.3	76.2
170.0-174.9 cm	24	87	58.11	13.209	2.343	46.2	47.1	48.4	52.9	65.3	68.6	96.8
175.0-179.9 cm	3	10	*	*	*	*	*	*	*	*	*	*
180.0-184.9 cm	—	—	—	—	—	—	—	—	—	—	—	—
185.0-189.9 cm	—	—	—	—	—	—	—	—	—	—	—	—
190.0-194.9 cm	—	—	—	—	—	—	—	—	—	—	—	—
195.0 cm. and over	—	—	—	—	—	—	—	—	—	—	—	—

NOTE: n = sample size; N = estimated number of youths in population in thousands; $\overline{X}$ = mean; s = standard deviation; $s_{\overline{x}}$ = standard error of the mean.

Table D-3. Weight in kilograms of youths aged 14 years at last birthday by sex and height group in centimeters: sample size, estimated population size, mean, standard deviation, standard error of the mean, and selected percentiles, United States, 1966-70

Sex and Height	n	N	$\overline{X}$	s	$s_{\overline{x}}$	Percentile						
						5th	10th	25th	50th	75th	90th	95th
Male								In Kilograms				
Under 130 cm	—	—	—	—	—	—	—	—	—	—	—	—
130.0-134.9 cm	—	—	—	—	—	—	—	—	—	—	—	—
135.0-139.9 cm	2	7	*	*	*	*	*	*	*	*	*	*
140.0-144.9 cm	3	13	*	*	*	*	*	*	*	*	*	*
145.0-149.9 cm	11	42	40.51	1.829	0.644	36.9	38.6	39.6	40.6	42.0	42.5	42.7
150.0-154.9 cm	45	135	43.63	6.277	1.182	36.2	37.0	39.0	41.4	48.0	51.7	55.3
155.0-159.9 cm	83	261	47.42	7.822	0.872	37.7	38.7	41.8	46.1	51.2	58.0	62.7
160.0-164.9 cm	96	299	52.28	6.785	0.584	42.5	44.0	47.5	52.1	56.3	61.5	65.1
165.0-169.9 cm	134	432	58.07	9.416	1.054	47.7	49.3	51.6	55.4	62.3	70.6	75.7
170.0-174.9 cm	144	435	62.37	11.516	1.095	49.7	51.0	55.0	59.4	65.6	79.2	86.3
175.0-179.9 cm	71	228	65.54	9.704	1.306	50.9	55.1	58.5	64.7	69.9	74.5	84.0
180.0-184.9 cm	25	81	72.44	13.014	2.298	59.6	60.0	65.1	69.4	77.0	83.0	94.3
185.0-189.9 cm	3	9	*	*	*	*	*	*	*	*	*	*
190.0-194.9 cm	1	3	*	*	*	*	*	*	*	*	*	*
195.0 cm. and over	—	—	—	—	—	—	—	—	—	—	—	—
Female												
Under 130 cm	—	—	—	—	—	—	—	—	—	—	—	—
130.0-134.9 cm	—	—	—	—	—	—	—	—	—	—	—	—
135.0-139.9 cm	1	2	*	*	*	*	*	*	*	*	*	*
140.0-144.9 cm	2	6	*	*	*	*	*	*	*	*	*	*
145.0-149.9 cm	17	52	42.00	5.879	1.683	32.0	35.3	36.3	42.3	47.5	49.5	51.1
150.0-154.9 cm	64	196	48.26	6.797	0.926	37.7	39.2	42.5	47.9	53.3	55.9	58.8
155.0-159.9 cm	157	508	51.35	7.705	0.520	41.2	43.4	46.3	49.6	55.6	62.2	64.3
160.0-164.9 cm	186	603	54.59	8.810	0.707	43.0	45.0	48.4	53.0	59.7	66.7	70.7
165.0-169.9 cm	114	372	58.46	10.185	0.955	45.9	47.5	52.1	56.8	61.8	70.5	76.4
170.0-174.9 cm	36	121	64.37	15.821	2.814	49.2	52.1	56.2	59.8	70.5	72.9	99.4
175.0-179.9 cm	7	28	61.33	5.496	2.620	51.7	52.0	57.7	59.8	64.6	70.2	70.6
180.0-184.9 cm	2	7	*	*	*	*	*	*	*	*	*	*
185.0-189.9 cm	—	—	—	—	—	—	—	—	—	—	—	—
190.0-194.9 cm	—	—	—	—	—	—	—	—	—	—	—	—
195.0 cm. and over	—	—	—	—	—	—	—	—	—	—	—	—

NOTE: n = sample size; N = estimated number of youths in population in thousands; $\overline{X}$ = mean; s = standard deviation; $s_{\overline{x}}$ = standard error of the mean.

Table D-4. Weight in kilograms of youths aged 15 years at last birthday by sex and height group in centimeters: sample size, estimated population size, mean, standard deviation, standard error of the mean, and selected percentiles, United States, 1966-70

Sex and Height	n	N	$\overline{X}$	s	$s_{\overline{x}}$	Percentile						
						5th	10th	25th	50th	75th	90th	95th
Male								In Kilograms				
Under 130 cm	—	—	—	—	—	—	—	—	—	—	—	—
130.0-134.9 cm	—	—	—	—	—	—	—	—	—	—	—	—
135.0-139.9 cm	—	—	—	—	—	—	—	—	—	—	—	—
140.0-144.9 cm	—	—	—	—	—	—	—	—	—	—	—	—
145.0-149.9 cm	1	2	*	*	*	*	*	*	*	*	*	*
150.0-154.9 cm	10	30	45.72	8.582	3.550	35.7	39.2	42.6	44.7	46.0	48.7	76.1
155.0-159.9 cm	34	99	52.81	10.552	1.695	40.3	43.1	46.7	49.2	56.7	69.6	76.3
160.0-164.9 cm	71	206	53.01	8.417	0.986	42.7	44.1	46.9	51.5	56.3	65.3	68.8
165.0-169.9 cm	132	404	57.72	8.503	0.819	48.0	48.8	53.1	56.4	61.3	67.1	73.3
170.0-174.9 cm	176	574	62.88	8.464	0.633	51.6	53.4	56.7	61.9	67.2	72.9	78.1
175.0-179.9 cm	118	374	65.80	9.457	1.045	53.1	55.6	59.7	64.3	69.5	80.2	89.2
180.0-184.9 cm	51	144	72.00	11.928	1.724	54.6	60.3	64.4	70.2	78.4	84.4	96.6
185.0-189.9 cm	14	48	74.21	15.035	5.200	58.3	58.5	62.9	70.7	84.6	92.4	110.8
190.0-194.9 cm	6	15	83.39	16.431	10.332	66.4	66.7	69.6	73.8	103.0	105.7	106.2
195.0 cm. and over	—	—	—	—	—	—	—	—	—	—	—	—
Female												
Under 130 cm	—	—	—	—	—	—	—	—	—	—	—	—
130.0-134.9 cm	—	—	—	—	—	—	—	—	—	—	—	—
135.0-139.9 cm	—	—	*	*	—	—	—	—	—	—	—	*
140.0-144.9 cm	2	5	*	*	*	*	*	*	*	*	*	*
145.0-149.9 cm	15	51	47.91	7.875	3.623	36.0	39.4	42.1	45.4	52.7	55.7	66.3
150.0-154.9 cm	69	242	49.69	8.895	1.190	39.1	40.6	44.3	48.1	52.8	60.5	68.3
155.0-159.9 cm	111	400	51.52	8.473	0.934	41.4	43.5	46.3	50.8	55.1	59.8	65.2
160.0-164.9 cm	137	509	57.03	10.828	0.875	45.1	47.3	50.2	55.0	60.2	71.7	77.7
165.0-169.9 cm	109	398	60.71	10.357	1.053	47.5	49.3	55.1	58.4	65.7	74.1	81.0
170.0-174.9 cm	49	188	65.27	10.730	1.880	49.7	53.6	57.2	61.2	71.6	85.3	86.4
175.0-179.9 cm	7	23	63.30	8.872	4.807	49.7	49.9	53.8	62.4	71.1	71.9	79.2
180.0-184.9 cm	3	26	*	*	*	*	*	*	*	*	*	*
185.0-189.9 cm	1	3	*	*	*	*	*	*	*	*	*	*
190.0-194.9 cm	—	—	—	—	—	—	—	—	—	—	—	—
195.0 cm. and over	—	—	—	—	—	—	—	—	—	—	—	—

NOTE: n = sample size; N = estimated number of youths in population in thousands; $\overline{X}$ = mean; s = standard deviation; $s_{\overline{x}}$ = standard error of the mean.

Table D-5. Weight in kilograms of youths aged 16 years at last birthday by sex and height group in centimeters: sample size, estimated population size, mean, standard deviation, standard error of the mean, and selected percentiles, United States, 1966-70

Sex and Height	n	N	$\overline{X}$	s	$s_{\overline{x}}$	Percentile 5th	10th	25th	50th	75th	90th	95th
Male						In Kilograms						
Under 130 cm	—	—	—	—	—	—	—	—	—	—	—	—
130.0-134.9 cm	—	—	—	—	—	—	—	—	—	—	—	—
135.0-139.9 cm	—	—	—	—	—	—	—	—	—	—	—	—
140.0-144.9 cm	—	—	—	—	—	—	—	—	—	—	—	—
145.0-149.9 cm	1	1	*	*	*	*	*	*	*	*	*	*
150.0-154.9 cm	4	12	*	*	*	*	*	*	*	*	*	*
155.0-159.9 cm	11	33	49.89	7.323	3.572	42.0	42.2	44.7	46.8	54.4	59.8	67.2
160.0-164.9 cm	32	108	53.09	6.459	1.273	44.2	44.9	48.2	51.4	58.0	60.9	66.1
165.0-169.9 cm	87	275	59.39	9.178	0.981	48.5	49.8	52.7	58.0	63.9	69.3	75.9
170.0-174.9 cm	166	552	62.66	7.556	0.629	51.6	53.8	57.5	61.6	67.1	73.1	78.0
175.0-179.9 cm	149	511	67.33	9.018	0.856	56.3	58.2	61.0	65.4	72.5	80.1	83.8
180.0-184.9 cm	72	227	72.38	12.485	1.993	58.3	59.3	64.4	68.9	76.5	90.2	96.9
185.0-189.9 cm	29	95	81.06	14.268	3.265	63.7	66.6	69.7	78.4	90.3	97.0	111.4
190.0-194.9 cm	3	10	*	*	*	*	*	*	*	*	*	*
195.0 cm. and over	2	7	*	*	*	*	*	*	*	*	*	*
Female												
Under 130 cm	—	—	—	—	—	—	—	—	—	—	—	—
130.0-134.9 cm	—	—	—	—	—	—	—	—	—	—	—	—
135.0-139.9 cm	—	—	—	—	—	—	—	—	—	—	—	—
140.0-144.9 cm	2	5	*	*	*	*	*	*	*	*	*	*
145.0-149.9 cm	10	33	52.58	8.198	3.191	43.9	44.1	44.9	51.0	54.5	72.0	72.1
150.0-154.9 cm	57	178	51.79	10.457	1.053	41.4	42.0	45.8	48.9	54.1	61.5	83.3
155.0-159.9 cm	117	354	53.20	7.766	0.734	44.0	45.6	48.4	51.6	56.4	61.9	69.0
160.0-164.9 cm	160	547	57.71	11.129	1.246	46.1	47.3	51.5	55.5	61.2	69.5	75.1
165.0-169.9 cm	122	450	61.72	11.998	0.802	47.1	48.8	53.3	59.1	67.3	78.7	86.7
170.0-174.9 cm	53	170	63.61	8.734	1.126	52.9	53.8	58.1	62.1	66.8	73.8	84.2
175.0-179.9 cm	14	45	72.55	15.012	5.224	58.6	58.8	61.7	65.9	80.6	99.1	105.5
180.0-184.9 cm	1	2	*	*	*	*	*	*	*	*	*	*
185.0-189.9 cm	—	—	—	—	—	—	—	—	—	—	—	—
190.0-194.9 cm	—	—	—	—	—	—	—	—	—	—	—	—
195.0 cm. and over	—	—	—	—	—	—	—	—	—	—	—	—

NOTE: n = sample size; N = estimated number of youths in population in thousands; $\overline{X}$ = mean; s = standard deviation; $s_{\overline{x}}$ = standard error of the mean.

Table D-6. Weight in kilograms of youths aged 17 years at last birthday by sex and height group in centimeters: sample size, estimated population size, mean, standard deviation, standard error of the mean, and selected percentiles, United States, 1966-70

Sex and Height	n	N	$\overline{X}$	s	$s_{\overline{x}}$	5th	10th	25th	50th	75th	90th	95th
Male								In Kilograms				
Under 130 cm	—	—	—	—	—	—	—	—	—	—	—	—
130.0-134.9 cm	—	—	—	—	—	—	—	—	—	—	—	—
135.0-139.9 cm	—	—	—	—	—	—	—	—	—	—	—	—
140.0-144.9 cm	—	—	—	—	—	—	—	—	—	—	—	—
145.0-149.9 cm	—	—	—	—	—	—	—	—	—	—	—	—
150.0-154.9 cm	1	3	*	*	*	*	*	*	*	*	*	*
155.0-159.9 cm	11	39	54.63	9.397	3.414	43.8	46.4	48.2	49.7	57.8	69.9	73.2
160.0-164.9 cm	25	81	57.75	6.503	1.355	49.7	51.1	52.5	56.9	61.6	70.1	70.8
165.0-169.9 cm	63	248	62.57	8.344	1.224	50.2	53.2	56.4	61.5	66.9	72.7	77.3
170.0-174.9 cm	115	396	67.06	11.163	0.704	53.3	55.5	59.5	64.6	71.9	80.9	91.6
175.0-179.9 cm	151	537	68.37	9.907	0.831	56.9	58.9	61.5	66.5	73.6	79.4	88.4
180.0-184.9 cm	80	297	73.31	12.454	1.335	59.6	61.0	65.1	71.2	78.4	91.8	102.7
185.0-189.9 cm	36	133	76.03	9.171	1.301	62.4	66.3	70.5	75.3	80.8	90.3	92.9
190.0-194.9 cm	7	25	81.40	10.985	7.588	62.9	62.9	67.8	87.3	90.3	90.6	90.6
195.0 cm. and over	—	—	—	—	—	—	—	—	—	—	—	—
Female												
Under 130 cm	—	—	—	—	—	—	—	—	—	—	—	—
130.0-134.9 cm	—	—	—	—	—	—	—	—	—	—	—	—
135.0-139.9 cm	—	—	—	—	—	—	—	—	—	—	—	—
140.0-144.9 cm	2	5	*	*	*	*	*	*	*	*	*	*
145.0-149.9 cm	8	26	43.49	3.939	1.604	38.6	38.8	40.1	45.1	45.7	51.1	51.2
150.0-154.9 cm	43	151	49.96	6.508	0.827	41.6	42.3	44.6	48.9	53.5	59.2	64.1
155.0-159.9 cm	103	385	54.71	9.903	0.775	44.4	45.5	48.7	53.2	57.7	61.6	76.2
160.0-164.9 cm	133	506	57.79	10.620	1.028	46.8	48.0	50.2	55.4	61.5	72.3	82.3
165.0-169.9 cm	116	433	60.63	10.117	1.182	47.9	50.3	55.1	59.3	65.1	69.4	71.6
170.0-174.9 cm	51	186	62.18	9.132	1.407	50.6	52.9	55.5	60.2	65.7	76.1	82.7
175.0-179.9 cm	12	47	65.76	8.405	2.229	54.9	56.7	60.1	61.7	75.2	75.9	83.0
180.0-184.9 cm	1	2	*	*	*	*	*	*	*	*	*	*
185.0-189.9 cm	—	—	—	—	—	—	—	—	—	—	—	—
190.0-194.9 cm	—	—	—	—	—	—	—	—	—	—	—	—
195.0 cm. and over	—	—	—	—	—	—	—	—	—	—	—	—

NOTE: n = sample size; N = estimated number of youths in population in thousands; $\overline{X}$ = mean; s = standard deviation; $s_{\overline{x}}$ = standard error of the mean.

Appendix E

Table E-1. Triceps skinfold of youths 12-17 years of age weighing less than 30 kilograms, by sex and age at last birthday: sample size, estimated population size, mean, standard deviation, standard error of the mean, and selected percentiles, United States, 1966-70

Sex and Age	n	N	$\overline{X}$	s	$s_{\overline{x}}$	Percentile 5th	10th	25th	50th	75th	90th	95th
Male						In Millimeters						
12 years	24	69	6.6	2.41	0.61	2.9	4.6	5.3	6.1	7.7	10.7	11.6
13 years	5	15	*	*	*	*	*	*	*	*	*	*
14 years	1	5	*	*	*	*	*	*	*	*	*	*
15 years	—	—	—	—	—	—	—	—	—	—	—	—
16 years	—	—	—	—	—	—	—	—	—	—	—	—
17 years	—	—	—	—	—	—	—	—	—	—	—	—
Female												
12 years	12	44	6.8	1.51	0.64	5.1	5.3	5.6	7.3	8.4	9.0	9.0
13 years	4	12	*	*	*	*	*	*	*	*	*	*
14 years	—	—	—	—	—	—	—	—	—	—	—	—
15 years	—	—	—	—	—	—	—	—	—	—	—	—
16 years	—	—	—	—	—	—	—	—	—	—	—	—
17 years	16	56	6.8	1.69	0.53	5.0	5.2	5.7	7.0	8.4	9.6	10.0

NOTE: n = sample size; N = estimated number of youths in population in thousands; $\overline{X}$ = mean; s = standard deviation; $s_{\overline{x}}$ = standard error of the mean.

From National Center for Health Statistics: Skinfold thickness of youths 12-17 years, United States. In Vital and health statistics, series 11, no. 132, National Health Survey, Department of Health, Education, and Welfare Publication (HRA) 74-1614, Washington, D.C., 1974, U.S. Department of Health, Education, and Welfare, Public Health Service.

Table E-2. Triceps skinfold of youths 12-17 years of age weighing 30-34.9 kilograms, by sex and age at last birthday: sample size, estimated population size, mean, standard deviation, standard error of the mean, and selected percentiles, United States, 1966-70

Sex and Age	n	N	$\overline{X}$	s	$s_{\overline{x}}$	Percentile 5th	10th	25th	50th	75th	90th	95th
Male						In Millimeters						
12 years	99	290	7.3	1.94	0.24	5.0	5.3	6.0	7.4	8.8	9.9	10.8
13 years	30	88	7.1	2.82	0.72	3.7	4.2	5.2	7.1	8.6	11.2	12.8
14 years	3	8	*	*	*	*	*	*	*	*	*	*
15 years	—	—	—	—	—	—	—	—	—	—	—	—
16 years	—	—	—	—	—	—	—	—	—	—	—	—
17 years	—	—	—	—	—	—	—	—	—	—	—	—
Female												
12 years	43	156	8.5	3.99	0.39	4.5	5.0	6.6	8.1	11.3	13.4	14.1
13 years	11	32	8.8	3.71	1.22	3.5	5.2	7.2	8.6	10.7	17.0	17.3
14 years	4	12	*	*	*	*	*	*	*	*	*	*
15 years	1	5	*	*	*	*	*	*	*	*	*	*
16 years	—	—	—	—	—	—	—	—	—	—	—	—
17 years	—	—	—	—	—	—	—	—	—	—	—	—

NOTE: n = sample size; N = estimated number of youths in population in thousands; $\overline{X}$ = mean; s = standard deviation; $s_{\overline{x}}$ = standard error of the mean.

Table E-3. Triceps skinfold of youths 12-17 years of age weighing 35-39.9 kilograms, by sex and age at last birthday: sample size, estimated population size, mean, standard deviation, standard error of the mean, and selected percentiles, United States, 1966-70

Sex and Age	n	N	$\overline{X}$	s	$s_{\overline{x}}$	Percentile 5th	10th	25th	50th	75th	90th	95th
Male						In Millimeters						
12 years	158	536	8.2	2.95	0.26	4.3	5.1	6.3	7.7	10.4	12.4	14.0
13 years	91	309	7.7	2.86	0.34	4.1	4.5	5.8	7.6	9.7	12.1	13.4
14 years	32	106	6.3	2.38	0.35	3.4	3.9	5.1	5.9	7.7	9.5	9.9
15 years	4	10	*	*	*	*	*	*	*	*	*	*
16 years	2	5	*	*	*	*	*	*	*	*	*	*
17 years	—	—	—	—	—	—	—	—	—	—	—	—
Female												
12 years	87	329	9.2	2.88	0.29	5.4	6.1	7.4	8.8	11.3	12.6	14.4
13 years	72	253	8.7	2.81	0.38	5.3	5.8	6.9	8.6	10.7	11.8	12.8
14 years	26	76	8.3	2.60	0.47	4.3	5.3	6.7	8.4	10.3	11.1	12.5
15 years	11	34	8.5	3.55	0.83	4.4	4.9	5.7	8.6	10.6	12.8	16.2
16 years	2	4	*	*	*	*	*	*	*	*	*	*
17 years	5	15	9.1	2.40	1.09	7.2	7.4	8.0	8.6	9.6	14.0	14.0

NOTE: n = sample size; N = estimated number of youths in population in thousands; $\overline{X}$ = mean; s = standard deviation; $s_{\overline{x}}$ = standard error of the mean.

Table E-4. Triceps skinfold of youths 12-17 years of age weighing 40-44.9 kilograms, by sex and age at last birthday: sample size, estimated population size, mean, standard deviation, standard error of the mean, and selected percentiles, United States, 1966-70

Sex and Age	n	N	$\overline{X}$	s	$s_{\overline{x}}$	Percentile						
						5th	10th	25th	50th	75th	90th	95th
Male						In Millimeters						
12 years	133	436	10.0	3.64	0.35	5.3	6.0	7.1	10.2	13.1	14.8	16.4
13 years	112	337	8.5	3.32	0.26	4.5	5.1	6.4	7.8	10.8	13.7	15.4
14 years	61	196	7.3	2.98	0.42	3.6	4.2	5.1	7.2	10.3	12.1	12.6
15 years	19	58	6.0	1.78	0.38	3.5	4.0	4.7	6.3	7.6	8.6	9.0
16 years	6	24	6.2	1.02	0.54	4.7	4.9	5.4	6.6	7.2	7.4	7.4
17 years	1	3	*	*	*	*	*	*	*	*	*	*
Female												
12 years	118	428	10.7	3.24	0.28	6.3	7.1	8.5	10.6	13.0	15.8	16.6
13 years	101	342	10.2	3.19	0.44	5.7	6.5	8.2	10.2	12.4	15.3	16.3
14 years	58	176	10.3	3.60	0.60	6.0	6.4	7.6	10.2	12.7	14.9	18.0
15 years	47	174	10.4	3.18	0.47	5.9	6.5	8.2	10.7	12.4	14.5	17.1
16 years	34	96	11.6	3.66	0.89	6.6	7.6	9.8	11.4	13.2	17.3	19.3
17 years	27	93	11.1	2.34	0.51	7.4	7.7	10.2	11.1	12.8	14.8	15.6

NOTE: n = sample size; N = estimated number of youths in population in thousands; $\overline{X}$ = mean; s = standard deviation; $s_{\overline{x}}$ = standard error of the mean.

Table E-5. Triceps skinfold of youths 12-17 years of age weighing 45-49.9 kilograms, by sex and age at last birthday: sample size, estimated population size, mean, standard deviation, standard error of the mean, and selected percentiles, United States, 1966-70

Sex and Age	n	N	$\overline{X}$	s	$s_{\overline{x}}$	Percentile						
						5th	10th	25th	50th	75th	90th	95th
Male						In Millimeters						
12 years	89	299	11.5	5.33	0.76	5.5	6.1	7.7	10.3	13.8	20.6	22.4
13 years	119	396	8.9	3.44	0.26	4.8	5.4	6.9	8.6	11.0	13.2	16.6
14 years	86	264	7.4	3.18	0.32	3.7	4.2	5.3	7.1	9.2	12.9	14.4
15 years	62	185	7.0	2.68	0.31	4.2	4.4	5.3	6.6	9.2	11.1	13.0
16 years	25	83	5.6	1.85	0.35	4.0	4.1	4.5	5.4	6.8	8.2	9.5
17 years	12	40	5.6	1.96	0.59	3.2	3.4	4.5	5.6	6.6	8.6	10.0
Female												
12 years	106	372	12.6	4.27	0.60	7.2	7.8	9.7	12.4	15.8	18.2	21.0
13 years	122	399	11.0	3.43	0.30	6.6	7.3	8.6	11.0	13.3	15.7	17.2
14 years	143	470	12.0	3.26	0.40	7.1	8.3	10.0	11.9	14.7	17.0	17.6
15 years	91	333	12.7	4.10	0.48	7.0	8.1	9.4	12.5	15.3	18.7	21.1
16 years	90	293	12.1	4.08	0.56	6.7	7.4	9.4	12.2	14.5	18.0	20.9
17 years	76	280	12.2	4.18	0.83	6.6	7.4	9.3	11.8	15.4	18.5	20.1

NOTE: n = sample size; N = estimated number of youths in population in thousands; $\overline{X}$ = mean; s = standard deviation; $s_{\overline{x}}$ = standard error of the mean.

Table E-6. Triceps skinfold of youths 12-17 years of age weighing 50-54.9 kilograms, by sex and age at last birthday: sample size, estimated population size, mean, standard deviation, standard error of the mean, and selected percentiles, United States, 1966-70

Sex and Age	n	N	$\overline{X}$	s	$s_{\overline{x}}$	Percentile						
						5th	10th	25th	50th	75th	90th	95th
Male						In Millimeters						
12 years	56	161	15.0	6.06	0.92	6.4	7.4	10.3	14.8	20.2	24.3	26.0
13 years	88	275	10.2	4.89	0.36	4.8	5.4	6.6	9.2	13.5	18.1	20.5
14 years	123	373	8.1	4.25	0.30	4.2	4.5	5.5	7.4	9.6	14.0	15.5
15 years	93	278	6.8	2.36	0.25	4.3	4.6	5.5	6.6	8.3	10.4	11.2
16 years	56	184	6.6	2.61	0.42	3.9	4.2	5.0	6.3	8.1	10.7	13.2
17 years	32	116	5.9	2.03	0.50	3.1	4.0	4.7	5.8	7.4	8.4	10.2
Female												
12 years	76	273	14.3	3.99	0.61	9.3	10.2	11.5	14.2	17.0	20.8	22.5
13 years	97	337	14.3	4.47	0.41	7.8	9.4	11.1	13.9	17.0	21.1	24.2
14 years	124	385	13.7	4.92	0.36	7.4	8.4	10.2	12.9	16.8	20.4	22.7
15 years	106	388	13.7	3.62	0.44	8.4	9.5	11.4	13.7	15.9	18.9	20.6
16 years	136	442	13.3	4.32	0.33	7.9	8.6	10.6	12.8	16.2	19.5	21.3
17 years	103	387	15.3	4.85	0.54	7.8	9.7	12.2	15.2	18.5	21.8	24.2

NOTE: n = sample size; N = estimated number of youths in population in thousands; $\overline{X}$ = mean; s = standard deviation; $s_{\overline{x}}$ = standard error of the mean.

Table E-7. Triceps skinfold of youths 12-17 years of age weighing 55-59.9 kilograms, by sex and age at last birthday: sample size, estimated population size, mean, standard deviation, standard error of the mean, and selected percentiles, United States, 1966-70

Sex and Age	n	N	$\overline{X}$	s	$s_{\overline{x}}$	Percentile						
						5th	10th	25th	50th	75th	90th	95th
Male						In Millimeters						
12 years	48	139	16.4	6.17	0.99	6.2	7.6	12.8	16.4	22.2	24.5	26.4
13 years	69	223	12.2	6.16	0.76	5.2	5.6	7.5	11.1	17.5	20.5	22.5
14 years	106	346	8.4	4.37	0.48	4.6	5.2	6.1	7.3	10.1	15.1	18.4
15 years	120	396	7.0	3.22	0.34	4.0	4.3	5.3	6.6	8.2	10.7	12.6
16 years	108	367	6.6	2.39	0.19	3.8	4.5	5.4	6.4	7.8	10.2	11.3
17 years	67	243	6.0	1.76	0.26	4.1	4.4	5.1	5.7	7.2	8.6	10.0
Female												
12 years	51	182	17.8	5.91	0.90	9.1	10.2	13.6	18.0	23.0	25.6	28.3
13 years	81	275	16.2	4.66	0.54	8.8	10.6	13.5	16.3	19.5	22.7	25.6
14 years	98	347	15.7	4.18	0.41	10.3	10.8	12.3	15.2	19.2	21.7	22.7
15 years	113	406	15.8	4.54	0.42	9.6	10.6	13.1	15.8	18.4	22.4	24.3
16 years	105	342	16.3	4.92	0.52	8.2	10.2	13.2	16.5	20.3	23.3	25.2
17 years	105	409	16.4	4.60	0.43	9.8	10.6	12.7	16.6	19.8	22.7	25.3

NOTE: n = sample size; N = estimated number of youths in population in thousands; $\overline{X}$ = mean; s = standard deviation; $s_{\overline{x}}$ = standard error of the mean.

Table E-8. Triceps skinfold of youths 12-17 years of age weighing 60-64.9 kilograms, by sex and age at last birthday: sample size, estimated population size, mean, standard deviation, standard error of the mean, and selected percentiles, United States, 1966-70

Sex and Age	n	N	$\overline{X}$	s	$s_{\overline{x}}$	Percentile						
						5th	10th	25th	50th	75th	90th	95th
Male						In Millimeters						
12 years	18	49	20.3	7.90	2.30	7.6	9.5	12.7	22.3	27.4	29.7	33.7
13 years	52	169	13.6	6.90	1.34	5.2	5.5	7.5	13.3	20.2	24.5	26.6
14 years	72	231	10.0	4.92	0.52	4.6	5.5	7.1	8.2	12.7	18.2	20.4
15 years	114	350	7.9	3.24	0.30	4.6	5.1	5.6	7.3	10.1	12.7	15.5
16 years	117	378	7.1	2.96	0.24	3.6	4.2	5.3	6.6	8.7	12.1	12.9
17 years	108	397	6.7	2.61	0.29	3.7	4.2	5.1	6.2	8.4	10.3	12.3
Female												
12 years	29	100	21.7	5.29	0.87	12.6	15.2	18.5	22.3	25.6	26.8	29.4
13 years	41	133	20.1	4.86	0.71	11.8	12.9	17.1	20.7	24.2	25.5	28.1
14 years	61	207	18.7	4.55	0.45	12.6	13.7	15.7	18.3	22.4	25.2	27.0
15 years	52	192	17.8	4.86	0.86	12.1	12.6	14.2	17.2	20.8	25.1	25.9
16 years	74	263	18.6	4.68	0.69	12.3	12.8	14.8	19.6	21.9	24.7	26.5
17 years	74	263	17.9	5.02	0.75	10.9	11.5	14.1	18.3	22.1	24.3	25.9

NOTE: n = sample size; N = estimated number of youths in population in thousands; $\overline{X}$ = mean; s = standard deviation; $s_{\overline{x}}$ = standard error of the mean.

Table E-9. Triceps skinfold of youths 12-17 years of age weighing 65-69.9 kilograms, by sex and age at last birthday: sample size, estimated population size, mean, standard deviation, standard error of the mean, and selected percentiles, United States, 1966-70

Sex and Age	n	N	$\overline{X}$	s	$s_{\overline{x}}$	Percentile						
						5th	10th	25th	50th	75th	90th	95th
Male						In Millimeters						
12 years	10	30	24.0	4.38	1.84	16.6	20.1	20.5	27.0	28.2	30.0	30.0
13 years	23	80	14.5	6.66	1.52	6.2	7.0	10.7	12.1	19.5	26.2	27.5
14 years	59	188	12.0	5.16	0.70	5.8	6.4	8.2	11.4	15.5	19.2	20.8
15 years	83	269	9.6	4.54	0.52	4.3	5.1	7.1	8.7	12.3	15.4	21.2
16 years	96	327	9.1	3.69	0.44	5.2	5.5	6.9	7.8	11.7	14.9	16.5
17 years	91	319	7.8	3.44	0.51	4.3	4.7	5.7	7.1	9.8	13.1	14.7
Female												
12 years	10	34	24.5	6.63	2.69	14.6	17.2	20.8	24.1	30.3	31.9	39.0
13 years	27	83	22.2	4.11	0.79	16.3	17.1	20.4	22.3	25.1	28.1	28.8
14 years	31	100	21.4	4.91	1.28	12.3	13.4	18.0	22.4	25.4	28.1	28.3
15 years	27	102	19.9	6.18	1.12	10.5	13.0	16.3	20.3	23.6	29.3	30.6
16 years	36	145	19.5	4.08	0.66	13.2	13.8	16.7	20.6	22.6	25.3	26.2
17 years	35	132	17.8	4.71	1.00	12.2	12.6	14.1	17.9	21.2	24.6	27.6

NOTE: n = sample size; N = estimated number of youths in population in thousands; $\overline{X}$ = mean; s = standard deviation; $s_{\overline{x}}$ = standard error of the mean.

Table E-10. Triceps skinfold of youths 12-17 years of age weighing 70-74.9 kilograms, by sex and age at last birthday: sample size, estimated population size, mean, standard deviation, standard error of the mean, and selected percentiles, United States, 1966-70

Sex and Age	n	N	$\overline{X}$	s	$s_{\overline{x}}$	Percentile						
						5th	10th	25th	50th	75th	90th	95th
Male							In Millimeters					
12 years	4	10	*	*	*	*	*	*	*	*	*	*
13 years	12	46	18.4	4.97	1.46	11.3	11.6	15.3	17.3	22.3	22.9	26.8
14 years	26	81	13.2	5.03	1.06	6.4	7.2	9.2	13.4	17.6	21.1	22.4
15 years	53	164	11.3	4.84	0.90	6.1	6.5	8.1	10.2	15.2	17.8	20.8
16 years	55	181	11.0	4.76	0.75	5.4	6.3	7.6	10.1	13.8	18.0	19.8
17 years	68	245	9.5	4.27	0.44	4.3	5.0	6.0	9.6	12.0	14.7	16.5
Female												
12 years	8	28	24.1	4.22	1.67	17.4	17.7	22.0	25.3	28.1	30.0	30.0
13 years	8	24	24.9	3.69	1.97	18.7	21.0	21.7	26.9	28.2	30.0	30.0
14 years	25	73	24.2	5.31	1.24	17.4	18.8	21.2	23.5	27.8	31.6	32.6
15 years	21	92	21.7	6.16	1.83	7.4	7.9	19.7	22.8	25.5	27.9	29.6
16 years	18	68	23.8	5.44	1.38	15.5	17.2	20.1	24.4	28.4	31.3	34.1
17 years	16	67	24.8	5.33	1.07	17.2	20.0	21.5	23.6	27.7	33.1	39.0

NOTE: n = sample size; N = estimated number of youths in population in thousands; $\overline{X}$ = mean; s = standard deviation; $s_{\overline{x}}$ = standard error of the mean.

Table E-11. Triceps skinfold of youths 12-17 years of age weighing 75-79.9 kilograms, by sex and age at last birthday: sample size, estimated population size, mean, standard deviation, standard error of the mean, and selected percentiles, United States, 1966-70

Sex and Age	n	N	$\overline{X}$	s	$s_{\overline{x}}$	Percentile						
						5th	10th	25th	50th	75th	90th	95th
Male							In Millimeters					
12 years	3	11	*	*	*	*	*	*	*	*	*	*
13 years	12	30	19.2	5.21	1.91	12.8	13.1	13.6	19.6	23.0	25.7	29.0
14 years	27	85	14.3	6.59	1.97	7.4	8.2	10.5	13.8	16.0	21.8	32.1
15 years	21	58	15.8	7.71	1.51	8.1	9.0	10.3	13.5	20.5	28.5	29.5
16 years	39	127	13.0	6.26	1.32	5.4	5.9	8.1	11.0	18.6	23.1	23.8
17 years	51	182	12.0	4.71	0.56	5.6	7.0	8.7	11.8	14.7	16.5	22.2
Female												
12 years	4	11	*	*	*	*	*	*	*	*	*	*
13 years	6	21	22.8	4.08	2.80	13.4	13.9	20.6	25.1	25.7	27.0	27.0
14 years	6	20	25.7	5.03	2.56	16.3	16.6	23.7	25.7	27.7	33.0	33.0
15 years	11	36	29.1	4.38	1.58	21.8	22.4	27.4	29.6	31.8	32.9	38.0
16 years	12	35	26.1	4.57	2.08	19.5	20.0	22.0	28.0	29.5	31.4	35.0
17 years	8	37	27.0	7.15	4.72	15.4	15.8	22.3	28.3	32.5	36.0	36.0

NOTE: n = sample size; N = estimated number of youths in population in thousands; $\overline{X}$ = mean; s = standard deviation; $s_{\overline{x}}$ = standard error of the mean.

Table E-12. Triceps skinfold of youths 12-17 years of age weighing 80-84.9 kilograms, by sex and age at last birthday: sample size, estimated population size, mean, standard deviation, standard error of the mean, and selected percentiles, United States, 1966-70

Sex and Age	n	N	$\overline{X}$	s	$s_{\overline{x}}$	Percentile						
						5th	10th	25th	50th	75th	90th	95th
Male						In Millimeters						
12 years	—	—	—	—	—	—	—	—	—	—	—	—
13 years	3	8	*	*	*	*	*	*	*	*	*	*
14 years	7	21	17.8	2.87	1.22	14.6	14.7	15.6	18.2	20.5	23.0	23.0
15 years	16	53	17.1	4.27	1.37	11.4	11.8	15.3	17.2	18.5	26.2	28.0
16 years	24	69	15.3	5.56	1.28	6.4	6.9	12.2	14.6	20.6	23.1	25.0
17 years	17	65	13.0	4.53	1.28	7.1	7.8	9.8	12.4	17.4	19.7	20.7
Female												
12 years	1	3	*	*	*	*	*	*	*	*	*	*
13 years	8	25	29.5	7.42	3.19	17.6	20.1	20.9	28.6	36.2	40.0	40.0
14 years	3	9	*	*	*	*	*	*	*	*	*	*
15 years	9	32	27.1	2.08	0.79	24.4	24.8	25.6	27.5	28.6	30.6	32.0
16 years	10	38	31.2	7.30	2.66	16.8	23.6	26.0	31.1	40.0	40.0	40.0
17 years	5	16	23.6	5.98	3.51	17.1	17.2	17.6	23.4	31.0	31.3	31.4

NOTE: n = sample size; N = estimated number of youths in population in thousands; $\overline{X}$ = mean; s = standard deviation; $s_{\overline{x}}$ = standard error of the mean.

Table E-13. Triceps skinfold of youths 12-17 years of age weighing 85-89.9 kilograms, by sex and age at last birthday: sample size, estimated population size, mean, standard deviation, standard error of the mean, and selected percentiles, United States, 1966-70

Sex and Age	n	N	$\overline{X}$	s	$s_{\overline{x}}$	Percentile						
						5th	10th	25th	50th	75th	90th	95th
Male						In Millimeters						
12 years	—	—	—	—	—	—	—	—	—	—	—	—
13 years	5	13	*	*	*	*	*	*	*	*	*	*
14 years	5	13	*	*	*	*	*	*	*	*	*	*
15 years	13	35	22.6	5.61	1.68	9.5	16.3	21.0	21.9	29.0	29.8	30.0
16 years	10	32	14.4	4.96	1.68	9.8	10.2	10.8	12.6	19.1	20.7	26.2
17 years	15	47	14.9	5.74	1.92	7.8	8.3	12.3	14.2	21.1	25.6	26.0
Female												
12 years	2	8	*	*	*	*	*	*	*	*	*	*
13 years	—	—	—	—	—	—	—	—	—	—	—	—
14 years	2	5	*	*	*	*	*	*	*	*	*	*
15 years	7	32	30.9	4.68	1.34	22.4	22.9	28.1	32.5	33.7	34.9	39.0
16 years	7	22	25.4	10.55	4.70	9.7	9.8	17.4	25.4	35.4	40.0	40.0
17 years	5	17	30.7	2.49	1.64	28.3	28.5	29.3	30.3	30.9	35.0	35.0

NOTE: n = sample size; N = estimated number of youths in population in thousands; $\overline{X}$ = mean; s = standard deviation; $s_{\overline{x}}$ = standard error of the mean.

Table E-14. Triceps skinfold of youths 12-17 years of age weighing 90-99.9 kilograms, by sex and age at last birthday: sample size, estimated population size, mean, standard deviation, standard error of the mean, and selected percentiles, United States, 1966-70

Sex and Age	n	N	$\overline{X}$	s	$s_{\overline{x}}$	Percentile						
						5th	10th	25th	50th	75th	90th	95th
Male						In Millimeters						
12 years	1	2	*	*	*	*	*	*	*	*	*	*
13 years	2	7	*	*	*	*	*	*	*	*	*	*
14 years	7	26	27.4	7.25	4.64	15.5	16.0	22.5	32.2	32.6	37.0	37.0
15 years	8	26	16.7	4.05	1.74	10.7	10.8	14.2	17.1	21.2	21.4	21.4
16 years	11	37	17.7	4.08	1.94	11.7	11.9	13.8	17.5	20.7	24.1	24.3
17 years	19	78	20.7	6.93	2.93	9.5	11.7	15.7	20.4	26.9	32.0	32.0
Female												
12 years	—	—	—	—	—	—	—	—	—	—	—	—
13 years	4	10	*	*	*	*	*	*	*	*	*	*
14 years	3	10	*	*	*	*	*	*	*	*	*	*
15 years	2	6	*	*	*	*	*	*	*	*	*	*
16 years	9	29	31.8	4.60	1.48	26.2	26.5	27.4	32.3	35.4	40.4	40.0
17 years	6	20	32.9	7.56	4.03	17.6	17.7	31.8	34.2	40.1	40.4	40.4

NOTE: n = sample size; N = estimated number of youths in population in thousands; $\overline{X}$ = mean; s = standard deviation; $s_{\overline{x}}$ = standard error of the mean.

Table E-15. Triceps skinfold of youths 12-17 years of age weighing 100 kilograms or more, by sex and age at last birthday: sample size, estimated population size, mean, standard deviation, standard error of the mean, and selected percentiles, United States, 1966-70

Sex and Age	n	N	$\overline{X}$	s	$s_{\overline{x}}$	Percentile						
						5th	10th	25th	50th	75th	90th	95th
Male						In Millimeters						
12 years	—	—	—	—	—	—	—	—	—	—	—	—
13 years	3	9	*	*	*	*	*	*	*	*	*	*
14 years	3	5	*	*	*	*	*	*	*	*	*	*
15 years	7	18	21.4	6.87	2.65	12.6	12.8	14.6	20.5	26.1	34.0	34.0
16 years	7	19	*	*	*	*	*	*	*	*	*	*
17 years	8	29	*	*	*	*	*	*	*	*	*	*
Female												
12 years	—	—	—	—	—	—	—	—	—	—	—	—
13 years	—	—	—	—	—	—	—	—	—	—	—	—
14 years	2	9	*	*	*	*	*	*	*	*	*	*
15 years	5	16	*	*	*	*	*	*	*	*	*	*
16 years	3	10	*	*	*	*	*	*	*	*	*	*
17 years	4	9	*	*	*	*	*	*	*	*	*	*

NOTE: n = sample size; N = estimated number of youths in population in thousands; $\overline{X}$ = mean; s = standard deviation; $s_{\overline{x}}$ = standard error of the mean.

Appendix F

From Gurney, J.M., and Jelliffe, D.B.: Am. J. Clin. Nutr.
26:912, 1973. © American Journal of Clinical Nutrition,
American Society for Clinical Nutrition.

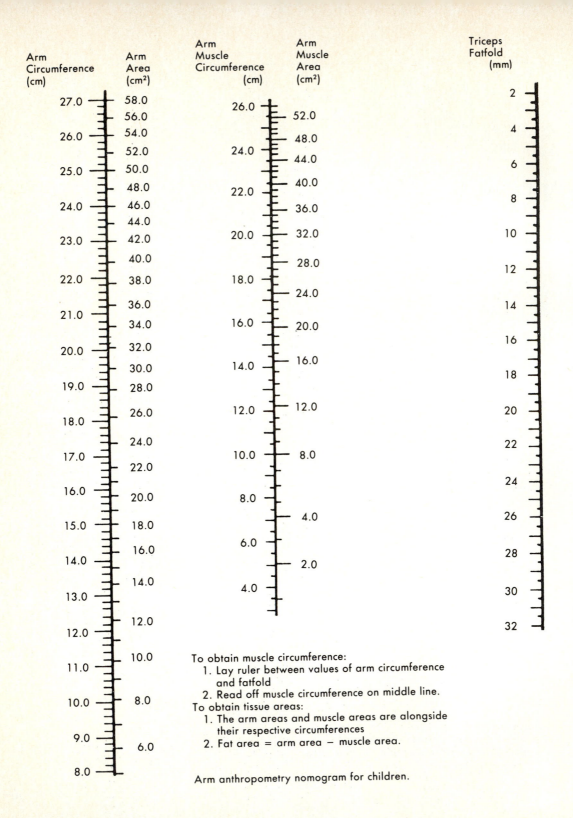

Arm Circumference (cm)	Arm Area (cm²)	Arm Muscle Circumference (cm)	Arm Muscle Area (cm²)	Triceps Fatfold (mm)

To obtain muscle circumference:
1. Lay ruler between values of arm circumference and fatfold
2. Read off muscle circumference on middle line.

To obtain tissue areas:
1. The arm areas and muscle areas are alongside their respective circumferences
2. Fat area = arm area − muscle area.

Arm anthropometry nomogram for children.

Arm Circumference (cm)	Arm Area (cm²)	Arm Muscle Circumference (cm)	Arm Muscle Area (cm²)	Triceps Fatfold (mm)

To obtain muscle circumference:
  1. Lay ruler between value of arm circumference and fatfold
  2. Read off muscle circumference on middle line.
To obtain tissue areas:
  1. The arm area and muscle area are alongside their respective circumferences
  2. Fat area = arm area − muscle area.

Arm anthropometry nomogram for adults.

Appendix G

Table G-1. Upper arm fat and muscle area standards (percentiles for estimates of upper arm fat area [mm²] and upper arm muscle area [mm²] for whites of the United States Health Examination Survey I of 1971 to 1974)

Age Group	Arm Muscle Area Percentiles (mm²)							Arm Fat Area Percentiles (mm²)						
	5	10	25	50	75	90	95	5	10	25	50	75	90	95
Males														
1-1.9	956	1014	1133	1278	1447	1644	1720	452	486	590	741	895	1036	1176
2-2.9	973	1040	1190	1345	1557	1690	1787	434	504	578	737	871	1044	1148
3-3.9	1095	1201	1357	1484	1618	1750	1853	464	519	590	736	868	1071	1151
4-4.9	1207	1264	1408	1579	1747	1926	2008	428	494	598	722	859	989	1085
5-5.9	1298	1411	1550	1720	1884	2089	2285	446	488	582	713	914	1176	1299
6-6.9	1360	1447	1605	1815	2056	2297	2493	371	446	539	678	896	1115	1519
7-7.9	1497	1548	1808	2027	2246	2494	2886	423	473	574	758	1011	1393	1511
8-8.9	1550	1664	1895	2089	2296	2628	2788	410	460	588	725	1003	1248	1558
9-9.9	1811	1884	2067	2288	2657	3053	3257	485	527	635	859	1252	1864	2081
10-10.9	1930	2027	2182	2575	2903	3486	3882	523	543	738	982	1376	1906	2609
11-11.9	2016	2156	2382	2670	3022	3359	4226	536	595	754	1148	1710	2348	2574
12-12.9	2216	2339	2649	3022	3496	3968	4640	554	650	874	1172	1558	2536	3580
13-13.9	2363	2546	3044	3553	4081	4502	4794	475	570	812	1096	1702	2744	3322
14-14.9	2830	3147	3586	3963	4575	5368	5530	453	563	786	1082	1608	2746	3508
15-15.9	3138	3317	3788	4481	5134	5631	5900	521	595	690	931	1423	2434	3100
16-16.9	3625	4044	4352	4951	5753	6576	6980	542	593	844	1078	1746	2280	3041
17-17.9	3998	4252	4777	5286	5950	6886	7726	598	698	827	1096	1636	2407	2888
18-18.9	4070	4481	5066	5552	6374	7067	8355	560	665	860	1264	1947	3302	3928
19-24.9	4508	4777	5274	5913	6660	7606	8200	594	743	963	1406	2231	3098	3652
25-34.9	4694	4963	5541	6214	7067	7847	8436	675	831	1174	1752	2459	3246	3786
35-44.9	4844	5181	5740	6490	7265	8034	8488	703	851	1310	1792	2463	3098	3624
45-54.9	4546	4946	5589	6297	7142	7918	8458	749	922	1254	1741	2359	3245	3928
55-64.9	4422	4783	5381	6144	6919	7670	8149	658	839	1166	1645	2236	2976	3466
65-74.9	3973	4411	5031	5716	6432	7074	7453	573	753	1122	1621	2199	2876	3327

From Frisancho, A.R.: Am. J. Clin. Nutr. **34:**2540, 1981. © American Journal of Clinical Nutrition, American Society for Clinical Nutrition.

Age Group	Arm Muscle Area Percentiles (mm²)							Arm Fat Area Percentiles (mm²)						
	5	10	25	50	75	90	95	5	10	25	50	75	90	95
Females														
1-1.9	885	973	1084	1221	1378	1535	1621	401	466	578	706	847	1022	1140
2-2.9	973	1029	1119	1269	1405	1595	1727	469	526	642	747	894	1061	1173
3-3.9	1014	1133	1227	1396	1563	1690	1846	473	529	656	822	967	1106	1158
4-4.9	1058	1171	1313	1475	1644	1832	1958	490	541	654	766	907	1109	1236
5-5.9	1238	1301	1423	1598	1825	2012	2159	470	529	647	812	991	1330	1536
6-6.9	1354	1414	1513	1683	1877	2182	2323	464	508	638	827	1009	1263	1436
7-7.9	1330	1441	1602	1815	2045	2332	2469	491	560	706	920	1135	1407	1644
8-8.9	1513	1566	1808	2034	2327	2657	2996	527	634	769	1042	1383	1872	2482
9-9.9	1723	1788	1976	2227	2571	2987	3112	642	690	933	1219	1584	2171	2524
10-10.9	1740	1784	2019	2296	2583	2873	3093	616	702	842	1141	1608	2500	3005
11-11.9	1784	1987	2316	2612	3071	3739	3953	707	802	1015	1301	1942	2730	3690
12-12.9	2092	2182	2579	2904	3225	3655	3847	782	854	1090	1511	2056	2666	3369
13-13.9	2269	2426	2657	3130	3529	4081	4568	726	838	1219	1625	2374	3272	4150
14-14.9	2418	2562	2874	3220	3704	4294	4850	981	1043	1423	1818	2403	3250	3765
15-15.9	2426	2518	2847	3248	3689	4123	4756	839	1126	1396	1886	2544	3093	4195
16-16.9	2308	2567	2865	3248	3718	4353	4946	1126	1351	1663	2006	2598	3374	4236
17-17.9	2442	2674	2996	3336	3883	4552	5251	1042	1267	1463	2104	2977	3864	5159
18-18.9	2398	2538	2917	3243	3694	4461	4767	1003	1230	1616	2104	2617	3508	3733
19-24.9	2538	2728	3026	3406	3877	4439	4940	1046	1198	1596	2166	2959	4050	4896
25-34.9	2661	2826	3148	3573	4138	4806	5541	1173	1399	1841	2548	3512	4690	5560
35-44.9	2750	2948	3359	3783	4428	5240	5877	1336	1619	2158	2898	3932	5093	5847
45-54.9	2784	2956	3378	3858	4520	5375	5964	1459	1803	2447	3244	4229	5416	6140
55-64.9	2784	3063	3477	4045	4750	5632	6247	1345	1879	2520	3369	4360	5276	6152
65-74.9	2737	3018	3444	4019	4739	5566	6214	1363	1681	2266	3063	3943	4914	5530

Appendix H

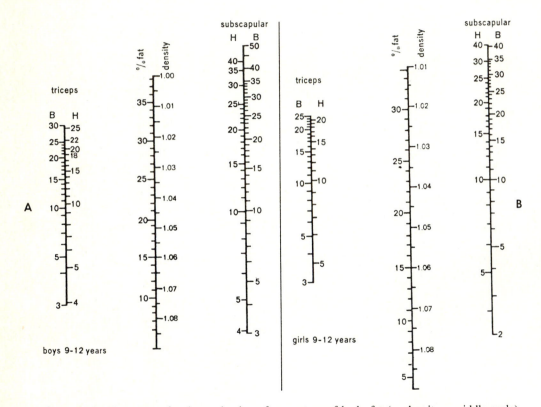

Fig. H-1. A, Nomogram for the evaluation of percentage of body fat (or density—middle scale) from two skinfolds: triceps—left; subscapular—right; external sides of both extreme scales = values for modified Best caliper (B), internal sides of extreme scales (H) = values for Harpenden caliper (and Lange's caliper resp.). The value of the percentage of body fat is read on the middle axis, on the cross-section point of the line connecting particular values on the scales for triceps and subscapular skinfolds. This nomogram refers to the boys 9-12 years old. **B,** Nomogram for the evaluation of percentage of body fat (or density—middle scale) from two skinfolds: triceps—left, subscapular—right, measured by Best or Harpenden (and Lange's caliper resp.). This nomogram refers to girls 9-12 years old. (From Pařízková, J.: Total body fat and skinfold thickness in children, Metabolism **10:**794-807, 1961. By permission of Grune & Stratton, Inc.)

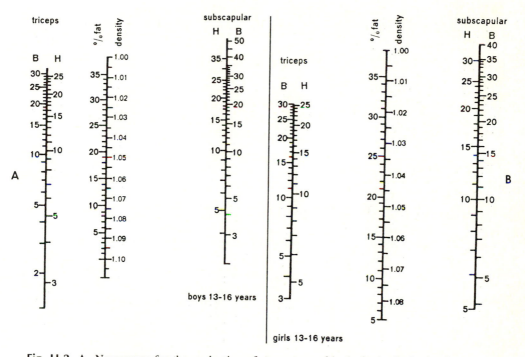

Fig. H-2. A, Nomogram for the evaluation of percentage of body fat (or body density—middle scale) from two skinfolds: triceps—left, subscapular—right, measured by Best or Harpenden (and Lange's caliper resp.). This nomogram refers to boys 13-16 years old. **B,** Nomogram for the evaluation of percentage of body fat (or body density—middle scale) from two skinfolds: triceps—left, subscapular—right, measured by Best or Harpenden (and Lange's caliper resp.). This nomogram refers to girls 13-16 years old. (From Pařízková, J.: Total body fat and skinfold thickness in children, Metabolism **10:**794-807, 1961. By permission of Grune & Stratton, Inc.)

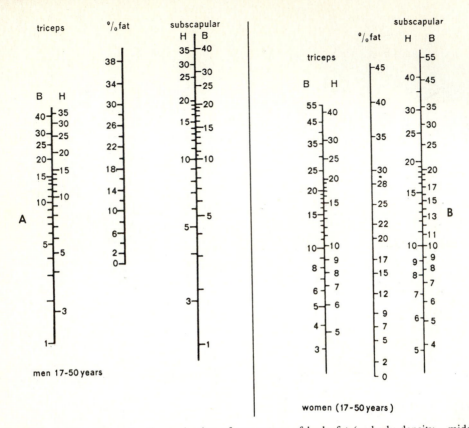

triceps %fat subscapular H B men 17-50 years

subscapular H B %fat triceps B H women (17-50 years)

Fig. H-3. A, Nomogram for the evaluation of percentage of body fat (or body density—middle scale) from two skinfolds: triceps—left, subscapular—right, measured by Best or Harpenden (and Lange's caliper resp.). This nomogram refers to men 17-50 years old. **B,** Nomogram for the evaluation of percentage of body fat (or body density—middle scale) from two skinfolds: triceps—left, subscapular—right, measured by Best or Harpenden (and Lange's caliper resp.). This nomogram refers to women 17-50 years old. (From Pařízková, J.: Total body fat and skinfold thickness in children, Metabolism **10:**794-807, 1961. By permission of Grune & Stratton, Inc.)

Appendix I

Table I-1. Body fat and skinfolds (the equivalent fat content, as a percentage of body-weight, for a range of values for the sum of four skinfolds [biceps, triceps, subscapular and supra-iliac] of males and females of different ages*)

Skinfolds (mm)	Males (Age in Years)				Females (Age in Years)			
	17-29	30-39	40-49	50+	16-29	30-39	40-49	50+
15	4.8	—	—	—	10.5	—	—	—
20	8.1	12.2	12.2	12.6	14.1	17.0	19.8	21.4
25	10.5	14.2	15.0	15.6	16.8	19.4	22.2	24.0
30	12.9	16.2	17.7	18.6	19.5	21.8	24.5	26.6
35	14.7	17.7	19.6	20.8	21.5	23.7	26.4	28.5
40	16.4	19.2	21.4	22.9	23.4	25.5	28.2	30.3
45	17.7	20.4	23.0	24.7	25.0	26.9	29.6	31.9
50	19.0	21.5	24.6	26.5	26.5	28.2	31.0	33.4
55	20.1	22.5	25.9	27.9	27.8	29.4	32.1	34.6
60	21.2	23.5	27.1	29.2	29.1	30.6	33.2	35.7
65	22.2	24.3	28.2	30.4	30.2	31.6	34.1	36.7
70	23.1	25.1	29.3	31.6	31.2	32.5	35.0	37.7
75	24.0	25.9	30.3	32.7	32.2	33.4	35.9	38.7
80	24.8	26.6	31.2	33.8	33.1	34.3	36.7	39.6
85	25.5	27.2	32.1	34.8	34.0	35.1	37.5	40.4
90	26.2	27.8	33.0	35.8	34.8	35.8	38.3	41.2
95	26.9	28.4	33.7	36.6	35.6	36.5	39.0	41.9
100	27.6	29.0	34.4	37.4	36.4	37.2	39.7	42.6
105	28.2	29.6	35.1	38.2	37.1	37.9	40.4	43.3
110	28.8	30.1	35.8	39.0	37.8	38.6	41.0	43.9
115	29.4	30.6	36.4	39.7	38.4	39.1	41.5	44.5
120	30.0	31.1	37.0	40.4	39.0	39.6	42.0	45.1
125	30.5	31.5	37.6	41.1	39.6	40.1	42.5	45.7
130	31.0	31.9	38.2	41.8	40.2	40.6	43.0	46.2
135	31.5	32.3	38.7	42.4	40.8	41.1	43.5	46.7
140	32.0	32.7	39.2	43.0	41.3	41.6	44.0	47.2
145	32.5	33.1	39.7	43.6	41.8	42.1	44.5	47.7
150	32.9	33.5	40.2	44.1	42.3	42.6	45.0	48.2
155	33.3	33.9	40.7	44.6	42.8	43.1	45.4	48.7
160	33.7	34.3	41.2	45.1	43.3	43.6	45.8	49.2
165	34.1	34.6	41.6	45.6	43.7	44.0	46.2	49.6
170	34.5	34.8	42.0	46.1	44.1	44.4	46.6	50.0
175	34.9	—	—	—	—	44.8	47.0	50.4
180	35.3	—	—	—	—	45.2	47.4	50.8
185	35.6	—	—	—	—	45.6	47.8	51.2
190	35.9	—	—	—	—	45.9	48.2	51.6
195	—	—	—	—	—	46.2	48.5	52.0
200	—	—	—	—	—	46.5	48.8	52.4
205	—	—	—	—	—	—	49.1	52.7
210	—	—	—	—	—	—	49.4	53.0

From Durnin, J.V., and Wormersley, J.: Body fat assessed from total body density and its estimation from skinfold thickness: measurements on 481 men and women aged from 16-72 years, Br. J. Nutr. **32**:77, 1974. © Cambridge University Press.
In two-thirds of the instances the error was within ±3.5% of the body-weight as fat for the women and ±5% for the men.
*Measurements made on the right side of the body.

Appendix J

METHOD FOR MEASURING CARDIORESPIRATORY FITNESS

1. a. Have patient sit quietly and relax for 3 to 5 minutes.
   b. Take pulse for 10 seconds. A 10-second time segment is easiest to measure and use.
   c. Record this pulse as the *resting heart rate* (RHR).
2. a. Have the patient, starting from a sitting position with arms folded in front, stand up and sit down in the chair twice every 5 seconds. Have patient continue for 3 minutes.
   b. At the end of 3 minutes or the period after which the patient can no longer continue, measure the pulse for 10 seconds. Record this as the *immediate post-test heart rate.*
   c. After 30 seconds following the test, take a pulse and record this as the *30-second recovery heart rate.*
   d. At 1 minute and 2 minutes following the test, take a pulse and record these as the *1-minute recovery heart rate* and the *2-minute recovery heart rate.*
   e. Monitor the pulse return toward RHR. It should be below 16 beats/10 sec by 5 minutes after the test.
   f. Multiply all of the recorded heart rates by 6 to obtain heart rates in beats per minute.

Using the box on p. 308 that gives the codes for each of the measured pulse rates, find the appropriate codes directly above the recorded heart rates and note them in the space provided. After doing this for all five test conditions, add the five codes together. Then using the box below that lists the fitness zones for cardiovascular health, determine whether the patient is in the danger zone, the safety zone, or the fitness zone. The sum of the five codes also can be used as a fitness score. The goal of a fitness program then would be to increase this fitness score.

Zones for Cardiovascular Health

Danger Zone

0-5 6-10 11-15 16-20 21-25 26-30 31-35

Safety Zone

36-40 41-45 46-50 51-55 56-60 61-65 66-70

Fitness Zone

71-75 76-81 82-85 86-90 91-95 96-100

From The Pipes fitness test and prescription, by Thomas Pipes and Paul A. Vodak. Copyright © 1978 by Thomas V. Pipes and Paul A. Vodak. Reprinted by permission of J.P. Tarcher, Inc., and Houghton Mifflin Company.

Coding Your Cardiovascular Health

	20	19	18	17	16	15	14	13	12	11	10	9	8	7	6	5	4	3	2	1	Code Score
										Codes											
Resting Heart Rate	44	48	52	56	60	62	64	66	68	70	72	74	76	78	80	84	88	92	96	100	———
Posttest Heart Rate	80	84	88	92	96	100	104	108	112	116	120	124	128	132	136	140	144	148	152	156	———
Second Recovery Heart Rate	64	68	72	76	80	84	88	92	96	100	104	108	112	116	120	124	128	132	136	140	———
1 Minute Recovery Heart Rate	56	60	64	68	72	76	80	84	88	92	96	100	104	108	112	116	120	124	128	132	———
2 Minute Recovery Heart Rate	56	60	64	68	72	76	80	84	88	92	96	100	104	108	112	116	120	124	128	132	———

Total Code Score ———

From The Pipes fitness test and prescription, by Thomas Pipes and Paul A. Vodak. Copyright © 1978 by Thomas V. Pipes and Paul A. Vodak. Reprinted by permission of J.P. Tarcher, Inc., and Houghton Mifflin Company.

Appendix K

Table K-1. Caloric expenditure during various activities*

Activity	Cal/min	Activity	Cal/min
Sleeping	1.2	Golf: foursome-twosome	3.7-5.0
Resting in bed	1.3	Horseshoes	3.8
Sitting, normally	1.3	Baseball (except pitcher)	4.7
Sitting, reading	1.3	Ping pong-table tennis	4.9-7.0
Lying, quietly	1.3	Calisthenics	5.0
Sitting, eating	1.5	Rowing: pleasure-vigorous	5.0-15.0
Sitting, playing cards	1.5	Cycling: 5-15 mph (10 speed)	5.0-12.0
Standing, normally	1.5	Skating: recreation-vigorous	5.0-15.0
Classwork, lecture (listen to)	1.7	Archery	5.2
Conversing	1.8	Badminton: recreational-competitive	5.2-10.0
Personal toilet	2.0	Basketball: half-full court (more for	6.0-9.0
Sitting, writing	2.6	fast break)	
Standing, light activity	2.6	Bowling (while active)	7.0
Washing and dressing	2.6	Tennis: recreational-competitive	7.0-11.0
Washing and shaving	2.6	Water skiing	8.0
Driving a car	2.8	Soccer	9.0
Washing clothes	3.1	Snowshoeing (2.5 mph)	9.0
Walking indoors	3.1	Handball and squash	10.0
Shining shoes	3.2	Mountain climbing	10.0
Making bed	3.4	Skipping rope	10.0-15.0
Dressing	3.4	Judo and karate	13.0
Showering	3.4	Football (while active)	13.3
Driving motorcycle	3.4	Wrestling	14.4
Metal working	3.5	Skiing	
House painting	3.5	Moderate to steep	8.0-12.0
Cleaning windows	3.7	Downhill racing	16.5
Carpentry	3.8	Cross-country: 3-8 mph	9.0-17.0

From Sharkey, B.J.: Physiology of fitness, Champaign, Ill., 1979, Human Kinetics Publishers, Inc. © 1979, Human Kinetics Publishers, Inc.

*Depends on efficiency and body size. Add 10% for each 15 lbs over 150, subtract 10% for each 15 lbs under 150. Use activity pulse rate (Fig. 6-4) to confirm the caloric expenditure. *Continued.*

Table K-1. Caloric expenditure during various activities—cont'd

Activity	Cal/min	Activity	Cal/min
Farming chores	3.8	Swimming	
Sweeping floors	3.9	Pleasure	6.0
Plastering walls	4.1	Crawl: 25-50 yds/min	6.0-12.5
Truck and automobile repair	4.2	Butterfly: 50 yds/min	14.0
Ironing clothes	4.2	Backstroke: 25-50 yds/min	6.0-12.5
Farming, planting, hoeing, raking	4.7	Breaststroke: 25-50 yds/min	6.0-12.5
Mixing cement	4.7	Sidestroke: 40 yds/min	11.0
Mopping floors	4.9	Dancing	
Repaving roads	5.0	Modern: moderate-vigorous	4.2-5.7
Gardening, weeding	5.6	Ballroom: waltz-rumba	5.7-7.0
Stacking lumber	5.8	Square	7.7
Chain saw	6.2	Walking	
Stone, masonry	6.3	Road-field (3.5 mph)	5.6-7.0
Pick-and-shovel work	6.7	Snow: hard-soft (3.5-2.5 mph)	10.0-20.0
Farming, haying, plowing with horse	6.7	Uphill: 5-10–15% (3.5 mph)	8.0-11.0-15.0
Shoveling (miners)	6.8	Downhill	
Walking downstairs	7.1	5-10% (2.5 mph)	3.6-3.5
Chopping wood	7.5	15-20% (2.5 mph)	3.7-4.3
Crosscut saw	7.5-10.5	Hiking: 40 lb pack (3.0 mph)	6.8
Tree felling (ax)	8.4-12.7	Running	
Gardening, digging	8.6	12 min mile (5 mph)	10.0
Walking upstairs	10.0-18.0	8 min mile (7.5 mph)	15.0
Pool or billiards	1.8	6 min mile (10 mph)	20.0
Canoeing: 2.5 mph-4.0 mph	3.0-7.0	5 min mile (12 mph)	25.0
Volleyball: recreational-competitive	3.5-8.0		

Appendix L

METHOD FOR DETERMINING APPROXIMATE DAILY ENERGY EXPENDITURE

A fairly good approximation of total daily energy expenditure can be calculated by adding together the following: (1) energy used in basal metabolism, (2) an additional percentage to account for the overall daily living pattern, (3) the energy used in recreational activity, and (4) the energy used in specific dynamic action (SDA).

Use the nomogram in Fig. L-1 to determine the basal energy expenditure. This takes into account the height, weight, surface area, age, and sex of the individual.

Then add the energy necessary to account for overall daily living pattern. Approximate increases are as follows:

Activity	Percent Above Basal
Bed rest (eating and reading)	10
Very light (sitting and standing activities, auto driving, lab work)	30
Light (office work)	40-60
Moderate (housework, gardening)	60-80
Heavy occupational (construction, walking with load uphill)	100

Modified from Krause, M.V., and Mahan, L.K.: Food, nutrition, and diet therapy, ed. 7, Philadelphia, 1984, W.B. Saunders, Co.

Basal energy expenditure multiplied by the percent over basal equals the energy in the daily living pattern. Basal energy expenditure plus the energy expended in the daily living pattern thus equals the energy spent daily in nonrecreational activity.

Using Appendix K, which gives the calories spent per minute of activity, calculate the energy spent in recreational activities. Using Fig. 6-4 determine the energy expenditure based on heart rate to account for the fact that the more fit the person is, the greater the energy expenditure for the same heart rate. Calories per minute multiplied by minutes of activity equals the calories spent in activity.

Now add together the three components of energy expenditure:

_____ Calories—basal energy expenditure
_____ Calories—daily living pattern expenditure
_____ Calories—recreational expenditure
This equals the daily energy expenditure.

The energy expenditure for SDA then is determined by multiplying the daily energy expenditure by 10%.

The total daily energy expenditure finally is calculated by adding the SDA to the daily energy expenditure.

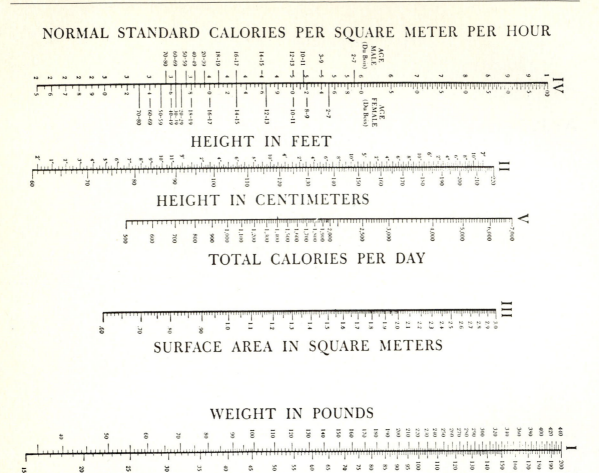

Fig. L-1. Place the chart on a flat, smooth table. Use only a ruler with a true straight edge. Do not draw lines on the chart but merely indicate their positions by the straight edge of the ruler. Locate the various points by means of needles (pin stuck through the eraser of a lead pencil). Locate the patient's normal weight on Scale I and his height on Scale II. The ruler joining these two points intersects Scale III at the patient's surface area. Locate the age and sex of the patient on Scale IV. A ruler joining this point with the patient's surface area on Scale III crosses Scale V at the *basal* energy requirement. To convert calories (kcal) to kj, multiply by 4.184. (From Boothby, W.M., Berkson, J., and Dunn, H.L.: Am. J. Physiol. **116:**468, 1936.)

Index